Comprehensive Food Allergy Management for Nurses

Julianne Doucette • Josie Howard-Ruben
Editors

Comprehensive Food Allergy Management for Nurses

Clinical Practices, Advocacy, and Support Strategies

Springer

Editors
Julianne Doucette
College of Nursing
Rush University
Chicago, IL, USA

Josie Howard-Ruben
Rush University College of Nursing
Chicago, IL, USA

ISBN 978-3-032-28646-8 ISBN 978-3-032-28647-5 (eBook)
https://doi.org/10.1007/978-3-032-28647-5

This Springer imprint is published by the registered company Springer Nature Switzerland AG
The registered company address is: Gewerbestrasse 11, 6330 Cham, Switzerland

Foreword

Nurses work at the frontline of health care. They provide critical and timely assistance; they are often the first people who hear a patient name, a pain, or worry. They offer support and information in vulnerable moments and help someone get the treatments they need.

When I was young, a beloved aunt was diagnosed with breast cancer. I was inspired by the nurses who surrounded her with care. Witnessing the way that they acted as advocates for all their patients became the introduction to an incredible profession that I wanted to join. I eventually earned a doctorate in nursing from Rutgers University and had my first teaching position within their School of Nursing. My colleagues in nursing have always impressed me with their incredible dedication and expertise.

More than 33 million people in the U.S. have food allergy, which can cause anaphylaxis, a type of life-threatening allergic reaction. Often, this disease of the immune system is not diagnosed until after a reaction, meaning that someone's understanding of their food allergy starts with a traumatic incident. Nurses are key to managing the patient journey during these incidents, or in their aftermath, as families regroup and figure out next steps. They provide critical education that can help avoid future reactions.

I am a food allergy patient myself. As someone who has experienced anaphylaxis, I have both an appreciation of the tremendous improvements we have made in understanding this disease, which is a silent epidemic, and a deep commitment to all that still needs to be done. Compared to other serious chronic diseases, food allergy research and innovation lags behind—a gap that I have dedicated my professional life to closing.

A food allergy cure is within reach. FARE is facilitating this breakthrough by removing research silos and encouraging multi-disciplinary research that combines immunology, gastroenterology, systems biology, rheumatology, oncology, therapeutic development, and artificial intelligence and machine learning. We are determining our future.

In the meantime, we have powerful tools for prevention while this pursuit continues. Scientific studies show the efficacy of early allergen introduction and an "eat early, eat often" approach in helping prevent the development of food allergy. This insight will accomplish little, unless it is amplified by the nurses and physicians who counsel expecting and new parents, and reinforced by government policy around providing training and nutritional support for families in need. Trusted voices and real conversations will be what evolve the strategies around feeding infants.

When it comes to managing existing food allergy, we face a similar challenge. We're in a moment of great advancement in terms of new treatments and novel ways to administer epinephrine, which is the only medication that can halt an anaphylactic reaction. But we can't create real impact without widespread awareness, as well as dedicated work on improving community access, affordability, and availability of food allergy support, and removing barriers.

Although American medical professionals often focus on the American landscape, food allergy is an international health crisis that affects 220 million people worldwide. To have full and lasting effects on how food allergy is managed, widespread collaboration is also key—as evident in recent efforts to create agreed-upon definitions of anaphylaxis, led by the Global Allergy and Asthma Excellence Network, and the work of the Codex Alimentarius Commission to shape global standards for food allergen labeling.

This handbook offers an informed, deeply thoughtful guide to food allergy in the contemporary moment, with attention given to a range of important and emerging topics such as the role of technology in diagnostics and the social and emotional impacts of food allergy. Although our understanding of food allergy is always evolving and improving, what remains constant is the value of nurses—as advocates, as teachers, and as compassionate allies. Thank you for your service to the food allergy community.

Biography

Sung Poblete PhD, RN, is the Chief Executive Officer of Food Allergy Research & Education (FARE). Her record of leadership spans for-profit and non-profit organizations including Fresenius Medical Care North America, Oxford Health Plans Foundation, and most recently, Stand Up To Cancer (SU2C), where she served as CEO for more than a decade. Dr. Poblete, who holds a doctorate in nursing, has received numerous high-level research grants from the Centers for Disease Control and Prevention, National Institutes of Health, National Science Foundation, and private foundations. She earned her degrees at Rutgers, The State University of New Jersey, where she still serves as a visiting associate professor at the School of Nursing, and where she is recognized in the Rutgers Hall of Distinguished Alumni.

For questions, please contact:
Jennifer (Jen) Webb, FARE
(Food Allergy Research & Education), FoodAllergy.org
jwebb@foodallergy.org

CEO of Food Allergy Research & Education (FARE) Sung Poblete
McLean, VA, USA

Contents

Introduction to IgE-Mediated Food Allergy

Julianne Doucette and Josie Howard-Ruben

Introduction

In generations past, food allergies were uncommon. You might have heard about someone allergic to bee stings, or perhaps to penicillin, and rarely would come across an adult with a seafood allergy, but knowing someone with a food allergy was not typical. Everyone had a peanut butter sandwich and a carton of milk for lunch. By the early 1990s, the prevalence of food allergies was more commonplace. In the past several decades, food allergy has emerged as a rising public health concern worldwide, reshaping the way clinicians, educators, and families approach nutrition, safety, and how they offer guidance on daily living for those affected. Once considered relatively rare, food allergies now affect an estimated 6–8% of children in the United States and up to about 10% of adults (Bartha et al., 2024; Gupta et al., 2018, 2019; Bottoms-McClain et al., 2026; Ng et al., 2026).

This book was designed to provide nurses and advance practice nurses (APNs) with the information they need to care effectively for people living with food allergies. We hope that you will find it to be a comprehensive, practical resource to help you to understand the diagnosis, management, and broader impact of IgE-mediated food allergy at home, school, and in other settings. Nurses and APNs in primary care, the inpatient setting, the community, or who work in schools are all at the frontline of identifying symptoms, coordinating care, educating families, and advocating for patient safety everywhere. As food allergy diagnostics and management strategies rapidly evolve, while it is challenging to do so, nurses caring

J. Doucette (✉)
College of Nursing, Rush University, Chicago, IL, USA
e-mail: Julianne_Doucette@rush.edu

J. Howard-Ruben
Rush University College of Nursing, Chicago, IL, USA
e-mail: josie_howard-ruben@rush.edu

J. Doucette, J. Howard-Ruben (eds.), *Comprehensive Food Allergy Management for Nurses*, https://doi.org/10.1007/978-3-032-28647-5_1

for people coping with food allergies need to stay informed about the latest evidence-based guidelines and recommendations to help inform patients and families and to meet the growing demand for safe, effective ongoing care. By staying abreast of the science surrounding food allergy, nurses can help patients understand how to manage their food allergies, including treatment and emergency management, and how to cope with food allergies effectively. The content provided in this book is educational and not intended as a guide to treatment but is meant to familiarize nurses with information to help them care for patients with knowledge and compassion, and to provide resources that can be used in practice.

Even as this book was in development, many changes occurred in the clinical management of food allergy, so there may be even more changes as we reach publication. While epinephrine auto-injector devices have been in use for years, recently an intranasal epinephrine device reached the marketplace, and the frontline role of epinephrine ("epi first, epi fast") has been emphasized. A sublingual form of epinephrine is likely to receive approval at some point in the near future, as updated trials on usability are completed. Palforzia (a peanut powder) treatment was approved by the FDA, to much fanfare, and a few years later, likely due to its time-intensive regimen and a slow market uptake, the product was discontinued. Omalizumab became the first anti-IgE monoclonal antibody introduced in the US to counter IgE-mediated food allergy, offering an entirely new approach to management of this condition. Early introduction guidelines for foods in infancy designed to prevent allergies have changed and have been increasingly promulgated by pediatric clinicians. In the US, food allergy labeling laws were updated with the FASTER Act implementation, changing the labeling requirements to nine major allergens (other countries have different labeling requirements). And unlike 20 years ago, online resources for people with food allergies are abundant, with support groups, access to information from experts, and patient advocacy organizations offering detailed information about food allergies.

The co-editors of this book are nurses with a personal connection to food allergies, since some of their own adult children have multiple, anaphylactic food allergies, and we dedicate this book to them. We have walked the anxiety-laden path of food allergy diagnosis, daily and emergency management, and everyday life including developmental milestones from infancy to adulthood as caregivers for our families. One of us is a pediatric nurse practitioner who has practiced in the field and now educates nurse practitioner students, and both are nursing faculty. Through our lived experiences, we have often learned things the hard way, so we are passionate about educating nurses on the many aspects of clinical care and daily living that patients with food allergies experience so they can help patients to live with greater ease and confidence. When our own children were first diagnosed, information about food allergies was not yet widely available, and patient and family education and support were not extensive. In the intervening years, the diagnosis and management of food allergy have undergone rapid change due to the explosion in scientific interest over the past 10 years or so. However, what nurses learn in basic education programs remains somewhat circumscribed to basic information about diagnosis of food allergies and the emergency management of anaphylaxis. The other authors of this text include nurses practicing in allergy care, food allergy parents, educators, or those who have food allergies themselves. We hope that this book will spark an interest in food allergy care, and the collective result will be a greater number of knowledgeable nurses involved in helping patients and families dealing with food allergy to be better prepared to manage this life-changing diagnosis. By providing evidence-based care and increased engagement in community outreach and advocacy, both locally, in their own practices, at schools, in larger communities, and globally, nurses can help transform the ability of people with food allergies to live fully and safely with this chronic condition.

Risk Factors and Causes of Food Allergy

Why are some people allergic to a food while others develop tolerance to all foods? Current scientific understanding suggests IgE-mediated food allergy is a chronic disease resulting from the interplay of a person's genetics, environmental exposures (pollutants, pesticides, microplastics, etc.) (Shi et al., 2026), perinatal influences, and epigenetic changes (Lee et al., 2024; Hui-Beckman & Kim, 2025; Hund et al., 2025; Sicherer & Sampson, 2018), so the reasons for the development of food allergy are complex. The prevailing thought is that some genetic predisposition, in combination with environmental factors, creates a milieu in which allergic disease develops. A "window of opportunity" in early life may exist which could allow us to shape aspects of the immune system and possibly prevent food allergies (e.g., early introduction) (DuToit et al., 2013; NASEM, 2017). Some recent work has explored the possibility for some role of the nervous system in food allergy, citing "bidirectional communication between mast cells and neurons, particularly with the enteric nervous system" (Houghton et al., 2024, p. 3327), but much more remains to be learned about the role of this neuro-immune interaction in the context of food allergy.

Potential risk factors for food allergy development include family members with atopic diseases such as eczema, food allergy, asthma, and/or allergic rhinitis; and possibly c-section births, early exposure to cow's milk, formula, and antibiotic exposure, all of which have been shown to cause changes to intestinal microbiota resulting in inflammation and intestinal dysfunction (Hui-Beckman & Kim, 2025; Lee et al., 2020, 2024). Additional maternal prenatal and postnatal risk factors may include smoking or vaping, secondhand smoke, air pollution, microbial exposure, pet/animal exposure, maternal nutrition and diet during breastfeeding, duration of breastfeeding, and age at introduction of complementary foods that include allergens (Hui-Beckman & Kim, 2025; NASEM, 2017). However, more investigation of all of these risk factors to understand how they impact the development of food allergies is needed.

Many theories have been proposed to explain the development of food allergies, but there is no single explanation. A prominent theory is the Lack dual-allergen exposure hypothesis, which suggests that sensitization to an allergen may first occur through a disrupted skin barrier, such as eczematous skin, early in life, before subsequent exposure to the allergen through the gastrointestinal system when food is consumed in larger amounts (Lack, 2012). Recent studies in an animal model have suggested that an IgE response can be mounted by the immune system after exposure through acute and chronic skin injury, resulting in a process called "remote priming," (Waizman et al., 2025), raising more questions about the role of non-intact skin in subsequent allergy development. Other theories, such as the hygiene hypothesis, suggest that better hygiene habits have resulted in less microbial exposure, which in turn may lead to the development of atopic diseases (Lee et al., 2024; Calvani et al., 2020). Vitamin D deficiency has also been implicated in the increased prevalence of allergic diseases (Calvani et al., 2020). Additional theories have been suggested, such as the microbiome depletion hypothesis, which focuses on low levels of gut bacterial metabolites, such as butyrate, in infancy, resulting in gut dysbiosis and immune system changes and the later development of food allergy (Di Costanzo et al., 2021). The epithelial barrier hypothesis implicates many environmental factors such detergents, cigarette smoke, dietary fatty acids, pollution, and microplastics, in inflammation and increased damage to epithelial barriers, contributing to immune system changes and is also a potential mechanisms of food allergy development (Ferraro et al., 2025).

Germane to this discussion is a recent systematic review and meta-analysis comprising 190 studies that included 2.8 million people, and which considered 342 risk factors associated with the development of food allergy (Islam et al., 2026). The findings supported that the causes of food allergy are multiple, and the solutions to preventing them will be multifactorial. The review classified risk factors as major and minor. Early in life antibiotic use, description of self as Black, allergic conditions diagnosed early in life, parental migration (moving to a new country), delayed introduction of complementary food, and family history of allergies were among some of the major risk factors determined. Minor risk factors included male sex, cesarean delivery, filaggrin gene changes, and being the firstborn child.

Often, parents worry that their behaviors have contributed to the development of their child's food allergy, but the state of the science does not currently point to any direct links between specific actions parents have taken and the development of allergies. If anything, as this recent meta-analysis concludes, the causes are multifactorial, and several different factors may have contributed to a person's food allergy. Diet, environment, genetic, and other factors may all be integrated in a new way of looking at why food allergies develop. Both modifiable and non-modifiable etiologies have been proposed, but there is still no clear-cut answer on why allergies develop in some people and not in others. Nurses can allay parents' concerns about this, especially mothers, who may experience guilt about how they fed their child or other exposures that may have occurred. There is still much to be learned to avert the development of food allergies, but to date, these factors remain poorly understood, and no firm conclusions can be made at the present time as to the definite cause or multiple causes of food allergy development (Di Costanzo et al., 2021; Ferraro et al., 2025; Hussain et al., 2019; Lee et al., 2020).

The Landscape of Food Allergy

A framework presented in chapter "Understanding the Diagnosis and Management of Food Allergy Part I: IgE-Mediated Food Allergy and Anaphylaxis" comprises the prevailing classification scheme for most adverse reactions to food. For a moment, though, we ask the reader to consider an additional perspective for food allergy classification that has recently emerged, which has been described as food allergy endotypes (Baker et al., 2025). This approach captures many of the nuances of how food allergies present, yet still sorts them into the broad categories of IgE-mediated and non-IgE-mediated classifications, based on disease mechanisms, as shown in Fig. 1 (Baker et al., 2025). In this book, we focus on IgE-mediated food allergy caused by proteins presented to the immune system through the gut or skin, and sometimes through the respiratory system, which may present in childhood or adulthood, and some of which are transient (children may grow out of them) or are persistent (they may continue for a lifetime). It is useful for the reader, however, to appreciate how food allergy presentations fit in the big picture of this novel perspective and how to think about the heterogeneity of food allergy presentations, not all of which will be discussed in this book. So while the majority of patients that nurses will care for may have IgE-mediated food allergies, there are other diagnoses to be aware of, and which would require different patient management and education.

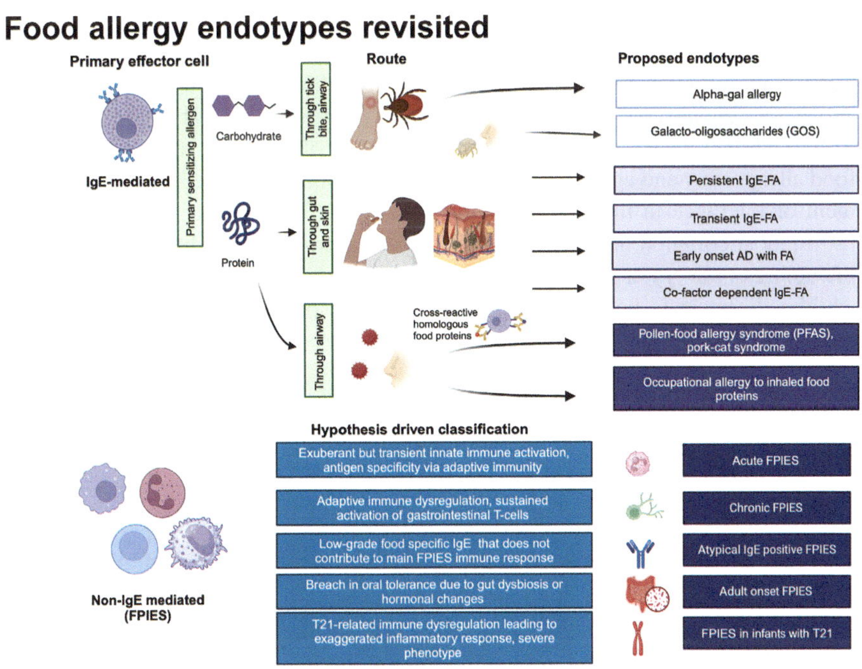

Fig. 1 Classification of FA endotypes. For IgE-FAs, endotypes are defined on the type of sensitizing allergen and route of sensitization. For FPIES, endotypes are proposed on the basis of our understanding of putative pathophysiologic mechanisms. T21, Trisomy 21. (Used with permission from: Elsevier https://doi.org/10.1016/j.jaci.2025.04.019)

IgE-Mediated Food Allergy

IgE-mediated food allergy is typically rapid in onset, can vary in severity, and is defined by the National Institute of Allergy and Infectious Diseases as "an adverse health effect arising from a specific immune response that occurs reproducibly on exposure to a given food" as stated in the original *Guidelines for the Diagnosis and Management of Food Allergy in the United States* (NIAID, 2010). Unlike food intolerances, which are non-immune in nature, IgE-mediated food allergies can lead to life-threatening reactions such as anaphylaxis (NIAID, 2010; National Academies of Sciences, 2017). While over 170 foods have been identified as causing these allergic reactions, and as noted below, there are common top allergens that are prevalent (FARE, 2024), with variations across geographic locations (see below). "Food" in this sense means those items eaten that are unprocessed (e.g., eggs or walnuts) as well as those that are processed (e.g., cookies or packaged meals), and includes food additives and dietary supplements.

Food allergies often develop in infancy or early childhood, though many persist into adulthood or even emerge later in life (See Fig. 2). Research shows those with persistent food allergies often have similar factors, such as early age at initial diagnosis and conditions such as atopic dermatitis, asthma, and/or allergic rhinitis (Elizur et al., 2012; Lee et al., 2024). It is unclear what the mechanism of persistence of food allergies entails versus the development of tolerance ("growing out of a food allergy") in later childhood, adolescence or adulthood. McIntyre et al. (2023) reported on the Food Allergy Research and Education (FARE) Food Allergy History Survey, an online data registry operated by FARE, finding that in a sample of 4505 survey participants, about one-third of children (as reported by caregivers), and one-fifth of adults relayed a history of the development of tolerance (or resolution) of a food allergy. Soy and egg were the most common foods associated with the development of tolerance in the overall sample, with soy (36%), wheat (29%), and meat (26%) most common in children. Adults experienced tolerance differently based on the timing of allergy onset. Top allergens that are persistent in the US population into adulthood appear to be shellfish 2.9%, milk 1.9%, peanut 1.8% and fin fish 1.2% (Lee et al., 2024).

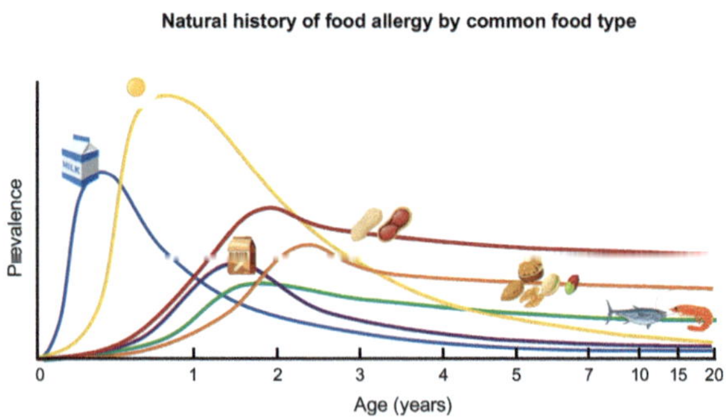

Fig. 2 Natural History of Food Allergy by Common Food Type. *Note.* (Used with permission from: Lee et al. (2024)). (Figure published under a Creative Commons Attribution 4.0 International License http://creativecommons.org/licenses/by/4.0/)

Obtaining an accurate diagnosis for IgE-mediated food allergy is paramount to determining which specific food is the culprit and assisting in both management decisions and follow-up planning. As with many medical conditions, the history remains a key component of the diagnostic process and should be correlated with skin testing, IgE-specific blood testing, and oral food challenges (gold standard) when a definitive diagnosis is necessary. If available, novel diagnostics such as the basophil activation test (BAT), component-resolved diagnostics (CRD), mast cell activation test (MAT), and microbiome analysis can add precision to the diagnosis (see chapter "Understanding the Diagnosis and Management of Food Allergy Part II: Diagnostics") (Hund et al., 2025).

IgE-Mediated Food Allergy Prevalence

Data collection methods for ascertaining the prevalence of food allergies vary, often including self-report, so there is some possibility for overestimation. The key points here, however, are that food allergies are increasingly diagnosed and are experienced not only by infants and children but also by adults. In adults, some food allergies were first diagnosed in childhood, while others presented in adulthood (Azzolino et al., 2024; Warren et al., 2023). Global prevalence estimates vary, ranging from 2% to 10% or more, reflecting differences in geography, migration, genetics, diet, diagnostic criteria, and reporting methods such as self-reported surveys versus clinician-diagnosed conditions (Bartha et al., 2024; Forero Molina et al., 2025; Hund et al., 2025). In some countries, data is not readily available for analysis.

The European Academy of Allergy and Clinical Immunology recently reiterated the increasing prevalence of food allergy, citing a range of 3–10% of children and as much as 10% of the adult population experiencing a food allergy diagnosis (Santos et al., 2023). A recent abstract describing a cross-sectional prevalence study of food allergy in children and adults illustrated the variability in food allergy diagnoses across the globe (Gupta et al., 2023), with the methodology for this international online self-report survey described elsewhere (Gupta et al., 2025). Prevalence estimates were reported by country, but overall, ranged from 2.35% to 8.71% in children, and 2.1% to 8.14% in adults, with individuals from Germany reporting the lowest prevalence (2.35%) in children and Japan reporting the lowest prevalence in adults (2.1%), while respondents in China reported the highest incidence in children (8.71%) and adults (8.14%). Respondents in the US ranked fourth in prevalence among children (4.32%) and third among adults (6.3%). In this study, peanuts, milk and dairy, and eggs emerged as the most prevalent allergens, but respondents in China reported shrimp to be the most prevalent food allergy.

Most Common IgE-Mediated Food Allergies

The most common allergens globally are cow's milk and egg (Feng et al., 2023; Forero Molina et al., 2025; Loh & Tang, 2018), but food allergens in different countries vary as noted above and likely reflect an array of environmental factors such as dietary patterns, cultural feeding practices, and other factors. For example, in the United States (US), the top nine foods labeled as food allergens include milk (dairy), egg, peanut, soy, wheat, tree nut (almond, cashew, hazelnut, macadamia, pistachio, pecan, walnuts, etc.), shellfish (crab, lobster, shrimp, etc.), fish (halibut, cod, salmon, etc.), and sesame (USFDA, 2025). Sesame was added to the list in 2023 under the Food Allergy Safety, Treatment, Education, and Research (FASTER) Act, reflecting the continued evolution of recognition and policy around food allergies in the US (USFDA, 2024). These top nine allergens account for 90% of all allergic reactions in the US (USFDA, 2025).

Priority food allergens that require labeling in Canada include milk, peanut, tree nuts, egg, fish, shellfish, including both crustaceans (crab, crayfish, lobster, prawns, and shrimp) and mollusks (clams, mussels, oysters and scallops, octopus, snail, and squid), wheat and triticale, sesame, soy, and mustard, as well as sulfites, which while not causing a true allergic reaction, can mimic the symptoms, especially in people with asthma (Health Canada, 2023). In the European Union, the list of food allergens includes celery, cereals that contain gluten, such as wheat, rye, barley, and oats, crustaceans, eggs, fish, lupin, milk, mollusks, mustard, tree nuts, peanuts, soybeans, sesame seeds, as well as sulfur dioxide and sulfites (European Food Information Council, 2025). Australia requires labeling for crustaceans, egg, fish, lupin, milk, mollusks, peanut, sesame, soy (also soya and soybean), tree nuts (which are specifically listed as almond, Brazil nut, cashew, hazelnut, macadamia, pecan, pistachio, pine nut, and walnut), wheat, and sulfites. Barley, oats, and rye must also be labeled if they contain gluten, and sulfites if they meet a threshold of greater than 10 mg/kg of food (Food Standards Australia New Zealand, 2022).

Food allergies are a global issue and require vigilance on the part of government agencies, industry, healthcare clinicians, and the greater population. Countries may have various requirements for labeling, and there may be additions to the above lists, based on the prevalence of allergies locally. New requirements for labeling may emerge as allergens are better understood (e.g., cross-reactivity and lipid transfer proteins). Many foods, but not all, require labeling, and understanding how to read labels will be discussed in greater detail in chapter "Understanding the Diagnosis and Management of Food Allergy Part III: Management of Food Allergy in the Outpatient Setting".

Disparities in IgE-Mediated Food Allergy

As we continue to learn more about the increased prevalence of food allergy, more evidence about the impact of healthcare disparities and social determinants of health has also been generated, bringing the collective challenge of living with food allergies into sharp focus. While more people are experiencing food allergy, disparities may not afford everyone access to up-to-date diagnostics and treatments. The rising prevalence of food allergies has major implications for physical and economic burdens on health systems, schools, families, and society at large. And while care for those with food allergy has changed rapidly in recent years, a web-based World

Allergy Organization survey of allergy treatment centers and members of the society across the world revealed that the availability of common diagnostic and treatment modalities varied across geographic regions (Arasi et al., 2025).

In the US, a survey conducted of over 50,000 US households in 2015–2016 was reported by Jiang et al. (2023), noting that Asian (10.5%), Black (10.6%), and Hispanic (10.6%) people of all ages reported a slightly higher incidence of food allergies than Whites (9.5%) (p. 10/15). The study reported extensively on the prevalence of food allergies with respect to race, ethnicity, income, and insurance, and the results require further study, but point to potential disparities in access to care, such as more instances of severe allergic reaction, multiple food allergies, and ED visits, in Black and Hispanic respondents.

Data on food allergy in children has also been reported separately. A meta-analysis of over two dozen surveys from 1988 to 2011, reporting on nearly 400,000 children based primarily on self-report, and which notably did not include oral food challenges, found that despite study heterogeneity, a steady increase in food allergy of 1.2% percentage points per decade was observed. Increase in prevalence varied by race with Blacks reporting the highest prevalence (2.1%) (Keet et al., 2014). Interestingly, the authors noted that Blacks had previously reported equal or lower rates of food allergy than Whites until the late 2000s, suggesting the possibility of underdiagnosis, perhaps due to access to specialty care.

In a study of over 800 children with provider-diagnosed food allergy, Mahdavinia et al. (2017) reported different presentations across groups. African American (AA) and Hispanic children (the authors' terms) both had significant differences in the prevalence of some allergens when compared to non-Hispanic White children, notably to corn, fish, and shellfish, while White children had statistically higher incidence of tree nut allergy. AA children also experienced a higher incidence of wheat allergy in comparison to White children, among other findings. Consistent with the disparity issues noted above, adverse events, including anaphylaxis and emergency department visits were also higher in the AA and Hispanic children. These disparities underscore the urgent need for culturally competent care and access to an accurate diagnosis and evidence-based management of food allergies. More about disparities related to food allergy is discussed in chapter "Disparities in Food Allergy".

Other IgE-Mediated Food Allergies

As noted earlier, in this book, we primarily focus on the IgE-mediated food allergies caused by the most common allergens. However, it is important for nurses to understand other diagnoses that are IgE-mediated, and they are presented briefly here.

Oral Allergy Syndrome

Oral allergy syndrome (OAS), otherwise known as pollen food allergy syndrome (PFAS), is also IgE-mediated, but is caused by cross-reactivity to proteins in foods that are similar to seasonal pollens, like ragweed, grass, birch, and mugmort (Bégin et al.,

2024). OAS typically results in an itchy mouth or throat after exposure to raw fruits or vegetables, such as bananas, cherries, or melon, and many others, or some vegetables and spices. Although anaphylaxis is possible in a small percentage of patients with this type of reaction, more often, symptoms are on the mild end of the spectrum.

Alpha-gal Syndrome

Alpha-gal syndrome (AGS) is also an IgE-mediated allergy, but there are some important differences in presentation from the top nine allergens (Thompson et al., 2025). It is notable that due to the lack of awareness of this condition, patients may experience a delay in diagnosis for several years as patients may not be referred appropriately. Unlike other top nine allergies, the offending antigen is a carbohydrate (oligosaccharide galactose-α-1-3) rather than a protein. This molecule is transmitted to humans via a tick bite, often the lone star tick in the US, although other ticks are implicated both inside and outside the US. Four to six weeks after the tick bite, a reaction may be triggered following consumption of non-primate mammalian red meat such as beef, pork, or lamb, or products derived from meat (e.g., gelatin), dairy products, or through exposure to personal care and medical products derived from animals, including heart valves or monoclonal antibodies, heparin, pancreatic enzymes (Commins, 2020; Emerson et al., 2026; Thompson et al., 2025).

AGS reactions, with symptoms such as urticaria or other skin symptoms, diarrhea, cramping and vomiting, and possibly anaphylaxis, occur from 2–6 h after ingestion, often occurring later in the evening following the dinner meal, although this time span can also vary, with reactions to drugs manifesting more rapidly. It is notable that B blood types seem to have a protective effect from developing AGS (Commins, 2020: Thompson et al., 2025). Patients are counseled to avoid provoking foods and certain medical products that are derived from mammalian tissue. Some patients may experience remission, but the overall course of this condition remains unknown, although greater awareness of the condition may provide more guidance in the future.

Food-Dependent, Exercise-Induced Anaphylaxis

Another uncommon IgE-mediated adverse reaction to food is food-dependent, exercise-induced anaphylaxis (FDEIA), which occurs when specific foods are eaten before exercise (Cox and Sicherer, 2020).

Non-IgE Mediated Food Allergies

Non IgE-mediated food allergies include such conditions as food protein-induced enterocolitis syndrome (FPIES), food protein-induced allergic proctocolitis (FPIAP), and food-protein-enteropathy (FPE). Instead of being IgE-mediated, other immune mechanisms cause these reactions. We will briefly review them here so that readers can appreciate the overall variability in adverse food reactions. These conditions are most commonly diagnosed in infants through age 2.

Food Protein-Induced Enterocolitis Syndrome (FPIES)

Food protein-induced enterocolitis is an uncommon non-IgE mediated food allergy with a delayed onset of symptoms. Any food may cause FPIES, but frequently milk and soy are the culprits, although the triggering food varies by geographic location and may include a wide variety of foods, including some fruits, grains, proteins, and vegetables (Baker et al., 2025). FPIES is cell-mediated (T cells and other cells) and causes a delayed inflammatory response in the gastrointestinal (GI) tract. FPIES often presents in infancy or childhood, but can also occur in adults.

Acute, chronic, atypical, and adult-onset presentations of FPIES occur (Beaudoin et al., 2025). Acute reactions, the most common presentation, occur within a couple of hours after food ingestion, and may include vomiting, watery or bloody diarrhea, dehydration, possibly hypotension and shock. The infant can look very unwell during this period after ingesting the offending food, but recovers by the next day. Chronic FPIES is more protracted, characterized by failure to thrive and GI symptoms, such as watery or bloody diarrhea and often vomiting, precipitated by ongoing ingestion of the triggering food. Diagnosis of FPIES is primarily made through an exploration of the clinical presentation based on the reported signs and symptoms, as there is no standard diagnostic test, although there are some findings that support the diagnosis. Immediate treatment for FPIES includes rehydration and antiemetic treatment (e.g., ondanseton), which can sometimes be managed at home or may require more intensive emergency care. Avoidance of the food suspected of causing the symptoms is essential to the management plan (Nowak-Węgrzyn et al., 2017). FPIES often resolves, and oral food challenges are conducted to determine resolution, although there are calls for more standardization of these dosing protocols (Baker et al., 2026).

Food Protein-Induced Allergic Proctocolitis (FPIAP)

Food protein-induced allergic proctocolitis (FPIAP) represents a non-IgE mediated delayed allergic reaction of the colon in response to ingestion of cow's milk or soy protein infants who are 1-4 weeks of age. Infants present with bloody stools which sometimes contain mucous, and possibly diarrhea. Symptoms can also include reflux, feeding issues, and irritability (Leney et al., 2025). While there are no confirmatory diagnostic tests, a presumptive diagnosis is made when symptoms improve after the removal of the suspected cause, with a return of symptoms when the food (usually milk) is reintroduced. In breastfed infants, milk is eliminated from the mother's diet, and in formula-fed babies, alternative hypoallergenic formulas are used. Resolution of bloody stool can occur within days, while mucus may persist for a month or so. The offending allergen can eventually be reintroduced roughly 6 months after symptomatic improvement, although the timeline may vary. Since FPIAP is believed to be a part of the allergic march, consideration should be given to when other food allergens should be introduced into the infant's diet to avoid the development of IgE-mediated food allergies.

Food Protein-Induced Enteropathy (FPE)

Food protein-induced enteropathy (FPE) is an uncommon non-IgE gastrointestinal food allergy that presents in infants. FPE is linked to cow's milk ingestion, resulting in malabsorption and failure to thrive, and featuring symptoms of diarrhea, weight loss, and possibly vomiting. FPE is diagnosed through biopsy of the small bowel, and is managed by elimination of the offending allergen, usually milk, from the diet, and will generally resolve by age 1–2. If the baby is not breastfeeding or needs supplementation, specialized formulas may be required (Barni et al., 2024).

Mixed IgE/Non-IgE Food Allergy

Several eosinophilic gastrointestinal disorders may be classified as having a mixed etiology, including eosinophilic esophagitis (EoE). Symptoms of EoE may include reflux, difficulty swallowing, and possible food impaction. Diagnosis is made by ruling out other causes, conducting a careful history, and esophageal biopsy for eosinophils (Cox and Sicherer, 2020).

Living with Food Allergies

Once a diagnosis is established, the patient and family coping with food allergies must adjust to living with food allergies. Living with food allergies can be very stressful due to the daily vigilance needed to stay safe. Routine activities such as grocery shopping, preparing food, dining out, and events such as parties and travel, which are usually fun, can cause tremendous anxiety for those with food allergies. Even some of the newer treatments for food allergy can provoke anxiety due to fear of injections, blood draws, or potential anaphylactic reactions during updosing of allergens to desensitize the immune system.

Traditionally, healthcare clinicians recommended that patients with food allergies avoid their allergen to decrease allergic reactions, but the science has evolved, and the guidance has changed to include recommendations for early allergen introduction as a primary prevention strategy, and to the expansion of novel treatment options, most notably immunotherapies and biologic therapies, with other options in the pipeline. Recently, FDA-approved treatments are available for accidental exposure to food allergens (see chapter "Understanding the Diagnosis and Management of Food Allergy Part III: Management of Food Allergy in the Outpatient

Setting"). Patients and families are participating in shared decision-making with healthcare clinicians, including nurses, to decide whether avoidance, oral immunotherapy (OIT), or even injectable biologic treatments are the right pathways to manage food allergy. These treatments will be explored along with other promising treatments in chapter "Understanding the Diagnosis and Management of Food Allergy Part III: Management of Food Allergy in the Outpatient Setting".

The Role of Nurses

Nurses play a pivotal role in the care continuum for patients with food allergies. In the outpatient setting, nurses often conduct the initial evaluation of suspected allergic reactions, provide anticipatory guidance, and coordinate referrals for allergy testing. In hospitals, bedside nurses monitor patients during food challenges or allergic reactions, administer emergency medications, and educate families prior to discharge, often from the emergency department or urgent care, as well as the inpatient setting. School nurses are responsible for developing and enforcing individualized healthcare plans, recognizing allergic reactions, and training staff on emergency response. However, despite the frequency of interaction with patients and families with food allergies, the content taught about the management of food allergies in medical and nursing curricula may be minimal. Bahna notes that medical students receive little training about food allergies, and for resident physicians, allergy rotations are not mandatory (Bahna, 2024).

With more knowledge about food allergies, nurses can play a transformative role in the care of patients and families coping with the many challenges associated with this diagnosis. Helping patients and caregivers to overcome epinephrine hesitancy is one example. Lack of confidence about when to use epinephrine can be overcome through education and coaching provided by nurses.

Advancing a nursing specialty or credential in food allergy care could be an important step that will benefit many of those living with food allergies. We also hope to motivate nurses who are pursuing advanced degrees to implement quality improvement projects relevant to patients and families with food allergies, and to engage in scientific inquiry to generate new knowledge through nursing research to help support patients and families. Because food allergy care spans multiple settings, nurses are uniquely positioned to serve as educators and advocates. They also bridge communication between families, physicians, pharmacists, nutritionists, psychologists, and educators, ensuring that the patient's safety and quality of life remain central.

The Need for Comprehensive Resources

Despite advances in allergy science and increasing public awareness, gaps remain in diagnosis, management, and education. Families frequently report feelings of fear, isolation, and uncertainty. Misconceptions about food allergy remain common among healthcare providers and the public, and practices such as over-restrictive diets or delayed epinephrine device use continue to pose risks. Nurses, therefore, must be well-prepared to deliver accurate education, advocate for evidence-based strategies, and empower patients and families to live safely and confidently.

This book is structured to address these gaps through a nursing-centered lens, with chapters covering clinical guidelines, social-emotional considerations, advocacy, and more. Each chapter combines evidence-based recommendations with practical strategies that nurses can apply directly in their practice.

Organization of the Book

The chapters that follow cover the following food allergy topics:

- *Understanding Diagnosis and Management of Food Allergy*—outlining current best practices in assessment, diagnostic testing, and evidence-based treatment.
- *Disparities in Food Allergy*—examining socioeconomic, racial, and cultural inequities in prevalence, diagnosis, and care.
- *Early Introduction of Food Allergens*—exploring landmark research (e.g., LEAP, EAT studies, and beyond) and its implications for prevention.
- *Food Allergy Management in Early Childhood Settings*—addressing the unique needs in preschools, daycares, and early education.
- *Food Allergy Management in Adolescents and Young Adults*—focusing on transitional care, self-management, and risk-taking behaviors.
- *Food Allergy Management in the Hospital Setting*—bridging inpatient clinical care with safe discharge planning.
- *Social Emotional Impact of Food Allergy*—exploring anxiety, stigma, and quality-of-life challenges for patients and families.
- *Role of Technology in the Management of Food Allergy*—highlighting emerging tools such as electronic health record alerts, telehealth, mobile apps, and diagnostic innovations.
- *Public Policy and Advocacy for People with Food Allergy*—outlining policy, legislation, and the importance of nurse-led advocacy.
- *Advancing Food Allergy Care: The Role of the Certified Allergy Nurse Educator*—discussing nurse-led training initiatives, simulation, and curriculum development for the proposed certified allergy nurse educator role.
- *Prior Authorization Recommendations*—providing practical tips for navigating insurance approvals for allergy testing and treatment.
- *Resources Page*—offering quick-reference tools and links, including resources from organizations around the globe.

Looking Ahead

Food allergy is a complex and rapidly evolving condition that intersects immunology, nutrition, psychology, public health, and policy. For nurses, staying informed is not only a professional responsibility but also a matter of patient safety and empowerment. Through this book, our goal is to provide a comprehensive, practical guide that equips nurses at any level and across specialties with the knowledge and confidence to care for patients with food allergies. By bridging clinical expertise with education, advocacy, and cultural awareness, nurses can lead the way in transforming food allergy care and improving quality of life for millions of patients and families worldwide. We hope you enjoy the book! (Cox and Sicherer, 2020; Giannetti, 2018).

References

Arasi, S., Morais-Almeida, M., Martin, B. L., Wing-Kin Wong, G., Ansotegui, I. J., Ebisawa, M., Custovic, A., Santos, A., Nowak-Wegrzyn, A., Stoddart, A., Deschildre, A., Cianferoni, A., Muraro, A., DunnGalvin, A., Vickery, B., Venter, C., Jones, C., Mazzuca, C., Warren, C., Munblit, D., et al. (2025). Food allergy severity across the world: A World Allergy Organization international survey. *The World Allergy Organization journal, 18*(11), 101123. https://doi.org/10.1016/j.waojou.2025.101123

Azzolino, D., Verdi, L., Perna, S., Baldassari, I., Cesari, M., & Lucchi, T. (2024). Food allergies in older people: An emerging health problem. *The World Allergy Organization Journal, 17*(9), 100967. https://doi.org/10.1016/j.waojou.2024.100967

Bahna, S. L. (2024). History of food allergy and where we are today. *The World Allergy Organization Journal, 17*(5), 100912. https://doi.org/10.1016/j.waojou.2024.100912

Baker, M. G., Wong, L. S. Y., Konstantinou, G. N., & Nowak-Wegrzyn, A. (2025). Food allergy endotypes revisited. *The Journal of Allergy and Clinical Immunology, 156*(1), 1–16. https://doi.org/10.1016/j.jaci.2025.04.019

Baker, M. G., Bird, J. A., Brown-Whitchorn, T., Cosper, A., Groetch, M., Horak, S., Leonard, S., Scurlock, A. M., Upton, J. E. M., Varshney, P., & Anvari, S. (2026). Standardizing oral food challenge protocols in food protein-induced enterocolitis syndrome (FPIES): A call for consensus. *Annals of Allergy, Asthma & Immunology: Official Publication of the American College of Allergy, Asthma, & Immunology, 136*(1), 16–24. https://doi.org/10.1016/j.anai.2025.10.005

Barni, S., Mori, F., Pecoraro, L., Saretta, F., Giovannini, M., Arasi, S., Liotti, L., Mastrorilli, C., Klain, A., Gelsomino, M., Castagnoli, R., Miraglia Del Giudice, M., & Novembre, E. (2024). Food protein-induced enteropathy: A revision for the clinician. *Frontiers in Pediatrics, 12*, 1417391. https://doi.org/10.3389/fped.2024.1417391

Bartha, I., Almulhem, N., & Santos, A. F. (2024). Feast for thought: A comprehensive review of food allergy 2021–2023. *Journal of Allergy and Clinical Immunology, 153*(3), 576–594. https://doi.org/10.1016/j.jaci.2023.11.918

Beaudoin, M., Mehra, A., Wong, L. S. Y., Vazquez-Ortiz, M., González-Delgado, P., & Nowak-Wegrzyn, A. (2025). An algorithm for the diagnosis and treatment of Food Protein-Induced Enterocolitis Syndrome (FPIES), 2024 Update. *Allergy, 80*(1), 362–365. https://doi.org/10.1111/all.16432

Bégin, P., Waserman, S., Protudjer, J. L. P., Jeimy, S., & Watson, W. (2024). Immunoglobulin E (IgE)-mediated food allergy. *Allergy, Asthma & Clinical Immunology, 20*(Suppl 3), 75. Published 2024 Dec 30. https://doi.org/10.1186/s13223-024-00930-7

Bottoms-McClain, L., Giri, A., & Ng, A. E. (2026 Jan). Diagnosed allergic conditions in adults: United States, 2024. *NCHS Data Brief, 545*, 1–11. https://doi.org/10.15620/cdc/174634

Calvani, M., Anania, C., Caffarelli, C., Martelli, A., Miraglia Del Giudice, M., Cravidi, C., Duse, M., Manti, S., Tosca, M. A., Cardinale, F., Chiappini, E., Olivero, F., & Marseglia, G. L. (2020). Food allergy: An updated review on pathogenesis, diagnosis, prevention and management. *Acta Bio-Medica: Atenei Parmensis, 91*(11-S), e2020012. https://doi.org/10.23750/abm.v91i11-S.10316

Commins, S. P. (2020). Diagnosis & management of alpha-gal syndrome: Lessons from 2,500 patients. *Expert Review of Clinical Immunology, 16*(7), 667–677. https://doi.org/10.1080/1744666X.2020.1782745

Cox, A. L., Sicherer, S. H. (2020). Classification of adverse food reactions. *Journal of Food Allergy, 2*(1), 3–6. https://doi.org/10.2500/jfa.2020.2.200022

Di Costanzo, M., De Paulis, N., & Biasucci, G. (2021). Butyrate: A link between early life nutrition and gut microbiome in the development of food allergy. *Life (Basel, Switzerland), 11*(5), 384. https://doi.org/10.3390/life11050384

Du Toit, G., Roberts, G., Sayre, P. H., Plaut, M., Bahnson, H. T., Mitchell, H., Radulovic, S., Chan, S., Fox, A., Turcanu, V., Lack, G., & Learning Early About Peanut Allergy (LEAP) Study Team. (2013). Identifying infants at high risk of peanut allergy: The Learning Early About Peanut Allergy (LEAP) screening study. *The Journal of Allergy and Clinical Immunology, 131*(1). https://doi.org/10.1016/j.jaci.2012.09.015

Elizur, A., Rajuan, N., Goldberg, M. R., Leshno, M., Cohen, A., & Katz, Y. (2012). Natural course and risk factors for persistence of IgE-mediated cow's milk allergy. *The Journal of Pediatrics, 161*(3), 482–487.e1. https://doi.org/10.1016/j.jpeds.2012.02.028

Emerson, A. G., Mundy, L., Murphy, B. A., & Stone, C. A. (2026). Cetuximab hypersensitivity in the setting of asymptomatic Alpha-Gal sensitization. *Head & Neck, 48*(3), E33–E36. https://doi.org/10.1002/hed.70030

European Food Information Council. (2025). *List of the 14 most common food allergens*. Retrieved August 5, 2025, from https://www.eufic.org/en/healthy-living/article/list-of-the-14-most-common-food-allergens

Feng, H., Xiong, X., Chen, Z., Xu, Q., Zhang, Z., Luo, N., & Wu, Y. (2023). Prevalence and influencing factors of food allergy in global context: A meta-analysis. *International Archives of Allergy and Immunology, 184*(4), 320–352. https://doi.org/10.1159/000527870

Ferraro, V. A., Zanconato, S., & Carraro, S. (2025). The epithelial barrier hypothesis in food allergies: The state of the art. *Nutrients, 17*(6), 1014. https://doi.org/10.3390/nu17061014

Food Allergy Research & Education. (2024). *Food allergy facts and statistics for the U.S.* Retrieved August 5, 2025, from https://www.foodallergy.org/resources/facts-and-statistics

Food Standards Australia New Zealand. (2022). *Allergen labelling for consumers*. Retrieved August 5, 2025, from https://www.foodstandards.gov.au/consumer/labelling/allergen-labelling

Forero Molina, M. A., Kram, Y. E., & Lanser, B. J. (2025). The global burden of food allergy. *Immunology and Allergy Clinics of North America, 45*(3), 325–337. https://doi.org/10.1016/j.iac.2025.04.002

Giannetti, M. P. (2018). Exercise-induced anaphylaxis: Literature review and recent updates. *Current Allergy and Asthma Reports, 18*(12), 72. https://doi.org/10.1007/s11882-018-0830-6. PMID: 30367321.

Gupta, R. S., Warren, C. M., Smith, B. M., Blumenstock, J. A., Jiang, J., Davis, M. M., & Nadeau, K. C. (2018). The public health impact of parent-reported childhood food allergies in the United States. *Pediatrics, 142*(6), 1. https://doi.org/10.1542/peds.2018-1235

Gupta, R. S., Warren, C. M., Smith, B. M., Blumenstock, J. A., Jiang, J., Davis, M. M., & Nadeau, K. C. (2019). Prevalence and severity of food allergies among us adults. *JAMA Network Open, 2*(1), e185630. https://doi.org/10.1001/jamanetworkopen.2018.5630

Gupta, R., Marvel, J., Tassinari, P., Mnif, T., Hleyhel, M., Vincent, B., Worm, M., & Fiocchi, A. (2023). Global prevalence of pediatric and adult IgE-mediated food allergies. Results: From the ASSESS FA study. *Annals of Allergy, Asthma & Immunology, 131*(5), S7–S8. https://doi.org/10.1016/j.anai.2023.08.039

Gupta, R., Mnif, T., Reed, S., Hleyhel, M., Dritsa, S., LeCalvé, P., Moussallem, A., Tassinari, P., Marvel, J., & Fiocchi, A. (2025). Methodology of the international cross-sectional prevalence and severity study of pediatric and adult IgE-mediated food allergies (ASSESS FA). *The World Allergy Organization journal, 18*(9), 101105. https://doi.org/10.1016/j.waojou.2025.101105

Health Canada. (2023). *Common food allergens*. Retrieved August 5, 2025, from https://www.canada.ca/en/health-canada/services/food-nutrition/food-safety/food-allergies-intolerances/food-allergies.html

Houghton, V., Eiwegger, T., Florsheim, E. B., Knibb, R. C., Thuret, S., & Santos, A. F. (2024). From bite to brain: Neuro-immune interactions in food allergy. *Allergy, 79*, 3326–3340. https://doi.org/10.1111/all.16366

Hui-Beckman, J. W., & Kim, B.-E. (2025). Origins of atopy and the role of the skin barrier in food allergy. *Immunology and Allergy Clinics of North America, 45*(3), 313–323. https://doi.org/10.1016/j.iac.2025.04.001

Hund, S. K., Sampath, V., Zhou, X., Thai, B., Desai, K., & Nadeau, K. C. (2025). Scientific developments in understanding food allergy prevention, diagnosis, and treatment. *Frontiers in Immunology, 16*, 1572283. https://doi.org/10.3389/fimmu.2025.1572283

Hussain, M., Bonilla-Rosso, G., Kwong Chung, C. K. C., Bäriswyl, L., Rodriguez, M. P., Kim, B. S., Engel, P., & Noti, M. (2019). High dietary fat intake induces a microbiota signature that promotes food allergy. *Journal of Allergy and Clinical Immunology, 144*(1), 157–170.e8. https://doi.org/10.1016/j.jaci.2019.01.043

Islam, N., Chu, A. W. L., Sheriff, F., et al. (2026). Risk factors for the development of food allergy in infants and children: A systematic review and meta-analysis. *JAMA Pediatrics*. https://doi.org/10.1001/jamapediatrics.2025.6105

Jiang, J., Warren, C. M., Brewer, A., Soffer, G., & Gupta, R. S. (2023). Racial, ethnic, and socioeconomic differences in food allergies in the US. *JAMA Network Open, 6*(6), e2. https://doi.org/10.1001/jamanetworkopen.2023.18162

Keet, C. A., Savage, J. H., Seopaul, S., Peng, R. D., Wood, R. A., & Matsui, E. C. (2014). Temporal trends and racial/ethnic disparity in self-reported pediatric food allergy in the United States. *Annals of Allergy, Asthma & Immunology: Official Publication of the American College of Allergy, Asthma, & Immunology, 112*(3), 222–229.e3. https://doi.org/10.1016/j.anai.2013.12.007

Lack, G. (2012). Update on risk factors for food allergy. *Journal of Allergy and Clinical Immunology, 129*(5), 1187–1197. https://doi.org/10.1016/j.jaci.2012.02.036

Lee, K. H., Song, Y., Wu, W., Yu, K., & Zhang, G. (2020). The gut microbiota, environmental factors, and links to the development of food allergy. *Clinical and Molecular Allergy, 18*(1), Article 5. https://doi.org/10.1186/s12948-020-00120-x

Lee, E. C. K., Trogen, B., Brady, K., Ford, L. S., & Wang, J. (2024). The natural history and risk factors for the development of food allergies in children and adults. *Current Allergy and Asthma Reports, 24*(3), 121–131. https://doi.org/10.1007/s11882-024-01131-3

Leney, M., Kahale, F., & Martin, V. M. (2025). Diagnosis and management of food protein-induced allergic proctocolitis. *Current Gastroenterology Reports, 27*(1), 76. https://doi.org/10.1007/s11894-025-01022-1

Linton, S., Hossenbaccus, L., Ellis, A.K. (2023). Evidence-based use of antihistamines for treat ment of allergic conditions. *Annals of Allergy, Asthma & Immunology, 131*(4), 412–420. https://doi.org/10.1016/j.anai.2023.07.019. Epub 2023 Jul 28. PMID: 37517656.

Loh, W., & Tang, M. L. (2018). The epidemiology of food allergy in the global context. *International Journal of Environmental Research and Public Health, 15*(9), 2043. https://doi.org/10.3390/ijerph15092043

Mahdavinia, M., Fox, S. R., Smith, B. M., James, C., Palmisano, E. L., Mohammed, A., Zahid, Z., Assa'ad, A. H., Tobin, M. C., & Gupta, R. S. (2017). Racial differences in food allergy phenotype and health care utilization among US children. *The Journal of Allergy and Clinical Immunology. In Practice., 5*(2), 352–357.e1. https://doi.org/10.1016/j.jaip.2016.10.006

McIntyre, A., Lee, K., & Singh, A. M. (2023). Adults and children report gaining natural tolerance to former food allergens at all ages regardless of age of food allergy onset. *Journal of Allergy and Clinical Immunology, 151*(2), AB30–AB30. https://doi.org/10.1016/j.jaci.2022.12.096

National Academies of Sciences, Engineering, and Medicine, Health and Medicine Division, Food and Nutrition Board, Committee on Food Allergies: Global Burden, Causes, Treatment, Prevention, and Public Policy. (2017). In M. P. Oria & V. A. Stallings (Eds.), *Finding a path to safety in food allergy: Assessment of the global burden, causes, prevention, management, and public policy*. National Academies Press. https://doi.org/10.17226/23658

Ng, A. E., Giri, A., & Bottoms-McClain, L. (2026). Diagnosed allergic conditions in children ages 0–17: United States, 2024. *NCHS Data Brief, 546*, 1–10. https://doi.org/10.15620/cdc/174635

NIAID-Sponsored Expert Panel, Boyce, J. A., Assa'ad, A., Burks, A. W., Jones, S. M., Sampson, H. A., Wood, R. A., Plaut, M., Cooper, S. F., Fenton, M. J., Arshad, S. H., Bahna, S. L., Beck, L. A., Byrd-Bredbenner, C., Camargo, C. A., Jr., Eichenfield, L., Furuta, G. T., Hanifin, J. M., Jones, C., Kraft, M., et al. (2010). Guidelines for the diagnosis and management of food allergy in the United States: Report of the NIAID-sponsored expert panel. *The Journal of Allergy and Clinical Immunology, 126*(6 Suppl), S1–S58. https://doi.org/10.1016/j.jaci.2010.10.007

Nowak-Węgrzyn, A., Chehade, M., Groetch, M. E., Spergel, J. M., Wood, R. A., Allen, K., Atkins, D., Bahna, S., Barad, A. V., Berin, C., Brown Whitehorn, T., Burks, A. W., Caubet, J. C., Cianferoni, A., Conte, M., Davis, C., Fiocchi, A., Grimshaw, K., Gupta, R., Hofmeister, B., et al. (2017). International consensus guidelines for the diagnosis and management of food protein-induced enterocolitis syndrome: Executive summary-workgroup report of the Adverse Reactions to Foods Committee, American Academy of Allergy, Asthma & Immunology. *The Journal of Allergy and Clinical Immunology, 139*(4), 1111–1126.e4. https://doi.org/10.1016/j.jaci.2016.12.966

Santos, A. F., Riggioni, C., Agache, I., Akdis, C. A., Akdis, M., Alvarez-Perea, A., Alvaro-Lozano, M., Ballmer-Weber, B., Barni, S., Beyer, K., Bindslev-Jensen, C., Brough, H. A., Buyuktiryaki, B., Chu, D., Del Giacco, S., Dunn-Galvin, A., Eberlein, B., Ebisawa, M., Eigenmann, P., Eiwegger, T., et al. (2023). EAACI guidelines on the diagnosis of IgE-mediated food allergy. *Allergy, 78*(12), 3057–3076. https://doi.org/10.1111/all.15902

Shi, Q., Gao, X., Zhang, S. et al. (2026). Environmental pollutants and food allergy: from traditional triggers to emerging hazards. *Clinical reviews in allergy & immunology, 69,* 13. https://doi.org/10.1007/s12016-026-09142-w

Sicherer, S. H., & Sampson, H. A. (2018). Food allergy: A review and update on epidemiology, pathogenesis, diagnosis, prevention, and management. *Journal of Allergy and Clinical Immunology, 141*(1), 41–58. https://doi.org/10.1016/j.jaci.2017.11.003

Thompson, C. C., Saracco, B., Pruthi, A., & Cerceo, E. (2025). Alpha-Gal Syndrome: Often hidden, under-recognized, and in need of attention-a rapid review. *International Journal of General Medicine, 18*, 3477–3488. https://doi.org/10.2147/IJGM.S519844

U.S. Food & Drug Administration (FDA). (2024). *The Faster Act: Sesame is the ninth major food allergen*. Retrieved August 28, 2025, from https://www.fda.gov/food/food-allergies/faster-act-sesame-ninth-major-food-allergen

U.S. Food & Drug Administration (FDA). (2025). *Food allergies*. Retrieved August 28, 2025, from https://www.fda.gov/food/nutrition-food-labeling-and-critical-foods/food-allergies

Waizman, D. A., Brown-Soler, I., Martin, A. L., Ma, Y., Zhou, K., Israni-Winger, K., Zhang, C., Medzhitov, R., Launay, P., Michieletto, M. F., Henao-Mejia, J., Palm, N. W., Craft, J., Eisenstein, A., & Wang, A. (2025). Skin damage signals mediate allergic sensitization to spatially unlinked antigen. *Science Immunology, 10*(106), eadn0688. https://doi.org/10.1126/sciimmunol.adn0688

Warren, C., Nimmagadda, S. R., Gupta, R., & Levin, M. (2023). The epidemiology of food allergy in adults. *Annals of Allergy, Asthma & Immunology: Official Publication of the American College of Allergy, Asthma, & Immunology, 130*(3), 276–287. https://doi.org/10.1016/j.anai.2022.11.026

Understanding the Diagnosis and Management of Food Allergy Part I: IgE-Mediated Food Allergy and Anaphylaxis

Sarah Pederson, Robyn Huey Lao, Mary Frances Vess, Josie Howard-Ruben, and Julianne Doucette

Care of the Patient with Food Allergy: Important Foundational Information for Nurses

Food allergies result from the complex interaction among body systems, including the immune, skin and mucosal, and gastrointestinal (GI) systems, as well as the influence of genetics and environmental conditions. A diagnosis of food allergies disrupts daily living, and the potential detrimental impact cannot be overstated, but it can be managed. From the day symptoms appear, or when the first reaction occurs, patients and/or caregivers seek a healthcare team to guide them. People with food allergy and/or their caregivers need to learn what the symptoms represent, understand what diagnostic test results mean, and then need to discover the knowledge, skills, and behaviors they need to master to live well with a food allergy diagnosis.

S. Pederson (✉)
Food Allergy Nursing Association, Great Neck, NY, USA

R. H. Lao
University of California Davis, Davis, CA, USA
e-mail: REHuey@health.ucdavis.edu

M. F. Vess
Children's Healthcare of Atlanta, Atlanta, Georgia, USA
e-mail: mary.vess@choa.org

J. Howard-Ruben
Rush University College of Nursing, Chicago, IL, USA
e-mail: josie_howard-ruben@rush.edu

J. Doucette
College of Nursing, Rush University, Chicago, IL, USA
e-mail: Julianne_Doucette@rush.edu

J. Doucette, J. Howard-Ruben (eds.), *Comprehensive Food Allergy Management for Nurses*, https://doi.org/10.1007/978-3-032-28647-5_2

Nurses can play an important role in providing support and education throughout the diagnostic process and help patients learn how best to cope with food allergies. By providing resources about daily activities, allergen avoidance, self-management strategies, emergency preparedness, and support and education for those who opt for active treatment, the nurse can be an engaged partner who helps to improve both quality of care and quality of life.

This chapter focuses on the diagnosis of food allergies and starts with basic scientific underpinnings of IgE-mediated allergies to help nurses understand how this process unfolds. The discussion assumes the outpatient setting, so in this chapter, there is a brief discussion of emergency management and a more extensive review of anaphylaxis.

Understanding IgE-Mediated Food Allergy and Other Adverse Effects from Foods

In chapter "Introduction to IgE-Mediated Food Allergy", a definition of food allergy was provided (NIAID-Sponsored Expert Panel, 2010). Various forms of adverse reactions to food can occur; however, not all food allergies are IgE-mediated. Adverse effects to foods have been classified as including immunological (hypersensitivities/food allergies), non-immunological (intolerances, such as lactose intolerances), and microbial reactions (caused by toxins and infection) (see Fig. 1). Below, we briefly discuss adverse reactions to foods so that nurses are familiar with their presentation. Our emphasis, throughout this book, however, is on IgE-mediated food allergies, including allergies to milk, eggs, fish, shellfish, tree nuts, peanuts, wheat, soybeans, and sesame.

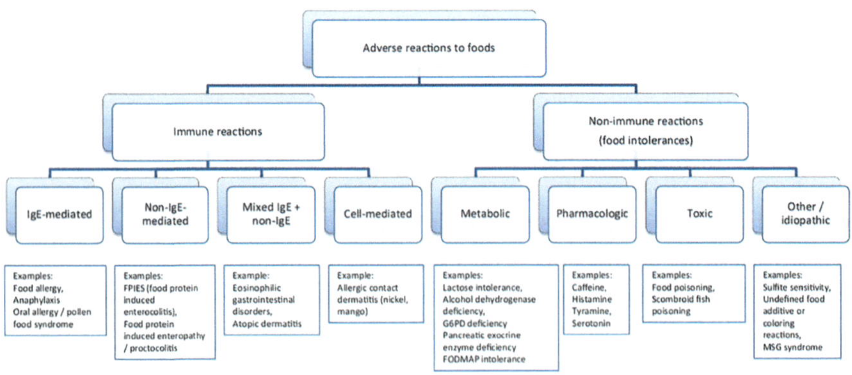

Fig. 1 Classification of adverse reactions to foods. Reactions are considered non-immunological or immunologic, with subtypes as pictured for each of these categories. Examples of each are provided. (Used with permission from: Cox and Sicherer 2020)

IgE-Mediated Food Allergy

IgE-mediated food allergy involves an abnormal response by the immune system that thwarts the development of oral tolerance, which is the ability to eat a food without an allergic response. IgE-mediated food allergies, known as Type I hypersensitivity reactions, are immune reactions to food that can cause immediate symptoms across multiple body systems. These symptoms can range from skin manifestations such as hives to multisystem involvement and include respiratory, cardiac, dermatologic (skin and mucosa), gastrointestinal, and even other symptoms (e.g., feeling of "impending doom," uterine contractions and cramping). Food allergies and food intolerance are two different entities, but the terminology might be confusing since the word tolerance is also used in the context of food allergies.

Tolerance has been described as the "state of healthy immunological nonresponsiveness (i.e., no symptoms occur, added by authors) to common food antigens" (Yu et al., 2016, p. 762). Disruption of the immune system in the person with food allergies prevents the development of oral tolerance. Although it is not completely understood, the development of oral tolerance is a complex process that involves both the gastrointestinal and innate and adaptive immune systems and typically occurs when foods are introduced in the diet. Usually, a normal gastrointestinal system recognizes these food proteins as harmless, ignores them, and a state of nonresponsiveness develops, as is the case with most people who do not develop food allergies.

In IgE-mediated food allergy, the patient reacts to food proteins (antigens), and reactions are typically immediate and occur within minutes to about 2 h after the allergen exposure (exceptions to this time frame are alpha-gal syndrome and food-dependent exercise-induced anaphylaxis, which are often delayed). Nurses should understand that anaphylaxis from food allergies may not have a single type of presentation; many body systems may be involved, and hives are *not* present in some cases. The need for prompt administration of epinephrine should be repeatedly reinforced with patients and caregivers when anaphylaxis is suspected, as they often question whether symptoms warrant epinephrine. Reactions may subside after treatment with epinephrine and then return without re-exposure to the allergen as long as 72 h later, in a biphasic reaction. Estimates of the incidence of biphasic reactions have varied from 1% to 20%, but a recent registry-based study suggested that the incidence was about 16.4% (Gupta et al., 2021), and this research confirmed the prevailing wisdom that the more severe the initial reaction, the more likely a biphasic reaction is to occur.

Traditionally, the advice has been to send patients to the emergency department after an anaphylactic episode and treatment with epinephrine/adrenaline, and this remains common practice. It should be made clear to patients and families that the reason for seeking this care is for continued observation, rather than because epinephrine was used, which seems to be frequently misunderstood and may contribute to epinephrine hesitancy. However, recent practice parameter updates have explored this issue in more detail and consider when home management of anaphylaxis might be safely considered under certain circumstances (Abrams et al., 2024; Golden et al., 2024) and will be discussed below. Patients and families can still be advised to summon emergency support (e.g., call 911) or get to an emergency facility, but this practice is evolving. Nevertheless, access to emergency care should be prioritized.

Other IgE-Mediated Food Reactions

Other IgE-mediated reactions to foods include acute urticaria and oral allergy syndrome (OAS) or pollen food allergy syndrome (PFAS). OAS and PFAS involve sensitivity to pollen (birch, grasses, ragweed, mugwort, etc.) which results in a reaction that is typically localized to the ears and/or mouth most often including itching but sometimes throat tightness, nausea or even hoarseness or difficulty swallowing after ingestion of raw fruits and/or vegetables, nuts, or herbs/spices (for example, bananas, melons, kiwi, almonds, and pitted fruits) (Varshney & Pongracic, 2020). Food-dependent exercise-induced anaphylaxis (FDEIA) may present with wheals and/or angioedema as well as respiratory or cardiovascular symptoms, although 1 in 6 may only exhibit wheals and/or angioedema (Kulthanan et al., 2022). FDEIA only occurs when certain foods (e.g., wheat) are eaten in time proximity (e.g., within approximately 4 hours after eating, although a range is reported) to physical exercise (Kulthanan et al., 2022; Srisuwatchari et al., 2023; Varshney & Pongracic, 2020). Diagnosis of this condition involves various challenges to confirm it and is not discussed in this chapter. Another IgE-mediated food allergy is alpha-gal syndrome, which is a hypersensitivity to a carbohydrate in meat rather than a food protein, and unlike most IgE-mediated reactions, has a delayed onset.

Other Adverse Reactions to Foods

In chapter "Introduction to IgE-Mediated Food Allergy", several other immune-mediated adverse reactions to food were discussed briefly. Food allergy responses with a mixed IgE etiology include atopic dermatitis and eosinophilic esophagitis. Non-IgE-mediated reactions to food include several gastrointestinal conditions, such as food protein-induced enterocolitis (FPIES) and food protein-induced allergic proctocolitis (FPIAP), and other conditions, which have a different pathophysiologic mechanism than IgE-mediated reactions and require different management strategies. Furthermore, non-IgE-mediated responses typically have a slower onset and are described as cell-mediated.

In contrast, food intolerances reflect the body's inability to digest a certain food, as in lactose intolerance, and typically cause gastrointestinal, skin, or respiratory symptoms. Food intolerances can also manifest in response to characteristics of the offending food that include pharmacologic properties, such as caffeine; toxic substances, such as scombroid (sometimes described as histamine poisoning); some host-dependent metabolic factors, such as lactose intolerance or various enzyme deficiencies; and others that may not fit into these categories.

Understanding all of these adverse reactions to food is foundational for nurses providing education and support to patients and families and helping them to understand a diagnosis of food allergies. Both the lay public and some health professionals may not appreciate the differences in these conditions, leading to misdiagnosis and either overreporting or underreporting of food allergies, as well as delays in treatment, so clearly describing the nature of the patient's diagnosis and providing the appropriate support and education is essential.

Inaccurate self-report and diagnosis of food allergies using broad food panels or other testing, such as IgG panels, can lead to unnecessary food restriction, unwarranted costs, anxiety and potentially more challenges for patients. As an example, tests measuring IgG are frequently marketed online to identify food intolerances, which patients may incorrectly interpret as true food allergies. As Kelso (2018) notes, these IgG antibodies are present in most healthy people, so the results do not support a diagnosis of food allergies. Other unproven tests, such as electrodermal testing using a galvanometer, cytotoxic testing, muscle testing, hair analysis, and other approaches have not been validated and may delay the use of evidence-based diagnostics to identify the actual diagnosis. An accurate diagnosis using an evidence-based approach is the first step in developing an individualized care plan for patients with food allergies and will be discussed in the next chapter.

What Is the Pathophysiology of IgE-Mediated Food Allergies?

The pathophysiology of IgE-mediated food allergies is multifaceted, and new discoveries are being made in basic science to explain many aspects of the disease. One question that remains unanswered is why some people are sensitized to foods and do not develop allergies, yet others do. Whether early introduction of foods, manipulation of the microbiome, or other interventions can help solve the problem of food allergies is still being discovered, and with time, new evidence will emerge. Armed with a basic understanding of how the immune system functions in food allergies, nurses can help patients and families to understand more about this complex disease.

Iglesia et al. (2024) describe two phases in food allergy development: the sensitization phase and the effector phase. In Fig. 2, the two phases are illustrated (Tedner et al., 2022). A person first becomes sensitized to a food protein (most food allergens are proteins) when the protein antigen is presented to the skin or mucosa directly, via ingestion to the gastrointestinal tract, or, less often, through inhalation to the respiratory tract (Sicherer & Sampson, 2018), and then is processed by cells (e.g., antigen-presenting cells, such as dendrites) and lymph nodes. Naïve T-cells become T-helper cells and produce cytokines, including interleukin-13 (IL-13) and others. These cytokines cause B cells to become plasma cells that differentiate to produce allergen-specific IgE (Borne et al., 2023; Iglesia, 2024; Tedner et al., 2022). This allergen-specific IgE then sensitizes mast cells and basophils by binding to FcεRI receptors on the mast cells, culminating in *sensitization*.

Upon subsequent exposure to the allergen, the allergic effector phase occurs, and the allergen connects or cross-links IgE-FcεRI on the sensitized mast cells and basophils in individuals who develop food allergies. Once this cross-linking occurs, effector cells (basophils and mast cells) degranulate and release histamine and other proinflammatory mediators such as leukotrienes, cytokines, and prostaglandins,

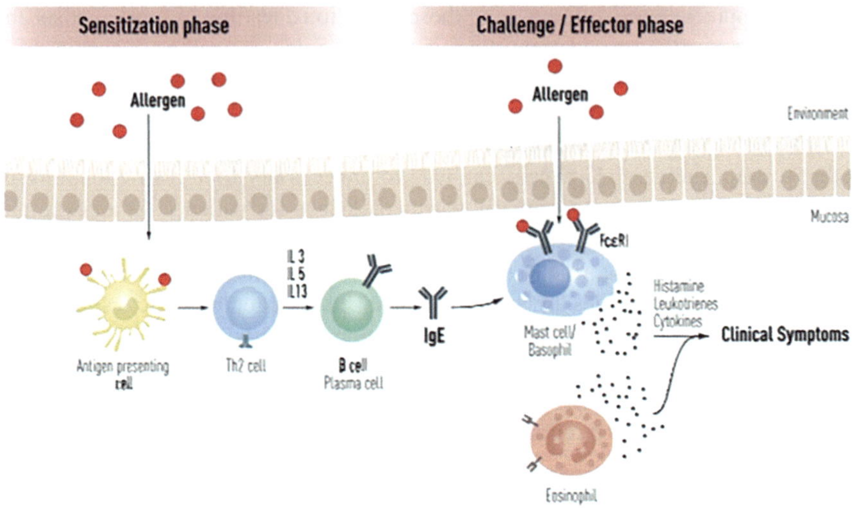

Fig. 2 Ig-E mediated food allergy pathophysiology. (Used with permission from: Tedner et al., 2022)

contributing to an allergic response that produces symptoms that can range from mild to severe (anaphylaxis) (Tedner et al., 2022).

Anaphylaxis and Food Allergy

Anaphylaxis is a severe, potentially life-threatening allergic reaction that requires immediate treatment. In this chapter, we will discuss the topic of anaphylaxis and the management in the outpatient setting. Care of the patient in the emergency department and inpatient setting will be discussed in chapter "Food Allergy Management in the Hospital Setting". Statistics suggest an increase in visits to the emergency department for anaphylaxis in recent years (Motosue et al., 2017).

A significant challenge in recognizing an allergic reaction is the inherent variability of presentations, in that reactions can look different in different people and even from one episode to the next. This unpredictability creates uncertainty for the patient and family, as well as for the nurse and healthcare team, and may contribute to a delay in epinephrine administration.

The patient may present with an immediate reaction within minutes to several hours after exposure to the allergen and a wide array of rapidly progressing symptoms, ranging from a few hives, an itchy mouth, red skin, or mild nausea to symptoms across multiple body systems (see Fig. 3). Often, two or more body systems are involved; however, symptoms in a single body system (e.g., cardiovascular or respiratory) may be consistent with anaphylaxis (NIAID, 2010). Skin and mucosal involvement are present in many cases, but anaphylaxis may occur without skin and mucosal symptoms (Dribin et al., 2025). However, as noted above, exceptions to this rapid onset timing are red meat allergy associated with tick bites, alpha-gal syndrome, where reactions may occur 2–6 h after ingestion and FDEIA.

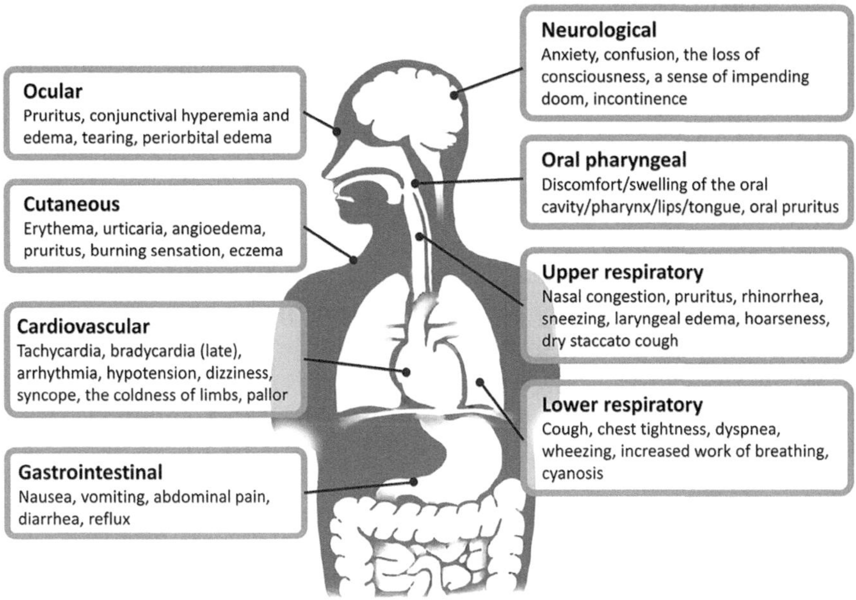

Fig. 3 Symptoms of food-induced allergic reactions. (Used with permission from: Wang et al., 2022)

Towards a Consensus Definition of Anaphylaxis

Over a dozen definitions of anaphylaxis have been published in the past several decades (Golden et al., 2024, p. 133) and the variability may have contributed to "both underdiagnosis and overdiagnosis" (Golden et al., 2024, p. 131). The nuances of these definitions point to the many variables that contribute to a diagnosis of anaphylaxis. An international expert panel (Global Allergy and Asthma Excellence Network [GA^{2}LEN]) recently created a consensus definition, overview, and clinical support tool on anaphylaxis, intended for clinicians (Dribin et al., 2025). The panel set out to reconcile differences between the National Institute of Allergy and Infectious Disease (NIAID), the Food Allergy and Anaphylaxis Network (FAAN) (Sampson et al., 2006), and the World Allergy Organization (WAO) (2020) (Cardona et al., 2020) guidelines, the latter which must still be validated.

The consensus definition of anaphylaxis, developed for use by healthcare professionals and the lay public, is that "*Anaphylaxis is a serious allergic (hypersensitivity) reaction that can progress rapidly and may cause death. It may involve the skin/mucosa (includes lip/tongue), respiratory (lungs, breathing), cardiovascular (heart, blood pressure), and/or gastrointestinal (stomach/gut) systems. Life-threatening anaphylaxis is characterized by respiratory and/or cardiovascular involvement and may occur without skin/mucosa involvement*" (Dribin et al., 2025, p. 410).

The Anaphylaxis Clinical Support Tool for Healthcare Professionals (See Fig. 4) presents three criteria that help determine when anaphylaxis is likely. The tool emphasizes that "anaphylaxis is likely" when any of the described criteria are fulfilled. In all criteria, whether there is no known allergen exposure, or a likely or

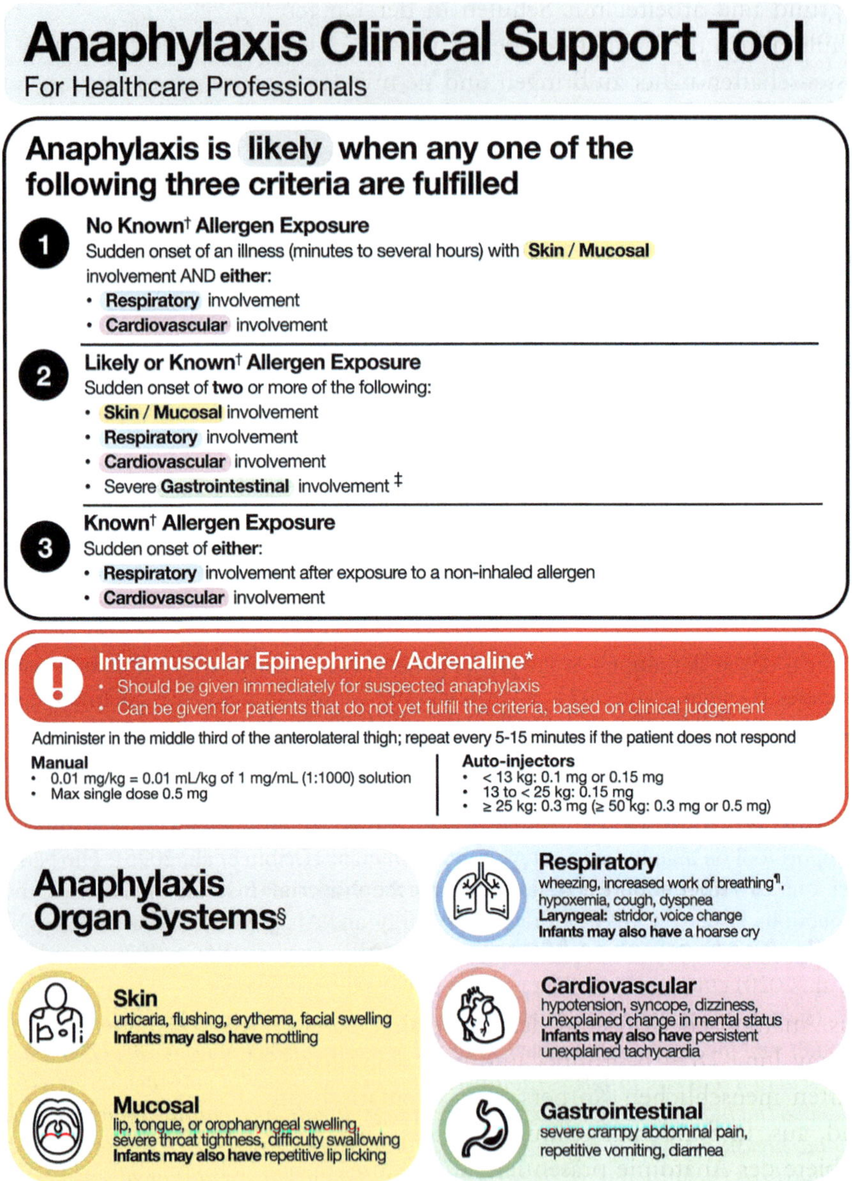

Fig. 4 Anaphylaxis clinical support tool for healthcare professionals. (Used with permission from: Dribin et al. 2025)

known exposure, respiratory and/or cardiovascular involvement warrant immediate treatment with epinephrine. The tool can be useful to characterize anaphylaxis, but as stated in the section labeled with an exclamation point, *"epinephrine should be given immediately for suspected anaphylaxis,"* and *"can be given for patients that do not yet fulfill the criteria, based on clinical judgment,"* supporting early use of epinephrine to prevent worsening of symptoms. A critical theme discussed in the consensus paper, "treatment with epinephrine should not be linked to anaphylaxis diagnosis (p. 410)," reiterates the need to err on the side of caution and give epinephrine regardless of meeting criteria.

Anaphylaxis Requires Immediate Epinephrine: Epi First, Epi Fast!

The most important point for nurses is to consider the clinical status of the patient, rather than focusing on whether patients meet specific criteria. These points are driven home in patient teaching about anaphylaxis, where a key message is not to delay epinephrine administration ("Epi first, epi fast"). Epinephrine is most effective when given early in a reaction, and there are few side effects from its use. In the case of an ingestion of a known allergen, with a prior history of anaphylaxis, epinephrine should be administered whenever symptoms develop, even if specific criteria are not met (Dribin et al., 2023). Respiratory, cardiovascular (which can include hypotension, dizziness, syncope, unexplained change in mental status) or severe gastrointestinal symptoms, as well as symptoms in multiple systems, require immediate treatment (Dribin et al., 2023).

Anaphylactic reactions are potentially life-threatening or fatal, fueling the anxiety many have about their food allergies. News reports draw attention to severe reactions, and most readers can recall a recent news story reporting on a fatal reaction as, unfortunately, they do occur. While the true incidence is unknown, several registries or databases exist and support the rare nature of this outcome, and available data on fatal reactions underscores their infrequency (Dorris, 2020; Dorris, 2025; Turner et al., 2017). However, since there is no way to predict the outcome of a food-induced reaction, any reaction must be taken seriously and managed optimally. Risk-taking or ignoring symptoms in this setting can result in devastating outcomes.

Anaphylaxis may resolve following the administration of a single dose of epinephrine. However, some patients may need two or more doses for symptom resolution either during initial treatment for anaphylaxis or for recurrent symptoms. Consensus definitions for biphasic, persistent and refractory reactions have been described (Dribin et al., 2020). A biphasic reaction recurs without re-exposure to the allergen within 1 to 48 hours after resolution of symptoms. Persistent reactions are characterized as those that last at least 4 and as long as 48 h. Refractory anaphylaxis reactions continue even after appropriate medical treatment, including epinephrine and necessary medical interventions such as intravenous fluids, and may raise the risk of fatality (Dorris, 2025; Golden et al., 2024). See discussion in chapter "Food Allergy Management in the Hospital Setting".

Assessing Anaphylaxis

Understanding the clinical presentation of anaphylaxis allows the nurse to accurately assess this rapidly evolving emergency and is useful in translating these symptoms for patients and families. Anaphylaxis may start with a few minor symptoms and can quickly involve the cardiovascular and respiratory or other systems. Insight into the various body systems affected will be reviewed here. Table 1 outlines the signs and symptoms, including information specific to infants, and a general discussion appears below.

Table 1 Potential anaphylaxis signs/symptoms

Organ system	Symptom	Sign	Infant
Skin/mucosa			
Skin	Pruritus, skin discomfort	Urticaria, erythema, flushing	Mottling
Mucosa	Mouth tingling, itchy mouth or throat, throat tightness,[a] discomfort	Facial swelling, conjunctival injection, chemosis, nasal congestion, rhinorrhea, throat clearing, lip swelling, tongue, soft palate, uvula swelling	Tongue thrusting or pulling, repetitive lip licking, ear tugging, eye rubbing
Respiratory			
General	Chest tightness, dyspnea	Cough, increased work of breathing, wheezing or bronchospasm, hypoxemia, apnea, cyanosis, pallor, reduced peak expiratory flow	–
Laryngeal	Throat tightness or discomfort	Voice change, hoarseness, stridor	Hoarse cry
Cardiovascular	Weak, dizzy, light-headed, palpitations, chest pain, blurred vision, difficulty hearing	Weak pulse, wide pulse pressure, syncope (collapse), cyanosis, pallor, arrhythmia, incontinence, bradycardia may occur in elderly and/or those in shock, hypotension,[b] shock, cardiac arrest	Persistent unexplained tachycardia, cyanosis
Gastrointestinal	Nausea, persistent crampy abdominal pain, dysphagia	Emesis, diarrhea, abdominal pain	Spitting up, hiccups, back arching
Neurologic[c]	Confusion, drowsy, headache	Unexplained change in mental status, lethargy, somnolence, seizure	Hypotonia, persistent and unexplained irritability, inconsolability, crying, decreased activity

(continued)

Table 1 (continued)

Organ system	Symptom	Sign	Infant
Other	Lower back pain in women due to uterine cramping, sense of impending doom, metallic taste, anxiety	–	–

With permission from: Dribin et al. (2025)
Signs/symptoms may occur before or during anaphylaxis. Modified from severity subgrading system for acute allergic reactions. 32
[a]Patient-reported throat tightness may indicate mucosal and/or laryngeal involvement—a distinction that is difficult to make in clinical practice without direct visualization of the laryngeal space
[b]Hypotension was as previously defined: [1,32] infants aged 1 month to <12 months, systolic blood pressure (SBP) <70 mm Hg; children aged 1–10 years, SBP less than [70 mm Hg + (2 × age in years)]; adults and children aged >10 years, SBP <90 mmHg; or decrease in SBP >30% from individual baseline
[c]May be secondary to other organ system involvement

Skin and Mucosa

The organ system in allergic reactions well-known among nurses and often featured in popular media is the skin as well as the mucosa. When writers want to signal that someone is having an allergic reaction, they typically depict someone who is scratching their red, inflamed skin (hives) or show significant swelling of the eyes and lips. Skin and mucosal signs and symptoms require careful assessment. Often, anaphylaxis does include urticaria (hives), pruritus, angioedema, and flushing, but this is not always the case. Dribin et al. (2025) reiterate that as many as 20% of patients with anaphylaxis **do not** exhibit skin/mucosal signs (p. 411, box). Other causes of skin manifestations unrelated to anaphylaxis can be viral hives, chronic hives, or even contact dermatitis. Ocular symptoms are also listed in Table 1 under skin/mucosa.

Patients often note oral or pharyngeal pruritus (itchy mouth or throat) as the first symptoms they experience during a reaction, though they are certainly not part of every reaction. Other symptoms can include throat tightness and objective signs as outlined in Table 1. Swelling in this area, often described by patients as a feeling of their throat closing, is often a source of psychological distress, as the patient fears being unable to breathe. It is important to note that patients can also experience conditions like pollen-food allergy syndrome or oral allergy syndrome, which while IgE-mediated, are often localized to the oral mucosa and can be lower risk. A history of tolerating the offending food when cooked or otherwise processed may be elicited in the assessment of the patient. However, about 3% of patients with these syndromes may report systemic symptoms (e.g., respiratory, skin, and gastrointestinal symptoms), and fewer may experience an episode of anaphylaxis (Carlson & Coop, 2019).

Gastrointestinal System

The gastrointestinal system is often involved at some point during an allergic reaction to ingested food. Abdominal pain or cramping, nausea, repetitive vomiting, and diarrhea are common symptoms. The severity and persistence of these symptoms varies, and management must be adjusted accordingly. Diarrhea may be a later symptom that follows other earlier indicators such as abdominal cramping. Like symptoms involving the skin, there are many other common causes of these gastrointestinal symptoms, such as viral illness and several non-IgE mediated food allergies and intolerances, so a thorough assessment is needed. Often, parents need reassurance that other illnesses can cause these symptoms.

Delayed gastrointestinal symptoms or persistent vomiting over several hours may be a sign of food protein-induced enterocolitis syndrome (FPIES). FPIES is a non-IgE-mediated food allergy that does not respond to antihistamines or epinephrine, and often requires antiemetics, corticosteroids and intravenous fluid replacement (Nowak-Wegrzyn et al., 2020).

Respiratory System

Hoarseness or stridor may indicate laryngeal edema and is often described by patients in the same way that they describe pharyngeal swelling—as throat pain, a sensation that their throat is closing or has a lump in it. They may experience dysphagia, voice changes, dyspnea, and feel the need to spit out their saliva. Swelling in the area could restrict breathing and therefore may necessitate prompt administration of intramuscular epinephrine. If a patient in the care of a medical team experiences these symptoms and is in distress, they may benefit from inhaled nebulized racemic epinephrine, the same treatment used for some croup patients, in addition to intramuscular or intranasal epinephrine treatment (Muraro et al., 2022).

Lower respiratory symptoms such as coughing, wheezing, dyspnea, and chest tightness may be more common in patients with asthma or with a history of wheezing but are also potential signs of anaphylaxis. Signs of hypoxia may be present. In addition to epinephrine, inhaled albuterol may help to alleviate symptoms in these patients.

Cardiovascular Symptoms

Tachycardia is common in patients experiencing an allergic reaction, and is an expected finding when epinephrine is administered. Heart rate and blood pressure should be closely monitored, along with capillary refill and general appearance in all patients who are experiencing an allergic reaction. Pallor or cold sweats would be concerning findings, as would hypotension and cyanosis.

Neurological Symptoms

Neurological symptoms can range from confusion, drowsiness, and headaches to changes in mental status and level of consciousness, and even seizures (Table 1). Other changes in behavior or mood such as increased anxiety, "feeling of impending doom," apathy, irritability, or lethargy should be considered potential indicators of a reaction. Seizures, syncope, or loss of consciousness are signs of end-organ dysfunction and should be treated aggressively as they may be indicative of a reaction that has progressed in severity to a life-threatening event, typically related to hypoxia and/or distributive shock. In infants, hypotonia and inconsolability are among the potential neurologic signs see (Table 1).

Other Symptoms

Other symptoms of note include shivering and uterine contractions that may result in abdominal or lower back pain and/or bleeding.

Symptoms in Pregnancy

Patients who are pregnant should be aware that allergic reactions feature typical symptoms, but may also include symptoms potentially affecting the uterus and fetus, such as itching in the vulvar or vaginal area, low back pain, uterine cramps, as well as fetal distress and the possibility of preterm labor (Simons & Schatz, 2012). Because of the increased risk of harm to mother and fetus, an oral food challenge should be avoided during pregnancy.

Can Severity of Allergic Reactions Be Predicted?

Patients and caregivers should know that there is no such thing as a "mild" food allergy, and whether future reactions will be mild or severe cannot be predicted, although some diagnostics point to the likelihood of clinical reactivity. The risk of anaphylaxis is always present, and patients should have epinephrine readily available, always carrying two doses. Delays in treatment with epinephrine can adversely impact outcomes. It is a myth that repeated food reactions worsen each time. Due to their unpredictability, reactions can vary each time a patient is exposed to an allergen.

The severity of reactions might depend on multiple factors, such as alcohol use, co-morbid diseases such as mast cell disorder, uncontrolled asthma, or infections, age-related factors (e.g., adolescents), co-factors (e.g., asthma, acute illness, exercise, psychological burdens or stressors, lack of sleep, premenstrual status, some medications [e.g., ACE inhibitors and NSAIDs]) (Cardona et al., 2020; Golden et al., 2024), and the amount of allergen ingested.

Several groups have reviewed evidence about risk factors for severe reactions. DuToit et al. (2024) noted they can include age, comorbidities, medications and more, and provide an in-depth discussion of these factors. Adolescence, for example, is often associated with risk-taking behavior and non-adherence to epinephrine carriage recommendations. Co-morbidities like poorly controlled asthma, underlying cardiovascular disease, or other forms of atopy, such as eczema or rhinitis may have an impact in some cases. However, a meta-analysis of studies exploring severe reactions in food allergy did not find asthma to be a risk factor if well-controlled (Turner et al., 2022), underscoring the need to adhere to asthma management plans, and highlighted that a past history of anaphylaxis may not be contributory. The value of various biomarkers in predicting severity of anaphylaxis was also questioned. Turner et al. (2022) called for longitudinal, population-based studies to help address the many unanswered questions raised by their review of the literature.

Preparedness for Systemic Allergic Reactions

For any patient with food allergies, basic emergency preparedness includes always carrying two doses of epinephrine, an emergency action or care plans (EAP), and if desired, medical emergency identification, such as wallet cards, or jewelry such as necklaces, bracelets or dog tags (Golden et al., 2024), or even articles of clothing for small children. More recently, medical alert systems have been adapted for food allergic emergencies so patients can alert emergency services with a watch or other electronic device.

Nurses can advocate for the development of EAPs for all patients with food allergies. Clinicians can devise EAPs that are tailored to each individual patient's food allergies and any applicable cofactors. See the chapter "Food Allergy Management in Early Childhood Settings" for an example of an EAP and the Resources Page for links to other plans and updated versions. Emergency action plans should be updated annually or when information changes.

Management of Anaphylaxis in the Community Setting

The advocacy groups Food Allergy Research and Education (FARE) (2024), Food Allergy and Anaphylaxis Connection Team (FAACT) (2025), and Kids with Food Allergies (KFA, 2025) feature many educational materials, including education about EAPs and teaching tools about anaphylaxis. Other international organizations, including Australian Society of Clinical Immunology and Allergy (ASCIA, 2025), Food Allergy Canada (2025), and Translating Emergency Knowledge for Kids (TREKK), also offer teaching materials. An additional new educational tool for patients and caregivers to learn about anaphylaxis is the Anaphylaxis Interactive Learning Guide (https://www.aaaai.org/tools-for-the-public/anaphylaxis) explaining anaphylaxis in children and adults recently developed by the American Academy of Allergy Asthma & Immunology (AAAAI, 2024). More information about educational materials is available on the Resources Page.

Epinephrine and some other medications used in the community will be reviewed here. A discussion on the management of patients in the emergency department and in the inpatient setting is included in chapter "Food Allergy Management in the Hospital Setting".

Epinephrine: The Only First-Line Treatment for Acute Anaphylaxis

Epinephrine is the most important medication for the treatment of systemic allergic reactions and the only first-line therapy for anaphylaxis. Epinephrine has its pharmacologic effect on α (alpha) and β (beta) receptors in both cardiovascular and smooth muscle. Epinephrine works on alpha receptors to cause vasoconstriction and helps to maintain cardiac function and prevent hypotension, while also reducing dermatologic symptoms like hives, redness and mucosal edema (Kemp et al., 2008). Its effect on beta receptors causes smooth muscle relaxation, helping to relieve bronchoconstriction and respiratory symptoms. In addition, these effects prevent mast cells and basophils from releasing additional mediators like histamine, and thereby worsening symptoms, which is important to understand and underscores the need for early administration. If a patient does not respond to a first dose of epinephrine, it should be repeated after 5–15 min (NIAID, 2010).

Nurses should be familiar with when and how to use epinephrine devices regardless of their practice setting, including autoinjectors for IM injections and nasal sprays. Nurses may also need to be familiar with epinephrine dosing if they work in a setting where vials are readily available for the treatment of reactions, including allergy practices, urgent care, emergency departments, hospitals, and outpatient surgery centers. If epinephrine needs to be drawn up from a vial, the nurse should choose a needle length that will ensure that the medication is delivered into the muscle (Golden et al., 2024). Nurses should also be aware that epinephrine is available in different strengths and should familiarize themselves with available medications in their practice setting (Institute for Safe Medication Practices Canada, 2016).

In the community setting, various epinephrine devices are available (see below and chapter "Food Allergy Management in Adolescents and Young Adults") designed for use by patients and families that are simple to use with appropriate training. For people with food allergies, epinephrine auto-injectors (EAIs) have been the mainstay for treatment of food allergy reactions, and now a nasal spray is also available. Epinephrine, which can be explained to patients as a form of adrenaline, is safe to administer and is very unlikely to cause adverse events when self-administered via an epinephrine device (auto-injector or newer devices like a nasal spray).

EAIs and prefilled-epinephrine injection devices for patient use are manufactured by several different companies in multiple dosage formulations. Availability of specific devices varies by country. In the United States, there are several FDA-approved epinephrine options. Among the available options are EPIPEN (epinephrine injection, USP) 0.3 mg and EPIPEN JR (epinephrine injection, USP) 0.15 mg.

Teva Pharmaceuticals also has standardized doses of 0.3 mg and 0.15 mg. The AUVI-Q is available in 0.3 mg, 0.15 mg, and 0.1 mg dosages (Asthma and Allergy Foundation, 2024), and offers audio instructions integrated into the device. According to the 2023 Anaphylaxis Practice Parameter, (Golden et al., 2024), there is some discussion among allergy specialty organizations about optimal epinephrine dosing recommendations, since there is a concern about underdosing with available EAI formulations based on weight. Nurses can refer to the practice parameter (Golden et al., 2024) for a full discussion, stay current with recommendations.

Intramuscular epinephrine injections (including EAIs) should only be injected into the anterolateral (outer) aspect of the thigh, and the device should be held in place for the number of seconds recommended by the manufacturer, which may vary. EAIs should not be injected into the buttocks, fingers, hands or feet, or used intravenously. If necessary, injections can be made through clothing. Nurses should teach patients to inspect the epinephrine solution and look for any signs of discoloration, cloudiness or particles. Typically, the epinephrine should appear clear and colorless so a significant change in clarity or color (e.g., pink, red, brown) would indicate some degradation, and the EAI should be replaced. EAIs should be protected from extreme temperatures and sunlight, and should be checked often to be sure no changes are visible.

Recently, an epinephrine (needle-free) nasal spray has been approved by the FDA formulated in 1 mg of epinephrine per spray dosage for 15 kg to less than 30 kg, and 2 mg of epinephrine for 30 kg or greater in a single dose format based on weight (ARS Pharmaceuticals Operations, 2025; 2026). Often, anecdotally, EAIs are not used due to the patient or caregiver's fear of giving an injection, the high cost of the medication, unavailability of the device, and other reasons. The epinephrine nasal spray device offers an alternative that mitigates the anxiety and fear related to injections and that does not require special temperature handling (See manufacturer website for instructions for use). On the horizon are other options for epinephrine delivery, such as a sublingual film the size of a postage stamp that would dissolve without water or swallowing. As a first step, a New Drug Application has been accepted by the FDA for this novel formulation with more expected official actions soon. Other technologies for epinephrine delivery are also on the drawing board, so needle-free options may become more common in the future.

Many resources including videos and print materials are available to illustrate usage of these devices. The proper way to use epinephrine injectors and nasal sprays using training devices should be reviewed regularly with patients and caregivers. A teach-back return demonstration session offers the opportunity to review technique, and to confirm that patients/caregivers have filled their prescription and are aware of guidance on proper storage, temperature control, and the need to review expiration dates and periodically check the device for discoloration. Several resources in this and other chapters provide patient education about use of epinephrine devices.

In the United States, it is common practice to recommend that two epinephrine devices be carried, and patients should be encouraged to do so when possible, keeping the device easily accessible. One systematic review indicated that slightly under 8% cases of anaphylaxis required two doses for symptoms to resolve, and about 2% required at least three doses in a pooled estimate (Patel et al., 2021). If symptoms do not improve, a second injection can be given at about 5–15 min, and a third injection infrequently may be needed. (See chapter "Food Allergy Management in the Hospital Setting" for more information about additional medical treatment).

While the prevailing advice is to immediately alert emergency services after epinephrine administration (e.g., call 911 or EMS), options for home management are emerging in the literature (Golden et al., 2024). When epinephrine is administered soon after symptoms appear, and symptoms resolve promptly, more recent thinking is that it is possible to remain at home if the response is sustained and the patient has access to another epinephrine device if needed, as well as a support person who can assist if help is necessary (Golden et al., 2024). Of course, this evolving practice may not apply to all and should be discussed by the patient and caregiver and the provider in a process of shared decision-making. For severe anaphylaxis that does not respond to epinephrine, or which progresses, and for those reactions requiring multiple injections, emergency services activation is essential (Golden et al., 2024).

The vital importance of epinephrine for treatment of anaphylaxis cannot be overstated, and early administration in the pre-hospital/community/school/home setting should be emphasized as it is the only treatment that may quickly stop an allergic reaction (See Fig. 5).

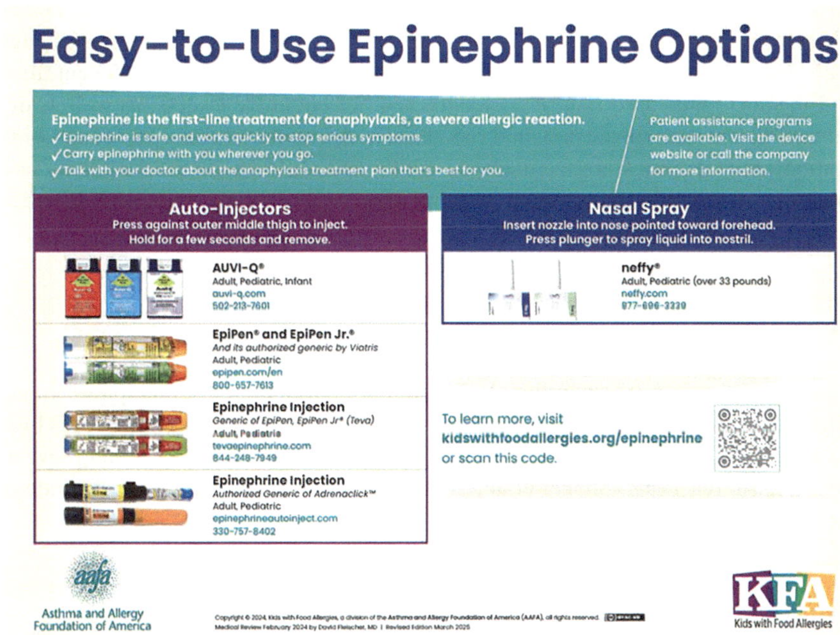

Fig. 5 Easy-to-use epinephrine options. (Used with permission from: https://kidswithfoodallergies.org/wp-content/uploads/2024/03/easy-to-use-epinephrine-options-handout.pdf. BY-NC-ND-4.0 Creative Commons license to the Asthma and Allergy Foundation of America and unaltered)

Antihistamines

As discussed in the pathophysiology section, histamine is a mediator released by mast cells and basophils responsible for many of the symptoms associated with allergic reactions; four histamine receptors have been identified (Reber et al., 2017), but H1 and H2 are most relevant in anaphylaxis. A major concern is that administration of antihistamines can delay epinephrine administration, so this is an important teaching point for patients and caregivers. Shaker et al. (2020) state that antihistamines should not be administered before or instead of epinephrine, as antihistamines will not reverse anaphylaxis. Antihistamines do not have the same pharmacologic effects as epinephrine (e.g., stabilization of mast cells) and they are slower acting, and should be considered to be adjunctive therapies (Linton et al, 2023). Cardona et al. (2020) underscore the second- or third-line role of antihistamines in treating anaphylaxis but acknowledge their usefulness in treating cutaneous symptoms, such as urticaria and itching.

H1 antagonists, like first-generation (e.g., diphenhydramine [Benadryl]) and second-generation (e.g., cetirizine [Zyrtec]) antihistamines are employed to manage symptoms during the treatment of allergic reactions. Although diphenhydramine, a first-generation antihistamine, is still commonly used, recent thinking suggests that second-generation antihistamines like cetirizine provide the same therapeutic effect with less or no sedation and a longer duration of action (Clark et al., 2025). Therefore, Wolfson et al. (2022, p. 3125) underscore the adverse effects associated with diphenhydramine, including not only sedation, but changes in concentration and memory; increased risk of accidents; risk for cognitive effects; as well as dry mouth, dizziness, hypotension, and risk of falls. A number of different second-generation antihistamines are available or adults and children. Some clinicians also prescribe H2 antihistamines such as famotidine as part of their anaphylaxis treatment, though this practice is not supported by any randomized, controlled trials.

Steroids

Like antihistamines, glucocorticoids are often used as adjunctive therapies for anaphylaxis, with the rationale that they limit biphasic reactions. However, there is little evidence to support their use in the management of acute anaphylaxis and preventing biphasic reactions (Shaker et al., 2020). If used, steroids should not precede or replace first-line treatment with epinephrine.

Bronchodilators

Cardona et al. (2020) state that in patients experiencing bronchoconstriction, short-acting beta 2 agonists (e.g., albuterol) can be prescribed, but again, are not a substitute for the appropriate use of epinephrine. With airway obstruction, albuterol can be administered via nebulizer.

Conclusion

This chapter offers an evidence-based overview of the classification of adverse reactions to food, the pathophysiology of IgE-mediated food allergy, signs and symptoms of anaphylaxis, and general management of food allergies in the outpatient setting. Nurses play an important role in reinforcing the importance of emergency preparedness through early recognition of anaphylaxis signs and symptoms and guiding prompt, accurate epinephrine administration as a first-line treatment. The chapter emphasizes the nurse's role in advocacy, patient safety, and empowering individuals to confidently manage food allergies and reduce the risk of adverse outcomes. Chapters "Understanding the Diagnosis and Management of Food allergy, Part II: Diagnostics" and "Understanding the Diagnosis and Management of Food Allergy, Part III: Management of Food Allergy in the Outpatient Setting" discuss diagnosis and management in more detail.

References

Abrams, E. M., Aquash, W., Fischer, D. A., et al. (2024). Anaphylaxis. *Allergy Asthma Clinical Immunology, 20*(Suppl 3), 62. https://doi.org/10.1186/s13223-024-00926-3

American Academy of Allergy, Asthma & Immunology. (2024). *Anaphylaxis interactive learning guide*. Retrieved August 5, 2025, from https://www.aaaai.org/tools-for-the-public/anaphylaxis

ARS Pharmaceuticals Operations. (2025). *Neffy*. Retrieved October 1, 2025, from https://neffypro.com/resources/#resource-library

ARS Pharmaceuticals. (2026). Retrieved from June 23, 2026, https://neffypro.com/dosing-and-usage/

Asthma and Allergy Foundation of America. (2024). *Epinephrine options poster*. Retrieved October 1, 2025, from https://secure.aafa.org/np/clients/aafa/product.jsp?product=397

Australasian Society of Clinical Immunology and Allergy (ASCIA). (2025). *Action plan for anaphylaxis*. https://www.allergy.org.au/images/stories/anaphylaxis/2025/ASCIA_Action_Plan_Anaphylaxis_General_2025.pdf

Bartra, J., Araujo, G., & Muñoz-Canoe, R. (2018). Interaction between foods and nonsteroidal anti-inflammatory drugs and exercise in the induction of anaphylaxis. *Current Opinion in Allergy and Clinical Immunology, 18*(4), 310–316. https://doi.org/10.1097/ACI.0000000000000461

Borne, G. E., Daniel, C. P., Wagner, M. J., Plaisance, C. J., Nolen, A., Kelkar, R. A., Ahmadzadeh, S., Myrcik, D., Shekoohi, S., Kaye, A. D., & Varrassi, G. (2023). Palforzia for Peanut Allergy: A narrative review and update on a novel immunotherapy. *Cureus, 15*(12), e50485. https://doi.org/10.7759/cureus.50485

Cardona, V., Ansotegui, I. J., Ebisawa, M., El-Gamal, Y., Fernandez Rivas, M., Fineman, S., Geller, M., Gonzalez-Estrada, A., Greenberger, P. A., Sanchez Borges, M., Senna, G., Sheikh, A., Tanno, L. K., Thong, B. Y., Turner, P. J., & Worm, M. (2020). World allergy organization anaphylaxis guidance 2020. *The World Allergy Organization Journal, 13*(10), 100472. https://doi.org/10.1016/j.waojou.2020.100472

Carlson, G., & Coop, C. (2019). Pollen food allergy syndrome (PFAS): A review of current available literature. *Annals of Allergy, Asthma & Immunology: Official Publication of the American College of Allergy, Asthma, & Immunology, 123*(4), 359–365. https://doi.org/10.1016/j.anai.2019.07.022

Clark, J. H., Meltzer, E. O, Naclerio, R. M. (2025). Diphenhydramine: It is time to say a final goodbye. *World Allergy Organization Journal, 18*(2), 101027. https://doi.org/10.1016/j.waojou.2025.101027

Cox, A. L., & Sicherer, S. H. (2020). Classification of adverse food reactions. *Journal of Food Allergy, 2*(1), 3–6. https://doi.org/10.2500/jfa.2020.2.200022

Dorris, S. (2020). Fatal food anaphylaxis: Registering a rare outcome. *Annals of Allergy, Asthma & Immunology: Official Publication of the American College of Allergy, Asthma, & Immunology, 124*(5), 445–446. https://doi.org/10.1016/j.anai.2020.02.001

Dorris, S. (2025). Fatal and near fatal anaphylaxis to food in children and young adults. *Immunology and Allergy Clinics of North America, 45*(3), 445–455. https://doi.org/10.1016/j.iac.2025.05.001

Dribin, T. E., Sampson, H. A., Camargo Jr, C. A., Brousseau, D. C., Spergel, J. M., Neuman, M. I., Shaker, M., Campbell, R. L., Michelson, K. A., Rudders, S.A. and Assa'ad, A.H. (2020). Persistent, refractory, and biphasic anaphylaxis: a multidisciplinary delphi study. *Journal of Allergy and Clinical Immunology, 146*, 1089–1096.

Dribin, T. E., Motosue, M. S., & Campbell, R. L. (2023). Overview of allergy and anaphylaxis. *Immunology and Allergy Clinics of North America, 43*(3), 435–451. https://doi.org/10.1016/j.iac.2022.10.009

Dribin, T. E., Muraro, A., Camargo, C. A., Jr., Turner, P. J., Wang, J., Roberts, G., Anagnostou, A., Halken, S., Liebermann, J., Worm, M., Zuberbier, T., Sampson, H. A., & GA(2)LEN Anaphylaxis Study Team. (2025). Anaphylaxis definition, overview, and clinical support tool: 2024 consensus report-a GA^{2}LEN project. *The Journal of Allergy and Clinical Immunology, 156*(2), 406–417.e6. https://doi.org/10.1016/j.jaci.2025.01.021

DuToit, G., Smith, P., Muraro, A., Fox, A. T., Roberts, G., Ring, J., & Worm, M. (2024). Identifying patients at risk of anaphylaxis. *The World Allergy Organization Journal, 17*(6), 100904. https://doi.org/10.1016/j.waojou.2024.100904

Food Allergy & Anaphylaxis Connection Team. (2025). https://foodallergyawareness.org

Food Allergy Canada. (2025). *Anaphylaxis emergency plan*. https://foodallergycanada.ca/tools-and-downloads/downloads/emergency-plan-forms/

Food Allergy Research and Education (FARE). (2024). *Food Allergy Facts and Statistics for the U.S.* https://www.foodallergy.org/sites/default/files/2024-07/FARE%20Food%20Allergy%20Facts%20and%20Statistics_April2024.pdf. Accessed on 28 Aug 2024.

Golden, D. B. K., Wang, J., Wasserman, S., Akin, C., Campbell, R. L., Ellis, A. K., Greenhawt, M., Lang, D. M., Ledford, D. K., Lieberman, J., Oppenheimer, J., Shaker, M. S., Wallace, D. V., Abrams, E. M., Bernstein, J. A., Chu, D. K., Horner, C. C., Rank, M. A., Stukas, D. R., Collaborators, & Wang, J. (2024). Anaphylaxis: A 2023 practice parameter update. *Annals of Allergy, Asthma & Immunology: Official Publication of the American College of Allergy, Asthma, & Immunology, 132*(2), 124–176. https://doi.org/10.1016/j.anai.2023.09.015

Gupta, R. S., Sehgal, S., Brown, D. A., Das, R., Fierstein, J. L., Casale, T. B., Nowak-Wegrzyn, A. H., & Blaver, L. A. (2021). Characterizing biphasic food-related allergic reactions through a US Food Allergy Patient Registry. *The Journal of Allergy and Clinical Immunology. In Practice, 9*(10), 3717–3727. https://doi.org/10.1016/j.jaip.2021.05.009

Iglesia, E. G. A., Kwan, M., Virkon, Y. V., & Iweala, O. I. (2024). Management of food allergies and food-related anaphylaxis. *Journal of the American Medical Association, 331*(6), 510–521. https://doi.org/10.1001/jama.2023.26857

Institute for Safe Medication Practices Canada. (2016). Changes in expression of strength: Elimination of ratios on single-entity injectable products. Retrieved on June, 22, 2026 from https://ismpcanada.ca/wp-content/uploads/ISMPCSB2016-02_ChangesInExpressionStrength.pdf

Kelso, J. M. (2018). Unproven diagnostic tests for adverse reactions to foods. *The Journal of Allergy and Clinical Immunology. In Practice, 6*(2), 362–365. https://doi.org/10.1016/j.jaip.2017.08.021

Kemp, S. F., Lockey, R. F., Simons, F. E., & World Allergy Organization ad hoc Committee on Epinephrine in Anaphylaxis. (2008). Epinephrine: The drug of choice for anaphylaxis. A statement of the World Allergy Organization. *Allergy, 63*(8), 1061–1070. https://doi.org/10.1111/j.1398-9995.2008.01733.x

Kids with Food Allergies. (2024). *Food allergy Action Plan for the treatment of anaphylaxis.* https://kidswithfoodallergies.org/living-with-food-allergies/food-allergy-treatment/allergy-anaphylaxis-action-plan/. Accessed on 8 Oct 2025.

Kids with Food Allergies (2025). Food Allergy Action Plan for the Treatment of Anaphylaxis. Retrieved on June 22, 2026 from https://kidswithfoodallergies.org/living-with-food-allergies/food-allergy-treatment/allergy-anaphylaxis-action-plan/

Kulthanan, K., Ungprasert, P., Jirapongsananuruk, O., Rujitharanawong, C., Munprom, K., Trakanwittayarak, S., Pochanapan, O., Panjapakkul, W., Maurer, M. (2022). Food-Dependent Exercise-Induced Wheals, Angioedema, and Anaphylaxis: A Systematic Review. *The Journal of Allergy and Clinical Immunology: In Practice, 10*(9), 2280–2296. https://doi.org/10.1016/j.jaip.2022.06.008. Epub 2022 Jun 22. PMID: 35752432.

Linton, S., Hossenbaccus, L., Ellis, A. K. (2023). Evidence-based use of antihistamines for treatment of allergic conditions. *Annals of Allergy, Asthma & Immunology, 131*(4), 412–420. https://doi.org/10.1016/j.anai.2023.07.019. Epub 2023 Jul 28. PMID: 37517656.

Motosue, M. S., Bellolio, M. F., Van Houten, H. K., Shah, N. D., & Campbell, R. L. (2017). Increasing emergency department visits for anaphylaxis, 2005–2014. *The Journal of Allergy and Clinical Immunology. In Practice, 5*(1), 171–175.e3. https://doi.org/10.1016/j.jaip.2016.08.013

Muraro, A., Roberts, G., Worm, M., Bilo, M. B., Brockow, K., Fernández Rivas, M., Santos, A. F., Zolile, Z. Q., Bellou, A., Beyer, K., Bindslev-Jensen, C., Cardona, V., Clark, A. T., DeMolay, P., Dubois, A. E. J., Dunn Galvin, A., Eigenmann, P., Halken, S., Harada, L., Lack, G., Jutel, M., Niggemann, B., Ruff, F., Timmermans, F., Vliet-Boerstra, B. J., Werfel, T., Dhami, S., Panesar, S., Akdis, C. A., Sheikh, A., & On Behalf of the EAACI Food Allergy and Anaphylaxis Guidelines Group. (2014). Anaphylaxis: Guidelines from the European Academy of Allergy and Clinical Immunology. *Allergy (Copenhagen, Denmark), 69*, 1026–1045.

Muraro, A., Worm, M., Alviani, C., Cardona, V., DunnGalvin, A., Garvey, L. H., Riggioni, C., de Silva, D., Angier, E., Arasi, S., Bellou, A., Beyer, K., Bijlhout, D., Bilò, M. B., Bindslev-Jensen, C., Brockow, K., Fernandez-Rivas, M., Halken, S., Jensen, B., Khaleva, E., European Academy of Allergy and Clinical Immunology, & Food Allergy, Anaphylaxis Guidelines Group. (2022). EAACI guidelines: Anaphylaxis (2021 update). *Allergy, 77*(2), 357–377. https://doi.org/10.1111/all.15032

NIAID-Sponsored Expert Panel, Boyce, J. A., Assa'ad, A., Burks, A. W., Jones, S. M., Sampson, H. A., Wood, R. A., Plaut, M., Cooper, S. F., Fenton, M. J., Arshad, S. H., Bahna, S. L., Beck, L. A., Byrd-Bredbenner, C., Camargo, C. A., Jr., Eichenfield, L., Furuta, G. T., Hanifin, J. M., Jones, C., Kraft, M., & Schwaninger, J. M. (2010). Guidelines for the diagnosis and management of food allergy in the United States: Report of the NIAID-sponsored expert panel. *The Journal of allergy and clinical immunology, 126*(6 Suppl), S1–S58. https://doi.org/10.1016/j.jaci.2010.10.007

Nowak-Wegrzyn, A., Berin, M. C., & Mehr, S. (2020). Food Protein-Induced Enterocolitis Syndrome. *The Journal of Allergy and Clinical Immunology: In Practice, 8*(1), 24–35. https://doi.org/10.1016/j.jaip.2019.08.020. PMID: 31950904.

Patel, N., Chong, K. W., Yip, A. Y. G., Ierodiakonou, D., Bartra, J., Boyle, R. J., & Turner, P. J. (2021). Use of multiple epinephrine doses in anaphylaxis: A systematic review and meta-analysis. *The Journal of Allergy and Clinical Immunology, 148*(5), 1307–1315. https://doi.org/10.1016/j.jaci.2021.03.042

Reber, L. L., Hernandez, J. D., & Galli, S. J. (2017). The pathophysiology of anaphylaxis. *The Journal of Allergy and Clinical Immunology, 140*(2), 335–348. https://doi.org/10.1016/j.jaci.2017.06.003

Robillard, K., & Varshney, P. (2025). Current food Allergy treatment options. *Immunology and Allergy Clinics of North America, 45*(3), 403–418. https://doi.org/10.1016/j.iac.2025.04.007

Sampson, H. A., Muñoz-Furlong, A., Campbell, R. L., Adkinson, N. F., Jr., Bock, S. A., Branum, A., Brown, S. G., Camargo, C. A., Jr., Cydulka, R., Galli, S. J., Gidudu, J., Gruchalla, R. S., Harlor, A. D., Jr., Hepner, D. L., Lewis, L. M., Lieberman, P. L., Metcalfe, D. D., O'Connor, R., Muraro, A., Rudman, A., & Decker, W. W. (2006). Second symposium on the definition and management of anaphylaxis: Summary report--Second National Institute of Allergy and Infectious Disease/Food Allergy and Anaphylaxis Network symposium. *The Journal of Allergy and Clinical Immunology, 117*(2), 391–397. https://doi.org/10.1016/j.jaci.2005.12.1303

Shaker, M. S., Wallace, D. V., Golden, D. B. K., Oppenheimer, J., Bernstein, J. A., Campbell, R. L., Dinakar, C., Ellis, A., Greenhawt, M., Khan, D. A., Lang, D. M., Lang, E. S., Lieberman, J. A., Portnoy, J., Rank, M. A., Stukus, D. R., Wang, J., Collaborators, Riblet, N., Bobrownicki, A. M. P., & Wang, J. (2020). Anaphylaxis-a 2020 practice parameter update, systematic review, and grading of recommendations, assessment, development and evaluation (GRADE) analysis. *The Journal of Allergy and Clinical Immunology, 145*(4), 1082–1123. https://doi.org/10.1016/j.jaci.2020.01.017

Sicherer, S. H., & Sampson, H. A. (2018). Food allergy: A review and update on epidemiology, pathogenesis, diagnosis, prevention, and management. *The Journal of Allergy and Clinical Immunology, 141*(1), 41–58. https://doi.org/10.1016/j.jaci.2017.11.003

Simons, F. E., & Schatz, M. (2012). Anaphylaxis during pregnancy. *The Journal of Allergy and Clinical Immunology, 130*(3), 597–606. https://doi.org/10.1016/j.jaci.2012.06.035

Srisuwatchari, W., Kanchanaphoomi, K., Nawiboonwong, J., Thongngarm, T., & Sompornrattanaphan, M. (2023). Food-dependent exercise-induced anaphylaxis: A distinct form of food allergy – An updated review of diagnostic approaches and treatments. *Foods (Basel, Switzerland), 12*(20), 3768. https://doi.org/10.3390/foods12203768

Tedner, S. G., Asarnoj, A., Thulin, H., Westman, M., Konradsen, J. R., & Nilsson, C. (2022). Food allergy and hypersensitivity reactions in children and adults – A review. *Journal of Internal Medicine, 291*, 283–302.

Translating Emergency Knowledge for Kids (TREKK) Network. (2023). *Canadian anaphylaxis plan for kids.* https://cms.trekk.ca/wp-content/uploads/2023/11/Anaphylaxis_Action_Plan_Redesign7_-_school_daycare_002_2.0.pdf

Turner, P. J., Jerschow, E., Umasunthar, T., Lin, R., Campbell, D. E., & Boyle, R. J. (2017). Fatal anaphylaxis: Mortality rate and risk factors. *The Journal of Allergy and Clinical Immunology. In Practice, 5*(5), 1169–1178. https://doi.org/10.1016/j.jaip.2017.06.031

Turner, P. J., Arasi, S., Ballmer-Weber, B., Baseggio Conrado, A., Deschildre, A., Gerdts, J., Halken, S., Muraro, A., Patel, N., Van Ree, R., de Silva, D., Worm, M., Zuberbier, T., Roberts, G., & Global Allergy, Asthma European Network (GA2LEN) Food Allergy Guideline Group. (2022). Risk factors for severe reactions in food allergy: Rapid evidence review with meta-analysis. *Allergy, 77*(9), 2634–2652. https://doi.org/10.1111/all.15318

Varshney, P., & Pongracic, J. (2020). Clinical manifestations of immunoglobulin E-mediated food allergy, including pollen-food allergy syndrome. *Journal of Food Allergy (East Providence, RI: Online), 2*(1), 22–25. https://doi.org/10.2500/jfa.2020.2.200002

Wang, L. J., Mu, S. C., Lin, M. I., Sung, T. C., Chiang, B. L., & Lin, C. H. (2022). Clinical manifestations of pediatric food allergy: A contemporary review. *Clinical Reviews in Allergy & Immunology, 62*(1), 180–199. https://doi.org/10.1007/s12016-021-08895-w

Wolfson, A. R., Wong, D., Abrams, E. M., Waserman, S., & Sussman, G. L. (2022). Diphenhydramine: Time to move on? *The Journal of Allergy and Clinical Immunology. In Practice, 10*(12), 3124–3130. https://doi.org/10.1016/j.jaip.2022.07.018

Yu, W., Freeland, D. M. H., & Nadeau, K. C. (2016). Food allergy: Immune mechanisms, diagnosis and immunotherapy. *Nature Reviews. Immunology, 16*(12), 751–765. https://doi.org/10.1038/nri.2016.111

Understanding the Diagnosis and Management of Food Allergy Part II: Diagnostics

Mary Frances Vess, Sarah Pederson, Robyn Huey Lao, Josie Howard-Ruben, and Julianne Doucette

Diagnosis of Food Allergy

A diagnosis of food allergy is made through understanding the patient's clinical history and interpreting appropriate and specific testing for each patient. Current options for diagnostic testing are skin prick testing (SPT) using allergen extracts, and in some cases actual food items; serum allergen-specific IgE (sIgE); and component-resolved diagnostics (CRD), featuring clinically important allergen components, when this laboratory test is available. Some patients also complete oral food challenges (OFC) (Bégin et al., 2024; Santos et al., 2023). A recent systematic review of studies representing nearly 25,000 patients with food allergies underscored the value of IgE sensitization in their diagnosis, but described nuances based on the allergen being assessed, with evidence for some allergens and specific diagnostics stronger than others (Riggioni et al., 2024). While SPTs, sIgE, and OFCs comprise the prevailing current approach to food allergy diagnosis, interpretation of the results is not always straightforward and requires the diagnostic expertise of a clinical team experienced in food allergy.

M. F. Vess
Children's Healthcare of Atlanta, Atlanta, GA, USA
e-mail: mary.vess@choa.org

S. Pederson (✉)
Food Allergy Nursing Association, Great Neck, NY, USA

R. H. Lao
University of California Davis, Davis, CA, USA
e-mail: REHuey@health.ucdavis.edu

J. Howard-Ruben
Rush University College of Nursing, Chicago, IL, USA
e-mail: josie_howard-ruben@rush.edu

J. Doucette
College of Nursing, Rush University, Chicago, IL, USA
e-mail: Julianne_Doucette@rush.edu

J. Doucette, J. Howard-Ruben (eds.), *Comprehensive Food Allergy Management for Nurses*, https://doi.org/10.1007/978-3-032-28647-5_3

Only foods identified as potential allergen culprits should be evaluated as a strategy to prevent false positives (Bégin et al., 2024; NIAID, 2010). Broad panels may yield findings that are not useful for clinical management and can have a negative impact. For example, patients may have false positives indicating sensitization to foods they have been safely eating. False positives can lead to limiting food options and unnecessary avoidance, which can impact nutrition and create anxiety, and even contribute to loss of tolerance if foods previously consumed safely are removed from the diet (Al Ghamdi et al., 2024). For this reason, it is important to consider which allergens require testing, although many practitioners still may order broad panels.

With OFCs, and rarely, skin prick testing (Liccardi et al., 2006), there is a risk of anaphylaxis. For this reason, clinicians use care in selecting those patients who need this type of testing (Wang, 2023). OFCs can also cause patient and family anxiety and involve a time-consuming process that may take hours to complete.

Basophil activation testing (BAT), mast cell activation testing (MAT), and epitope analysis are among the newer diagnostic modalities being actively studied and currently available in some settings which may reduce the need for OFC (Patel et al., 2023). Future testing modalities could deploy alternative biologic samples (e.g., buccal swabs, saliva, stool), new technologies, and even artificial intelligence (Boyd & Santos, 2025).

Clinical History

Sicherer and Sampson (2018) underscore that the clinical history is the "most important single test" in the diagnosis of food allergies (p. 45). Allergy clinicians should always begin by obtaining an allergy-focused history, which includes reviewing diet, symptoms, other atopic conditions, occupational exposures, and more as outlined by Santos et al. (2023). Since food allergies may present differently in different patients, clinical history is an essential element in the differential diagnosis of an IgE-mediated food allergy (Chinthrajah et al., 2015; Boyd & Santos, 2025). Detailed information about a patient's diet and associated symptoms serves as the basis upon which diagnostic testing is ordered and interpreted, as providers will use this clinical history to determine the "pre-test probability" of an allergy so the right tests are ordered (Santos et al., 2023). Clinical history, documentation of reproducible symptoms to a food, and tailored testing together help the allergy provider to make a diagnosis and to rule out many other conditions associated with similar symptoms.

During an allergy-focused clinical history, nurses and other healthcare providers will explore the topics presented below when evaluating the patient (Anvari et al., 2019; Muraro et al., 2014; NIAID-Sponsored Expert Panel, 2010; Santos et al., 2023; Santos et al., 2025; Sicherer & Sampson, 2018; Skypala et al., 2015).

Signs and Symptoms Ask the patient or caregiver about the signs or symptoms they have observed in reaction to the food, including a discussion of skin and mucosal, gastrointestinal, respiratory, neurological, or cardiovascular symptoms. When did these symptoms first appear? Ask if the patient had hives, and how they would characterize them. What did they experience after eating, drinking, or coming into contact (touching, inhalation exposure through cooking or heating, etc.) with the food?

Noting the route of exposure can be helpful to consider based on the symptoms experienced, and is also relevant for occupational exposure. For infants, the caregiver should be asked about feeding (breast milk or formula) and any complementary foods consumed. How soon after the exposure did the symptoms occur? Were they immediate? Within an hour or two? Or did the symptoms appear later? How long did it take for the symptoms to resolve? Discuss whether any treatment was given, and if so, was it effective? What was done to alleviate the symptoms? Did the symptoms come back after they were resolved? Where did the reaction happen?

Acute signs or symptoms may no longer be present during the patient encounter, but if the exam is occurring shortly after a reaction, the symptoms could reflect those discussed in the section on anaphylaxis (chapter "Understanding the Diagnosis and Management of Food Allergy. Part I: IgE-Mediated Food Allergy and Anaphylaxis"). Other conditions, such as asthma, dermatitis, or allergic rhinitis, may be noted. Assessment would include inspection of the skin and mucosa, the respiratory system, and the cardiovascular system.

Since infants are unable to explain what they are feeling, careful assessment is needed, but many common food allergy symptoms, such as behavioral changes, clinging, inconsolability, sleepiness, flushing, dysphonia, drooling, regurgitation, and incontinence of urine and stool, could occur in a healthy baby (Simons & Sampson, 2015). Symptoms in infants and children that are noteworthy, and may be different than those experienced by adults, include tongue thrusting; eye, ear, and nose rubbing (Pistiner et al., 2021); tugging at ears; and arching the back (Carlisle & Lieberman, 2021). Young children may exhibit itchy ears or mouth, hoarseness due to laryngeal involvement (Dribin et al., 2025), or experience throat sensations, and lips feeling big (Pistiner et al., 2021). Also see chapters "Understanding the Diagnosis and Management of Food Allergy Part I: IgE-Mediated Food Allergy and Anaphylaxis", "Food Allergy Management in Early Childhood Settings" and "Food Allergy Management in the Hospital Setting"

Dietary History Skypala et al. (2015) recommend a structured approach to gathering a dietary history and have developed tools for adult and pediatric patients that can help guide this process, including a diary table provided in the supplementary information of the journal article. The diary includes the columns: food, symptom type, speed of onset, amount provoking reaction, raw or cooked, and whether the symptoms occur every time the food is eaten. In the adult patient, there may be a history of safely consuming a food for years before an allergic reaction, since allergies can develop at any age.

Offending Foods Ask the patient or caregiver to name the food(s) they think caused the reaction. Does this happen whenever they eat the food? Was the food previously consumed without causing any allergic signs or symptoms? How much was eaten? Does the amount consumed seem to make a difference? Was the food raw, cooked, or how was the food prepared? Was the food something that had been eaten before without symptoms? Is there a label available to review ingredients? What ingredients are noted?

Other Relevant History of Atopy Is the patient allergic to any environmental or other allergens? Is there any atopic disease? Review the patient's history for other

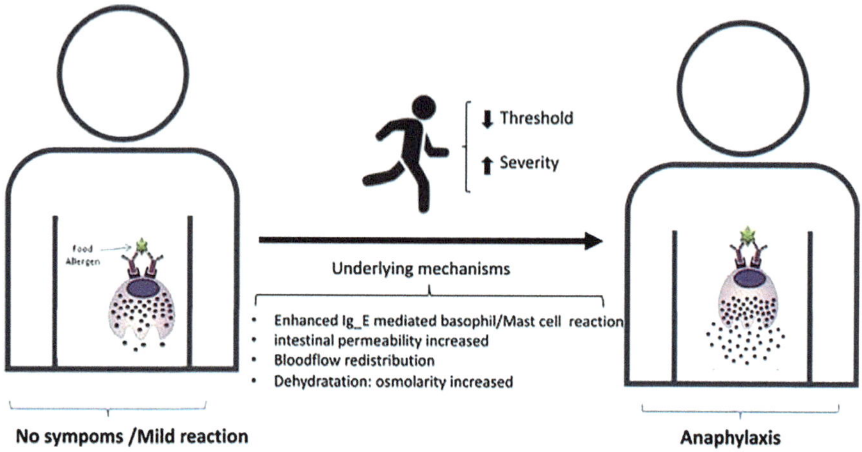

Fig. 1 Exercise acts as a cofactor in food anaphylaxis. (Used with permission from: Bartra et al. 2023)

atopic conditions, such as asthma, eczema, and allergic rhinitis. Any family history of atopic disease?

Extrinsic Factors/Intrinsic Factors/Cofactors Various factors may worsen an allergic response and have been classified as intrinsic (e.g., asthma or other host factors), extrinsic (e.g., behaviors), or have been described as cofactors. Cofactors are conditions that somehow change the response to a food in an allergic reaction. Bartra et al. (2023) postulate that cofactors make reactions more severe or can decrease the amount of food "dose" that will cause a reaction, such as when a patient reacts to a food normally tolerated after exercise. Figure 1 depicts the impact of cofactors on allergic reactions. Exercise, NSAIDs, alcohol, other medications, sleep deprivation, and estrogen have all been implicated. To explore whether any of these factors are relevant, patient assessment can include the following questions: Had the patient recently been exercising or exerting themselves? Have they recently been ill with a viral infection or other illness? Was alcohol consumed in proximity to the reaction? If so, what kind? What medications had been administered recently, including aspirin or NSAIDs? Any hormonal factors, such as menses?

Diagnostic Tests for IgE-Mediated Food Allergy

Several food allergy diagnostic algorithms have been published (Bégin et al., 2024; Foong & Santos, 2021; Santos et al., 2025), and this recent version, based on updated clinical guidelines from the European Academy of Allergy and Clinical Immunology (EAACI) depicts a comprehensive stepwise approach that is useful to understand the big picture in the diagnosis of food allergy. Clinical history, SPTs, specific IgE, component testing when available, oral food challenges, and emerging diagnostic tests are shown (Fig. 2).

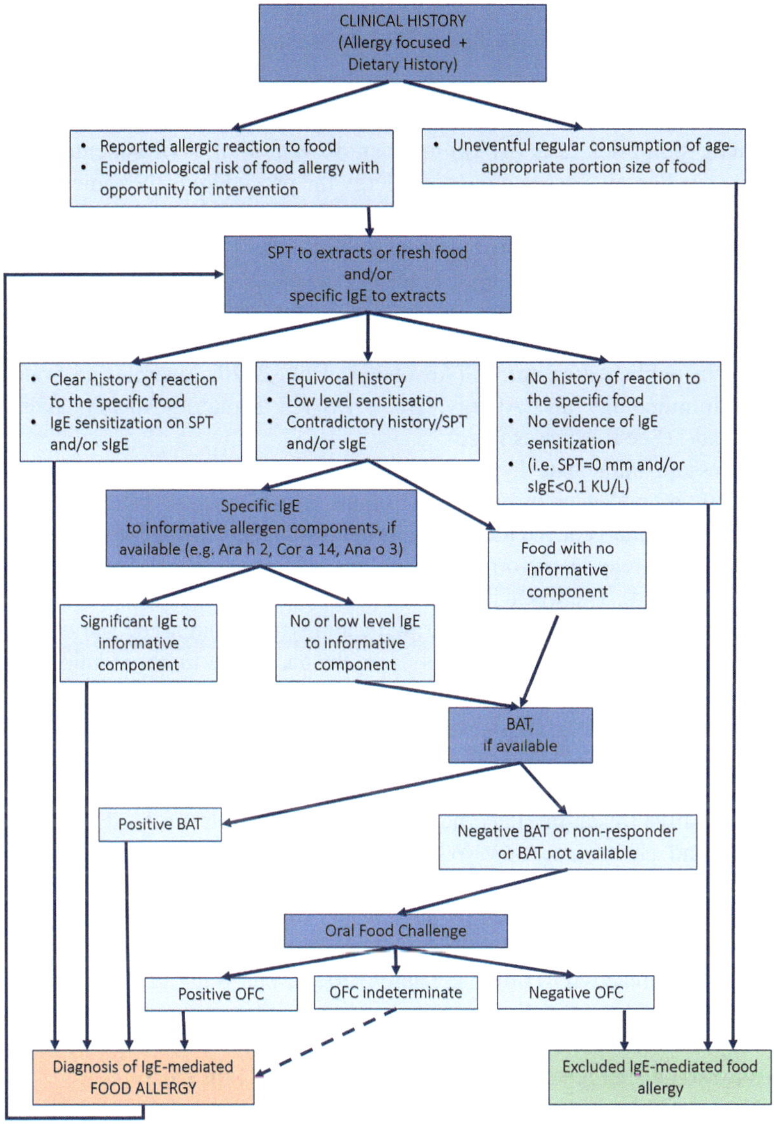

Fig. 2 IgE-Mediated Food Allergy Diagnostic Algorithm for the recommended diagnostic approach to the patient withIg E-mediated food allergy. Skin prick test and/or specific IgE are first-line tests; oral food challenges can be done at any point of the diagnostic process from here. Specific IgE to allergen components should be done, if available, for foods that IgE to allergen components have been shown to be more specific than IgE to allergen extract and should be requested in conjunction with IgE to allergen extract to provide a more complete picture of sensitization. The basophil activation test can be used, in equivocal cases, before referral for an oral food challenge, if available. BAT, basophil activation test; SPT, skin prick test; OFC, oral food challenge. (Used with permission from: Santos et al. 2025. Published under CC BY 4.0 https://creativecommons.org/licenses/by/4.0/) Note. From An algorithm for the diagnosis and management of IgE-mediated food allergy, 2024 update. By Santos, A. F., Riggioni, C., Du Toit, G., & Skypala, I. (2025). In Allergy, 80(2), 629–632. https://doi.org/10.1111/all.16321 © 2024 The Author(s)

Skin Prick Testing

Many nurses working in allergy offices, or some general pediatric and other specialty practices in areas without access to allergists, may already be familiar with performing skin prick tests (SPTs) to diagnose venom or environmental allergies. When using allergen extracts, for food allergy the procedure is the same, regardless of the allergen being tested. Clinicians use a device designed to apply allergy extracts percutaneously (via prick or puncture) or intradermally on the arm or back. Many variables, including the type of testing device, the technique applied in conducting the test, careful storage of extracts, and variations in measurement, are among the factors that can affect the integrity of SPT results. Guidance on SPTs is available in published resources (Ansotegui et al., 2020; Australasian Society of Clinical Immunology and Allergy, 2025; BSACI Pediatric Allergy Skin Prick Testing, n.d.) (See Resources Page).

SPTs assess immediate hypersensitivity and sensitization to allergens (Anvari et al., 2019), as evidenced by activation of mast cells in the skin. When the patient is sensitized to the allergen, and the mast cells bind with allergen-specific IgE, mast cells degranulate and release preformed histamines, causing a wheal and flare reaction (Bégin et al., 2024). The wheal is the localized swelling around the site of the allergen SPT resulting from increased vascular permeability and fluid at the site of the allergen, while the flare, which is redness or erythema, is due to vasodilation (Carr & Saltoun, 2012). A positive result, a wheal with a mean diameter of 3 mm or greater than the negative control (NIAID-Sponsored Expert Panel; Boyce et al., 2010), signals that the patient has been sensitized to an allergen and that IgE is present on the mast cells and is associated with an increased likelihood of clinical reactivity.

Both positive (histamine) and negative (saline) controls are used to assess skin reactivity and ensure accuracy. While histamine control skin reactions peak at 8–10 minutes, allergen reactions should be read at 10–15 minutes (Ansotegui et al., 2020). Wheal measurement cutoffs have been established for some allergens. For example, a wheal ≥8 mm has a 95% positive predictive value (PPV) for peanut allergy clinical reactivity (Boyd & Santos, 2025), but Wang (2023) cautions that cutoffs may vary across studies due to heterogeneity of study populations, allergens, and study characteristics. Table 1 provides selected positive and negative predictive values for some allergen diagnostics (Foong et al., 2021, p. 73).

SPTs are highly sensitive, but offer less specificity (Wang, 2023), so a limitation of the SPT is the risk for false positives. A patient can be sensitized to an allergen as indicated by sIgE, but not have any allergic symptoms after consuming it (tolerant), which is the rationale for testing only for foods that have caused symptoms as evidenced by clinical history (Al Ghamdi et al., 2024; Sampson et al., 2014), and not panels of multiple allergens (NIAID, 2010). However, it is noted that a case can be made for testing for additional major allergens which may be suspected, for example, testing for tree nut allergy in a child who is allergic to peanuts (Sicherer & Sampson, 2018, p.48). While SPTs cannot forecast how severe an allergy might be, they may be useful in ruling out an IgE-mediated allergy due to a high negative predictive value (NPV). However, it is possible to be allergic even with a negative

Table 1 Diagnostic cutoffs for specific IgE and skin prick testing with 95% positive predictive value

Foods	Specific IgE 95% PPV	Specific IgE 50% NPV	Skin prick test 95% PPV
Cow's milk[a]	15 kU/L (32 also reported) Infants ≤2 years: 5 kU/L	2 kU/L	≥8 mm Infants ≤2 years: 6 mm
Egg[a]	7 kU/L Infants ≤2 years: 2 kU/L	2 kU/L	≥7 mm Infants ≤2 years: 4–5 mm
Peanut	15–34 kU/L	2 kU/L if history of reaction 5 kU/L is no history of reaction	≥8 mm Infants ≤2 years: 4 mm
Fish	20 kU/L	–	
Tree nuts	20 kU/L		≥8 mm for walnut ≥12 mm for cashew
Sesame	50 kU/L (86% PPV)		≥8 mm

Note. Used with permission Foong et al. (2021)
NPV negative predictive value, *PPV* positive predictive value
[a]These numbers were derived from uncooked milk and direct egg and do not apply to baked milk or baked egg

result. In cases where an extract of the allergen in question is not available, nurses may be called upon to perform a skin prick test using fresh food, called a "prick-to-prick" (PTP) test (Terlouw et al., 2024).

An important consideration for some allergy testing, notably SPTs and oral food challenges, is the need to stop certain medications (e.g., H1 and H2 antihistamines and antidepressants with H2 antihistamine activity) for a specified number of days before the test is scheduled because they may affect reactivity. Several lists of medications to avoid in advance of testing have been published, and each setting should provide patient teaching about holding specific medications (Ansotegui et al., 2020; Australasian Society of Clinical Immunology, 2025; Sampson et al., 2024). Medications may need to be held from 2 to 11 days based on the pharmacokinetics of the drug. Cetirizine, for example, should be withheld for 3–5 days. Before performing the skin prick testing procedure, nurses should confirm that patients have withheld any antihistamine and other relevant medications for the specified duration based on the standard practice in their office. In addition, if the patient has experienced recent anaphylaxis, there are varying practices about how long to wait to conduct SPT testing, so the allergy specialist should be consulted for scheduling (Pitt et al., 2022; Kraft et al., 2024).

Ansotegui et al. (2020) outline several precautions for SPTs and other Type I skin testing, including availability of a provider who can manage and treat systemic anaphylaxis with appropriate equipment and medications, appropriate technique and placement of SPT, careful clinical assessment before testing, documentation of medication use, and care in conducting the procedure with accuracy and safety.

Specific IgE

Specific IgE is a blood test that measures circulating allergen-specific IgE for allergens and is central to the diagnostic work-up for food allergies. No special handling of specimens is needed, so the test can be performed on stored blood samples. While often used alongside SPTs, sIgE may be used alone for patients unable to stop prescribed medications that may interfere with results, when patients have dermatologic conditions or dermatographism (Boyd & Santos, 2025), or when SPT might not be well-tolerated by the patient (e.g., aversion to needles). Specific IgE tests also have the advantages of wide availability and no need to withhold antihistamines for a time period before a blood draw since antihistamines do not affect the results.

Specific IgE testing indicates allergic sensitization, but diagnosis of food allergies requires clinical correlation with these results to avoid overdiagnosis and unnecessary dietary restriction. A person with food allergies may have antibodies to a food (a positive test), since they have been sensitized and produce antibodies to an allergen, but show no signs of clinical reactivity (Foong & Santos, 2021; Parrish, 2023), so testing should be confined to foods that have provoked symptoms. Patients may infrequently have a negative result, but still exhibit symptoms of a food allergy, so additional testing is warranted. Cutoff values for sIgE are available that have a 95% PPV for food-induced reactions, and an IgE $\geq$ 0.35ku/L is considered "positive," but the results need to be interpreted by an expert in food allergy, considering symptoms and other patient-related factors (See Table 1). A higher sIgE level suggests a greater chance of a reaction, but cannot predict severity. Parrish (2023) provides a through discussion of the potential negative effects of sIgE food allergy panels.

Component-Resolved Diagnostic Testing

Component-resolved diagnostic (CRD) testing uses a blood sample in a molecular approach to analyze the individual components of an allergen by measuring IgE to those components. For example, in the case of peanut allergy, the component Ara h 2 (storage protein) correlates with clinical reactivity (allergic symptoms) but does not seem to correlate with the severity of an allergy (Sampson et al., 2024). Other components, such as Ara h 8, may indicate cross-reactivity to pollens (Foong et al., 2021). At present, only some components are available, and how this approach fits into the overall diagnosis of food allergies continues to evolve. These "components" of the allergen are puzzle pieces that make up the allergenic protein and can provide some additional details in understanding of the allergy since some of the proteins are more likely to cause an allergic reaction. Sampson et al. (2024) note that CRDs are not always useful in predicting reactivity, so testing must be individualized for each patient.

Oral Food Challenges (OFC)

The oral food challenge (OFC), the intentional feeding of increasing amounts of a specific food allergen under medical supervision, is often described as the gold standard for diagnosing IgE-mediated food allergy. Many situations may warrant OFCs, including when other testing leaves questions about the diagnosis, if there is a possibility that the allergy has resolved (development of tolerance), if questions about cross-reactive foods are unanswered, to determine thresholds for clinical reactivity, and in the research setting (Bird et al., 2020; Upton & Bird, 2020). The OFC effectively serves to confirm a food allergy, or to rule it out. However, safe conduct of OFCs requires many resources, including adequate and appropriately trained staff, emergency medications, and rigorous protocols.

Nurses play a vital role before, during, and after OFCs through providing education, practical support and instructions. Patients and caregivers should be informed of the need to withhold antihistamines (Bird et al., 2020) and other medications that could alter symptoms and impact the assessment of the challenge outcome. Other medications may worsen the severity of any reaction resulting from the challenge, such as beta blockers and ACE inhibitors, while drugs like systemic glucocorticoids may also affect OFC result interpretations (Sampson et al., 2024). Sampson et al. provide an extensive list of medications to be avoided provided in an appendix to their paper, and nurses should familiarize themselves with this list.

Guidance on food intake prior to the OFC is often provided by nurses. Sampson et al. (2024) recommend that the patient not eat for several hours before the challenge (2–4 h) so that the stomach is empty to improve absorption of the food. However, a small low-fat snack can be given 2 h before the challenge for young children, or if longer fasting is not possible (Bird et al., 2020). In addition, the patient should not eat the offending allergen (if still in the diet) for several weeks prior to the challenge. Nurses should be familiar with the doses, based on the patient's age and the milligrams of allergen protein in the food preparation being consumed, as well as the allergy clinician preferred timing of the doses.

In the research setting, one dosing schedule for a double-blind placebo-controlled food challenge outlined by Sampson et al. (2024) is 3, 10, 30, 100, 300, 1000, and 3000 mg of the specific food protein with a specified interval between doses. However, in the office setting for diagnostic challenges, the dosing may be variable. The goal is for the patient to consume an entire age-appropriate serving size of the allergen that is divided into doses which can range in number (e.g., three or more). Literature suggests many allergist use either a four to six-dose oral food challenge protocol for in-office open OFCs (Macdougall et al., 2025) or combine the first few doses outlined above to create a 5-dose regimen (Sampson et al., 2024).

Previous guidance suggested that dosing be administered in 15–20 min intervals, but newer recommendations (Sampson et al., 2024) note that the time lapse between consuming the allergen and experiencing a reaction depends upon the allergen being evaluated, with milk having a shorter period to reaction, and some foods not eliciting reactions for longer periods of time. Abbreviated intervals may allow for overlap, in that an earlier dose causes a reaction after a subsequent dose is administered. In the clinical setting, dosing is recommended to be at least 20–30 min apart, and perhaps longer, depending on the circumstances (Sampson et al., 2024, p. 13). In either case, OFCs can last many hours, and patients and families should be prepared to spend the day in the testing location, so planning for long periods of waiting is needed. In the absence of support from a mental health professional, nurses often play a crucial role in supporting patients and family and helping to allay the anxiety they may be experiencing prior to or during the challenge. Bird et al. (2020) provide many useful resources for OFCs, including age-specific portion sizes, written consents, and instructional handouts designed to educate and support patients and families before and after a challenge.

Most practices require that patients bring the food or foods they will consume during the challenge with them, and nurses are often responsible for both answering questions about acceptable foods and sharing recommendations. In the case of baked egg and baked milk challenges, specific recipes may be provided to the patient or their caregiver. Ideally, offices will provide precise recipes for home preparation that require careful measurement and adherence to the ingredients listed.

Nurses, particularly those in leadership roles within a practice, may be asked to ensure a practice's emergency preparedness. Though allergy practices are often already equipped to manage anaphylaxis or allergic reactions related to immunotherapy or other procedures, there may be additional considerations to review prior to conducting food challenges. The setting for OFCs may vary, but in any case, emergency medications (e.g., epinephrine, H1 and H2 antihistamines, albuterol, vasopressors, steroids, IV fluids) and equipment (e.g., airways, bag-mask kit, oxygen and nasal cannula, pulse oximeter, nebulizer) must be immediately accessible, and the staff in attendance must have the necessary skills to address any reaction (Bird et al., 2020; Macdougall et al., 2025). Intravenous access may be advised for those patients who have experienced a severe reaction in the past, those with severe asthma, and for those where access may be challenging (Sampson et al., 2024).

Ensuring sufficient availability of qualified clinicians, medications (with pre-calculated doses based on patient weight), equipment, and documentation procedures is a minimum requirement. Nurses and providers involved in food challenges should be re-trained regularly on their practice's protocol for anaphylaxis management optimally using hands-on simulation or practice drills. (See chapter "Understanding the Diagnosis and Management of Food Allergy Part I: IgE-Mediated Food Allergy and Anaphylaxis" for more on recognizing and treating anaphylaxis).

In 2024, the American Academy of Allergy, Asthma, and Immunology (AAAAI) and the European Academy of Allergy and Clinical Immunology (EAACI) published updated recommendations for food challenges based on expert consensus and analysis of the literature (PRACTALL Consensus Report). These new guidelines offer practical information and address the safety of OFCs (Sampson et al., 2012, 2024). Criteria for OFC progression are provided, using a color-coded system of green, orange, and red, to characterize patient response across multiple body systems. For example, when describing a skin reaction, a few areas of skin redness would be green, erythema of less than half of the body surface area would be orange, and generalized redness over more than 50% of the body would be red. Symptoms would need to be reviewed in totality. The challenge should be stopped if one red symptom is present or two orange symptoms from different body systems. Sampson et al. (2024) provide a comprehensive overview of the challenge criteria. Deferring OFCs is recommended for patients with a serious cardiovascular or respiratory condition and should not be conducted with a pregnant patient due to the risk to mother and baby (Bird et al., 2020).

In addition to challenging patients to foods they have avoided due to concern for an IgE-mediated food allergy, practices may also conduct food challenges for a non-IgE-mediated food allergy called food protein-induced enterocolitis syndrome (FPIES). This text will not discuss the specifics of FPIES in detail; however, it is important to note that the symptoms and protocols for managing an FPIES reaction are different from those for anaphylaxis, but include intravenous fluids, ondansetron, and corticosteroids (Bird et al., 2020; Ibrahim et al., 2025; Sampson et al., 2024).

Nurses also play an important role in providing or emphasizing key elements of post-challenge guidance as part of the discharge instructions, which should include an instructional handout and review of an emergency treatment plan and prescriptions.

Novel Diagnostics

Additional diagnostic tests are used in some countries and in research settings and may be more widely available in the future. Researchers are still working to identify and understand novel biomarkers that can more accurately characterize a patient's food allergy. Below are some examples of novel diagnostic tests emerging in the clinical setting.

Basophil Activation Test

The basophil activation test (BAT) is a newer cellular assay for allergies. When basophils are activated in an allergic response, upregulation of CD63 occurs in concert with degranulation and histamine release. The BAT measures degranulation markers associated with histamine release (e.g., CD63 and CD203c) on basophils in a whole blood sample (Ansotegui et al., 2020). The peripheral blood sample is exposed to increasing amounts of an allergen concentration, using flow cytometry (Passanisi et al., 2021).

Sensitivity and specificity for the BAT compare favorably to other allergy diagnostics with reported high specificity and sensitivity, as well as high positive (PPV) and negative predictive value (NPV) (Foong et al., 2021). Some evidence to support its use in identifying clinical reactivity thresholds has also been documented (Marini-Rapoport et al., 2025). The BAT has demonstrated good accuracy in peanut allergy, with the ability to differentiate between patients with allergies and those who were sensitized but tolerant and may reduce the need for food challenges, with the exception of some patients (about 10%) whose basophils did not respond (Boyd

& Santos, 2025), so the BAT may be a useful step prior to implementing an OFC. Testing with other allergens (e.g., tree nuts) has also shown promise (Marini-Rapoport et al., 2025; Opper et al., 2025).

Advantages of the BAT are that it can be a safer alternative to actual exposure of the patient to the allergen in an SPT or oral food challenge, so allergic reactions may be averted. The BAT also requires only a small amount of blood and is not affected by any medications, so antihistamines and other drugs do not need to be withheld. However, basophils in whole blood must be tested within 4–24 h due to their short life span. In addition, special equipment and training are needed (Opper et al., 2025). More research, validation, and development of standardization of the BAT is needed to determine its optimal use in the overall algorithm of food allergy diagnosis, but this approach appears to offer another valuable diagnostic approach.

Mast Cell Activation Test

Mast cells play a significant role in allergic response, so they are another potential target in diagnostic testing. The mast cell activation test is also a cellular assay, but in contrast to the BAT, uses the patient's plasma or serum to sensitize mast cells grown in culture and then exposes them to an allergen in vitro (Foong & Santos, 2021; Santos et al., 2021). Various sources of mast cells, both human- and mouse-derived, have been used in this test. Flow cytometry is also used to analyze these samples. MAT does not need fresh blood, and samples can be frozen, easing some logistical issues associated with the BAT. However, Foong et al. (2021) note that MAT is less sensitive than BAT, and may differ in its predictive value, and also has an overall higher cost than BAT, sIgE, and SPTs (p. 76). More research is needed to establish the optimal use and method for MAT testing in both the research and clinical settings.

Conclusion

Due to the imperfect nature of the existing diagnostic methods for food allergy, it is essential for patients and families to work with a clinician who has experience in food allergy, including allergists who are experts in diagnosing food allergy. The consequences of misdiagnosis can be significant both for those who are incorrectly advised to avoid a food allergen as well as for those who are told a food is safe to eat when in fact they are allergic. Furthermore, nurses working with families during this diagnostic period must keep in mind that for many families, the sometimes lengthy process of completing allergy testing can be a scary and frustrating time. Particularly with young children, the diagnosis may also change over time, so repeat testing may be advised to see if a child has outgrown their allergy or in some cases developed a new one. Clinical history informs both the need for and in some cases the interpretation of the existing standard diagnostic methods of SPT, sIgE, and oral food challenges. It is important that clinicians and families have completed all of the testing for various food allergens prior to considering and initiating treatments, as some of the treatments such as omalizumab can alter the accuracy of further testing. As diagnostic methods continue to improve, it is likely that in the near future there will be new testing options to ease the current difficulties associated with making an accurate food allergy diagnosis.

References

Al Ghamdi A., Abrams E, M., Carr, S., Hanna, M, A., Herman, S, M., Lavine, E., Kim, H., Vander Leek, T. K, Mack, D. P. (2024). Canadian Society of Allergy and Clinical Immunology position statement: panel testing for food allergies. *Allergy, Asthma & Clinical Immunology, 20*(1),61. https://doi.org/10.1186/s13223-024-00937-0

Ansotegui, I. J., Melioli, G., Canonica, G. W., Caraballo, L., Villa, E., Ebisawa, M., Passalacqua, G., Savi, E., Ebo, D., Gómez, R. M., Luengo Sánchez, O., Oppenheimer, J. J., Jensen-Jarolim, E., Fischer, D. A., Haahtela, T., Antila, M., Bousquet, J. J., Cardona, V., Chiang, W. C., Demoly, P. M...Zuberbier, T. (2020). IgE allergy diagnostics and other relevant tests in allergy, a World Allergy Organization position paper. *The World Allergy Organization journal, 13*(2), 100080. https://doi.org/10.1016/j.waojou.2019.100080

Anvari, S., Miller, J., Yeh, C. Y., & Davis, C. M. (2019). IgE-mediated food allergy. *Clinical Reviews in Allergy & Immunology, 57*(2), 244–260. https://doi.org/10.1007/s12016-018-8710-3

Australasian Society of Clinical Immunology and Allergy. (2025). *Skin prick testing guide for diagnosis of allergic disease*. Retrieved August 8, 2025, from https://www.allergy.org.au/hp/papers/skin-prick-testing/

Bartra, J., Turner, P. J., & Muñoz-Cano, R. M. (2023). Cofactors in food anaphylaxis In adults. *Annals of Allergy, Asthma & Immunology: Official Publication of the American College of Allergy, Asthma, & Immunology, 130*(6), 733–740. https://doi.org/10.1016/j.anai.2023.03.017

Bégin, P., Waserman, S., Protudjer, J. L. P., et al. (2024). Immunoglobulin E (IgE)-mediated food allergy. *Allergy, Asthma and Clinical Immunology, 20*(Suppl 3), 75. https://doi.org/10.1186/s13223-024-00930-7

Bird, J. A., Leonard, S., Groetch, M., Assa'ad, A., Cianferoni, A., Clark, A., Crain, M., Fausnight, T., Fleischer, D., Green, T., Greenhawt, M., Herbert, L., Lanser, B. J., Mikhail, I., Mustafa, S., Noone, S., Parrish, C., Varshney, P., Vlieg-Boerstra, B., Young, M. C., & Nowak-Wegrzyn, A. (2020). Conducting an oral food challenge: An update to the 2009 adverse reactions to Foods Committee Work Group Report. *The Journal of Allergy and Clinical Immunology. In Practice., 8*(1), 75–90.e17. https://doi.org/10.1016/j.jaip.2019.09.029

Boyd, H., & Santos, A. F. (2025). Novel diagnostics in food allergy. *The Journal of Allergy and Clinical Immunology, 155*(2), 275–285. https://doi.org/10.1016/j.jaci.2024.12.1071

British Society for & Clinical Immunology (BSACI). (n.d.). *Paediatric allergy skin prick testing*. https://www.bsaci.org/wp-content/uploads/2024/10/paedSPTnew_V2.pdf

Carlisle, A., & Lieberman, J. (2021). Clinical management of infant anaphylaxis. *Journal of Asthma and Allergy, 14*, 821–827. https://doi.org/10.2147/JAA.S286692

Carr, T. F., & Saltoun, C. A. (2012). Chapter 2: Skin testing in allergy. *Allergy and Asthma Proceedings, 33*(Suppl 1), 6–8. https://doi.org/10.2500/aap.2012.33.3532

Chinthrajah, R. S., Tupa, D., Prince, B. T., Block, W. M., Rosa, J. S., Singh, A. M., & Nadeau, K. (2015). Diagnosis of food allergy. *Pediatric Clinics of North America, 62*(6), 1393–1408. https://doi.org/10.1016/j.pcl.2015.07.009

Dribin, T. E., Muraro, A., Camargo, C. A., Jr., Turner, P. J., Wang, J., Roberts, G., Anagnostou, A., Halken, S., Liebermann, J., Worm, M., Zuberbier, T., Sampson, H. A., & GA(2)LEN Anaphylaxis Study Team. (2025). Anaphylaxis definition, overview, and clinical support tool: 2024 consensus report-a GA^{2}LEN project. *The Journal of Allergy and Clinical Immunology, 156*(2), 406–417.e6. https://doi.org/10.1016/j.jaci.2025.01.021

Foong, R. X., Santos, A, F. (2021). Biomarkers of diagnosis and resolution of food allergy. *Pediatr Allergy Immunol, 32*:223–233. https://doi.org/10.1111/pai.13389

Foong, R. X., Dantzer, J. A., Wood, R. A., & Santos, A. F. (2021). Improving diagnostic accuracy in food allergy. *The Journal of Allergy and Clinical Immunology. In Practice, 9*(1), 71–80. https://doi.org/10.1016/j.jaip.2020.09.037

Ibrahim, T., Argiz, L., Infante, S., Arasi, S., Nurmatov, U., & Vazquez-Ortiz, M. (2025). Oral food challenge protocols in food protein-induced enterocolitis syndrome: A systematic review. *The Journal of Allergy and Clinical Immunology. In Practice., 13*(4), 814–832. https://doi.org/10.1016/j.jaip.2024.12.033

Kraft, M. T., Coletta, C., Mikhail, I., Prince, B. T., Scherzer, R., Eisner, M., & Mustillo, P. (2024). The sensitivity of food allergy skin testing soon after food-induced anaphylaxis. *The Journal of Allergy and Clinical Immunology in Practice (Cambridge, MA), 12*(5), 1384–1386.e2. https://doi.org/10.1016/j.jaip.2024.01.041

Liccardi, G., D'Amato, G., Canonica, G. W., Salzillo, A., Piccolo, A., & Passalacqua, G. (2006). Systemic reactions from skin testing: Literature review. *Journal of Investigational Allergology & Clinical Immunology, 16*(2), 75–78.

Macdougall, J., Shah, D., & Bird, J. A. (2025). Oral food challenges: The standard of diagnosis. *Immunology and Allergy Clinics of North America, 45*(3), 355–365. https://doi.org/10.1016/j.iac.2025.04.004

Marini-Rapoport, O., Bhowmik, M., & Patil, S. U. (2025). Basophil activation test for the improved diagnosis of peanut and tree nut allergy. *Current Allergy and Asthma Reports, 25*(1), 19. https://doi.org/10.1007/s11882-025-01200-1

Muraro, A., Werfel, T., Hoffmann-Sommergruber, K., Roberts, G., Beyer, K., Bindslev-Jensen, C., Cardona, V., Dubois, A., du Toit, G., Eigenmann, P., Fernandez Rivas, M., Halken, S., Hickstein, L., Høst, A., Knol, E., Lack, G., Marchisotto, M. J., Niggemann, B., Nwaru, B. I., Papadopoulos, N. G., & EAACI Food Allergy and Anaphylaxis Guidelines Group. (2014). EAACI food allergy and anaphylaxis guidelines: Diagnosis and management of food allergy. *Allergy, 69*(8), 1008–1025. https://doi.org/10.1111/all.12429

NIAID-Sponsored Expert Panel; Boyce JA, Assa'ad A, Burks AW, Jones SM, Sampson HA, Wood RA, Plaut M, Cooper SF, Fenton MJ, Arshad SH, Bahna SL, Beck LA, Byrd-Bredbenner C, Camargo CA Jr, Eichenfield L, Furuta GT, Hanifin JM, Jones C, Kraft M, Levy BD, Lieberman P, Luccioli S, McCall KM, Schneider LC, Simon RA, Simons FE, Teach SJ, Yawn BP, Schwaninger JM (2010). Guidelines for the diagnosis and management of food allergy in the United States: report of the NIAID-sponsored expert panel. *J Allergy Clin Immunol. 126*(6 Suppl):S1–58. https://doi.org/10.1016/j.jaci.2010.10.007. PMID: 21134576; PMCID: PMC4241964.

Opper, C., Bannon, M., & Devonshire, A. L. (2025). Diagnosis of immunoglobulin E-mediated food allergy. *Immunology and Allergy Clinics of North America, 45*(3), 339–354. https://doi.org/10.1016/j.iac.2025.04.003

Parrish, C, P. (2023). A review of food allergy panels and their consequences. *Annals of Allergy, Asthma & Immunology, 131*(4), 421–426. https://doi.org/10.1016/j.anai.2023.04.011

Passanisi, S., Lombardo, F., Crisafulli, G., Salzano, G., Aversa, T., & Pajno, G. B. (2021). Novel diagnostic techniques and therapeutic strategies for IgE-mediated food allergy. *Allergy and Asthma Proceedings, 42*(2), 124–130. https://doi.org/10.2500/aap.2021.42.200129

Patel, N., Shreffler, W. G., Custovic, A., & Santos, A. F. (2023). Will oral food challenges still be part of allergy care in 10 years' time? *The Journal of Allergy and Clinical Immunology. In Practice, 11*(4), 988–996. https://doi.org/10.1016/j.jaip.2023.02.010

Pistiner, M., Mendez-Reyes, J. E., Eftekhari, S., Carver, M., Lieberman, J., Wang, J., & Camargo, C. A. (2021). Caregiver-reported presentation of severe food-induced allergic reactions in infants and toddlers. *The Journal of Allergy and Clinical Immunology in Practice (Cambridge, MA), 9*(1), 311–320.e2. https://doi.org/10.1016/j.jaip.2020.11.005

Pitt, J., Shopper, C., Dowling, P., Miller, C., Sherman, A., & Aljubran, S. (2022). Current practices in delaying testing for IgE-mediated food allergy after anaphylaxis. *The Journal of Allergy and Clinical Immunology. Global, 1*(4), 312–313. https://doi.org/10.1016/j.jacig.2022.05.010

Riggioni, C., Ricci, C., Moya, B., Wong, D., van Goor, E., Bartha, I., Buyuktiryaki, B., Giovannini, M., Jayasinghe, S., Jaumdally, H., Marques-Mejias, A., Piletta-Zanin, A., Berbenyuk, A., Andreeva, M., Levina, D., Iakovleva, E., Roberts, G., Chu, D., Peters, R., du Toit, G., & Santos, A. F. (2024). Systematic review and meta-analyses on the accuracy of diagnostic tests for IgE-mediated food allergy. *Allergy, 79*(2), 324–352. https://doi.org/10.1111/all.15939

Sampson, H. A., Gerth van Wijk, R., Bindslev-Jensen, C., Sicherer, S., Teuber, S. S., Burks, A. W., Dubois, A. E., Beyer, K., Eigenmann, P. A., Spergel, J. M., Werfel, T., & Chinchilli, V. M. (2012). Standardizing double-blind, placebo-controlled oral food challenges: American Academy of Allergy, Asthma & Immunology-European Academy of Allergy and Clinical Immunology PRACTALL consensus report. *The Journal of Allergy and Clinical Immunology, 130*(6), 1260–1274. https://doi.org/10.1016/j.jaci.2012.10.017

Sampson, H. A., Aceves, S., Bock, S. A., James. J., Jones, S., Lang, D., Nadeau, K., Nowak-Wegrzyn, A., Oppenheimer, J., Perry, T. T., Randolph, C., Sicherer, S. H., Simon, R. A., Vickery, B. P., Wood. R. Bernstein, D., Blessing-Moore J., Khan. D., Lang, D., Nicklas, R., Oppenheimer, J., Portnoy, J., Randolph, C., Schuller, D., Spector, S., Tilles, S. A., Wallace, D., Sampson, H. A., Aceves, S., Bock, S. A., James, J., Jones, S., Lang, D., Nadeau, K., Nowak-Wegrzyn, A., Oppenheimer, J., Perry, T. T., Randolph C., Sicherer, S. H., Simon, R, A., Vickery, B. P., Wood, R. (2014). Joint task force on practice parameters; practice parameter workgroup; Food allergy: a practice parameter update-2014. *Journal of Allergy and Clinical Immunology, 134*(5), 1016–25.e43. https://doi.org/10.1016/j.jaci.2014.05.013. Epub 2014 Aug 28. PMID: 25174862.

Sampson, H. A., Arasi, S., Bahnson, H. T., Ballmer-Weber, B., Beyer, K., Bindslev-Jensen, C., Bird, J. A., Blumchen, K., Davis, C., Ebisawa, M., Nowak-Wegrzyn, A., Patel, N., Peters, R. L., Sicherer, S., Spergel, J., Turner, P. J., Yanagida, N., & Eigenmann, P. A. (2024). AAAAI-EAACI PRACTALL: Standardizing oral food challenges-2024 update. *Pediatric Allergy and Immunology: Official Publication of the European Society of Pediatric Allergy and Immunology, 35*(11), e14276. https://doi.org/10.1111/pai.14276

Santos, A. F., Alpan, O., & Hoffmann, H. J. (2021). Basophil activation test: Mechanisms and considerations for use in clinical trials and clinical practice. *Allergy, 76*(8), 2420–2432. https://doi.org/10.1111/all.14747

Santos, A. F., Riggioni, C., Agache, I., Akdis, C. A., Akdis, M., Alvarez-Perea, A., Alvaro-Lozano, M., Ballmer-Weber, B., Barni, S., Beyer, K., Bindslev-Jensen, C., Brough, H. A., Buyuktiryaki, B., Chu, D., Del Giacco, S., Dunn-Galvin, A., Eberlein, B., Ebisawa, M., Eigenmann, P., Eiwegger, T., & Skypala, I. (2023). EAACI guidelines on the diagnosis of IgE-mediated food allergy. *Allergy, 78*(12), 3057–3076. https://doi.org/10.1111/all.15902

Santos, A. F., Riggioni, C., Du Toit, G., & Skypala, I. (2025). An algorithm for the diagnosis and management of IgE-mediated food allergy, 2024 update. *Allergy, 80*(2), 629–632. https://doi.org/10.1111/all.16321

Sicherer, S. H., & Sampson, H. A. (2018). Food allergy: A review and update on epidemiology, pathogenesis, diagnosis, prevention, and management. *The Journal of Allergy and Clinical Immunology, 141*(1), 41–58. https://doi.org/10.1016/j.jaci.2017.11.003

Simons, F. E., & Sampson, H. A. (2015). Anaphylaxis: Unique aspects of clinical diagnosis and management in infants (birth to age 2 years). *The Journal of Allergy and Clinical Immunology, 135*(5), 1125–1131. https://doi.org/10.1016/j.jaci.2014.09.014

Skypala, I. J., Venter, C., Meyer, R., deJong, N. W., Fox, A. T., Groetch, M., Oude Elberink, J. N., Sprikkelman, A., Diamandi, L., Vlieg-Boerstra, B. J., & Allergy-focussed Diet History Task Force of the European Academy of Allergy and Clinical Immunology. (2015). The development of a standardised diet history tool to support the diagnosis of food allergy. *Clinical and Translational Allergy, 5*, 7. https://doi.org/10.1186/s13601-015-0050-2

Terlouw, S., van Boven, F. E., Borsboom-van Zonneveld, M., de Graaf-In 't Veld, T., Gerth van Wijk, R., van Daele, P. L. A., van Maaren, M. S., Kuijpers, J. H. S. A. M., Veenbergen, S., & de Jong, N. W. (2024). Comparison of skin prick test and prick-to-prick test with fruits and vegetables in the diagnosis of food allergy. *Clinical and Translational Allergy, 14*(7), e12375. https://doi.org/10.1002/clt2.12375

Upton, J., E., M., Bird, J., A. (2020). Oral food challenges: special considerations. *Annals of Allergy, Asthma & Immunology, 124*(5), 451–458. https://doi.org/10.1016/j.anai.2020.02.008

Wang, J. (2023). Food challenges: Patient selection, predictors, component testing, and decision points. *Journal of Food Allergy (East Providence, RI: Online), 5*(2), 38–42. https://doi.org/10.2500/jfa.2023.5.230010

Understanding the Diagnosis and Management of Food Allergy Part III: Management of Food Allergy in the Outpatient Setting

Robyn Huey Lao, Mary Frances Vess, Sarah Pederson,
Josie Howard-Ruben, and Julianne Doucette

Introduction

For many children and adults, food allergies are a lifelong issue (the "classic phenotype" of food allergy), and lifestyle modifications and new behaviors must be adopted to allow for safe eating and a good quality of life (Baker & Sampson, 2018, p. 246). While many food allergies are persistent from childhood, there are some that may resolve as a child grows older. Milk and egg allergies, for example, seem to resolve more than others, but still do not resolve for many people. Allergies like tree nuts, fish and shellfish often persist (Lee et al., 2024), and many people will develop new-onset food allergies beyond childhood and into adulthood. More recently, early introduction of food allergens in the infant diet has emerged as a potential preventive strategy for averting food allergies from developing in the first place. This approach to prevention of food allergies is discussed in chapter "Early Introduction of Food Allergens".

For some patients, the ability to tolerate baked allergens, due to the changes of the protein structure during heating, may suggest future tolerance. Dietary

R. H. Lao (✉)
University of California Davis Medical Center, Davis, CA, USA
e-mail: REHuey@health.ucdavis.edu

M. F. Vess
Children's Healthcare of Atlanta, Atlanta, GA, USA
e-mail: Mary.Vess@choa.org

S. Pederson
Food Allergy Nursing Association, Great Neck, NY, USA

J. Howard-Ruben
Rush University College of Nursing, Chicago, IL, USA
e-mail: josie_howard-ruben@rush.edu

J. Doucette
College of Nursing, Rush University, Chicago, IL, USA
e-mail: Julianne_Doucette@rush.edu

J. Doucette, J. Howard-Ruben (eds.), *Comprehensive Food Allergy Management for Nurses*, https://doi.org/10.1007/978-3-032-28647-5_4

advancement therapies (e.g., milk and egg ladders) may play a role in children with those allergies as a means for developing tolerance, although a systematic review of studies using this approach yielded weak support (Lambert et al., 2017; Gallagher et al., 2024). Anagnostou et al. (2024) likewise observed that well-designed studies to support this approach do not currently exist and suggested that well-controlled studies are needed. Further, these authors suggest that tolerance of baked milk and baked egg may suggest a "transient allergy phenotype," or one that is likely to be outgrown (p. 2469). Mack (2023) stresses that many variables must be considered and that standardization of protocols, including heating time, specific recipe or commercial products, and other factors must be addressed. However, this information highlights that there is much to be learned about food allergy phenotypes and how they may be managed in the future (Baker & Sampson, 2018).

With the current state of knowledge, for most patients, managing food allergies still requires strict avoidance of the allergens. Well-informed nurses can be instrumental in helping patients and families to develop resilience and to acquire the new knowledge, skills, and behaviors needed to manage life with food allergies, including the critical skills of avoidance and emergency management. Living with food allergies requires learning about many aspects of avoidance and emergency management across many situations. Sicherer and Sampson (2018) have provided a good overview and outline some food allergy management issues, including topics to discuss with patients and caregivers to help them to implement avoidance and emergency management strategies effectively. In this chapter, we discuss strategies for avoidance, and in the chapter "Understanding the Diagnosis and Management of Food Allergy Part I: IgE-Mediated Food Allergy and Anaphylaxis" recognition of anaphylaxis and emergency management, including administration of epinephrine, is discussed.

Allergen Avoidance

For decades, the treatment for IgE-mediated food allergies has been limited to the avoidance of the offending allergen(s), as well as recognition and rapid treatment of a suspected allergic reaction. Every patient and family should have access to an emergency action plan, such as the examples provided in the chapter "Food Allergy Management in Early Childhood Settings".

Avoiding allergens requires a careful approach to any situation where food is present, including the home, the workplace, school and the community. For food allergies to be safely navigated, allergen avoidance requires extensive patient and caregiver education to help reduce the risk of exposures. Patients and families need a full understanding of the foods containing specific allergens and recommended dietary restrictions. Careful label reading, avoidance of cross-contact, optimal cleaning and food preparation strategies, and due diligence when eating in any setting, are all required. Providing online resources, suggestions for support groups, and connecting patients with others with the same allergies can enhance the education provided by nurses and help to normalize experiences for patients and families. Many of the web sites in the Resources pages provide extensive lists of foods and non-food items to avoid with specific allergies, and nurses can point patients and caregivers to these sites to educate them on allergen avoidance. One example is the Living with Food Allergies page at Kids with Food Allergies (2026). Downloadable guides for all top allergens are available (e.g., "A Guide to Managing Tree Nut Allergy").

Understanding Food Labels

Reading labels and recognizing allergens is a major aspect of avoidance. Reading every label, every time, whenever food is purchased or prepared, is a cardinal rule of allergen avoidance. Labeling can change, so it must be emphasized that the label on the packaging of the product currently in hand (not the web site ingredient list) must be scrutinized. Knowing a product is usually safe is the first step, but reading every package label must be a consistent practice, as even the same product, sourced from a different facility or in a different size or formulation, can have different labeling.

Required Labeling in the US

In the US, according to the Food Allergen Labeling and Consumer Protection Act of 2004 (FALCPA), major food allergens must be labeled on packaged foods and dietary supplements manufactured in or imported into the country. Originally, this included eight major allergens, but with the passage of the Food Allergy Safety, Treatment, and Education Act (2021), labeling requirements for food allergens were updated (FDA, 2025). Now, nine major allergens require labeling, including peanuts, tree nuts (e.g., almonds, cashews, hazelnuts, macadamia, pecans, pistachios, walnuts, etc.), soy, milk and dairy, eggs, sesame, wheat, finfish, and crustacean shellfish (crab, lobster, shrimp). However, mollusks (clams, mussels, oysters, and scallops) do not require labeling in the US, nor do other allergens such as celery, lupine, and mustard. Certain items classified by the FDA as tree nuts no longer require labeling with this recent revision, such as coconut, chestnut, ginkgo nut, and shea nut (FARE, 2025). Other exceptions are meat, poultry, catfish, and some processed egg products, which are governed by the US Department of Agriculture (USDA), and alcohol, which falls under the Tobacco Tax and Trade Bureau.

Manufacturers can provide either:

- an ingredient list on the label with the common or usual name of the allergen in the ingredient list,
- or an ingredient list with a "contains" statement immediately after or next to the list,
- or in parentheses following the name of the allergen ingredient in the ingredient list.

Different label formats require that every part of the label ingredients be read before consumption of the product. Any markings on the front of a package

By its common or usual name in the ingredient list
Example:

Ingredients: Brown rice flour, sesame seeds, potato starch, flax seeds, olive oil, amaranth, quinoa, salt

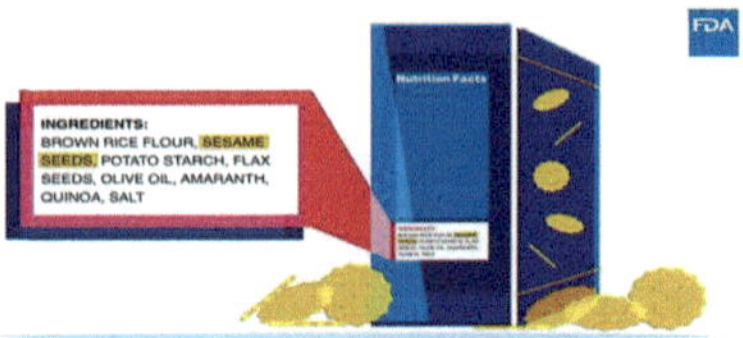

OR

In a "Contains" statement immediately after or next to the list of ingredients:

Example:

Ingredients: Potatoes, canola oil, spices (sesame, wheat), salt, garlic powder, sugar, natural flavoring

CONTAINS: Wheat, Sesame

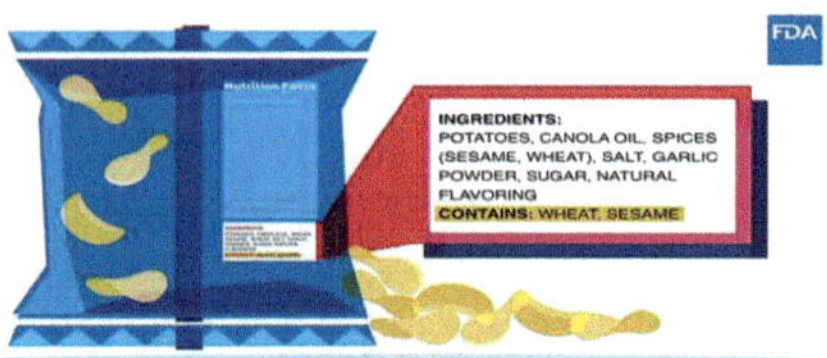

OR

In parentheses following the name of the ingredient in the ingredient list
Example: Tahini paste (sesame, canola oil), water, garlic, lemon juice, parsley, salt

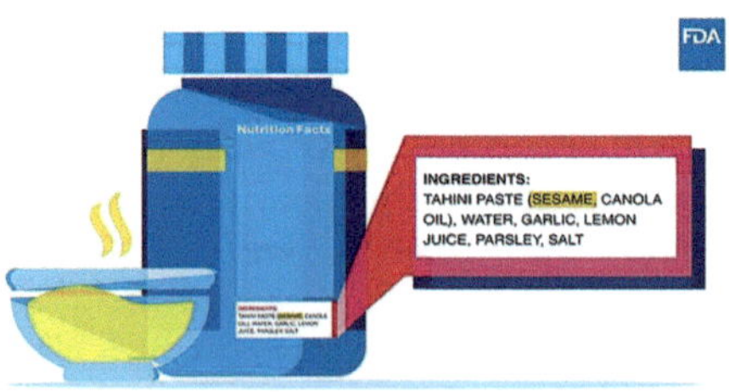

Fig. 1 Food Allergen Labeling with Examples. (Used with permission from: the Food and Drug Administration (2024). *The FASTER Act: Sesame is the ninth major food allergen*. Accessed June 1, 2026 from https://www.fda.gov/food/food-allergies/faster-act-sesame-ninth-major-food-allergen. Open access)

(e.g., nut-free) are marketing information and not currently regulated, but a "Nutrition Info" box is under consideration. A mock-up of this label online does not address food allergies, but addresses saturated fat, sodium and added sugars, so it would be a separate label on the food packaging (Fig. 1).

Allergy Labeling Outside the US

Across the globe, allergen labeling laws differ, with some countries requiring labeling for additional allergens beyond the top nine. Other variations in labeling practices are also noted (Ham et al., 2025). When traveling, awareness of the local requirements for labeling is needed, since there may be variations among countries. Most, however, do adhere to the Codex Alimentarius (Chang et al., 2023) (See chapter "Public Policy and Advocacy for People with Food Allergy").

Precautionary Labeling

Food allergen labeling can be confusing, so several key points can be shared with patients and caregivers. First, every part of the ingredients section on the package must be read, as described above. Additional precautionary allergy labeling (PAL) is not regulated in the EU and US, so some terms used on labels, such as "may contain traces," "may contain," "processed in a facility with," and "manufactured on shared equipment with," are voluntary. Originally intended to address the presence of unintended allergens, these statements are not standardized, so the degree of risk is not currently quantified. Discussions about how to decipher "may contain" and "shared facility" labeling can include whether patients are also advised to avoid these items. Precautionary labeling is also discussed in the chapters "Food Allergy Management in Adolescents and Young Adults" and "Public Policy and Advocacy for People with Food Allergy". In addition, the chapter "Public Policy and Advocacy for People with Food Allergy" discusses more about labeling laws. Finally, since there are over 170 foods and other items (e.g., chemicals and even insect infestations) that can provoke a reaction, not all potential allergens will be labeled, and in some cases, a more detailed assessment of ingredients is needed.

Educating Patients and Families About Labels

Nurses can teach families how to recognize their allergens and other terms for their allergens on food labels. Butter is a dairy product, for example, and if allergic to milk, butter is also an allergen. One helpful educational tool is to provide a list of terms for applicable allergens such as whey (milk) or casein (milk) and tahini (sesame), and many allergy web sites offer this information. Patients may not know that lactose-free items still contain milk, for example. Literacy level should be assessed and patient education materials provided in preferred language at an appropriate level.

Purchasing Safe Food

Learning to read labels (every label, every time) is an important skill for safe food shopping. While some products will be trusted brands, there are variations even among products by the same manufacturer, so labels must always be checked. Manufacturers use different facilities and co-packers, for example, so exposure to allergens can vary from one time to the next. Some people with food allergies or their caregivers contact manufacturers to verify safety and to confirm that there is no cross-contact with allergens in the manufacturing process. Families can stock up on safe foods in the freezer and pantry to always have back-up foods available.

Medications and Over-the-Counter Products

Medications, despite containing food allergens as excipients or inactive ingredients such as corn, polyethylene glycol, sugars etc., do not fall under the current food allergy labeling laws in the US. Although legislation requiring labeling of major allergens in medication has been introduced in the US, the bipartisan ADINA Act, it has not been passed into law (H.R. 3821, 2025). Bahna (2023) and Kelso (2014) provide the most comprehensive peer-reviewed information on this topic to date, describing excipients that are included in pharmaceutical and other medical products. Some of the items mentioned include vaccines (discussed below), interferons, dry powder inhalers, emulsions, hormone and other injections, oral medications, supplements and over-the-counter medications. Bahna (2023) also lists dermatologic topicals, nasal drops, suppositories, and dental preparations as medication products where food allergens, such as lactose (from milk) and gelatin (from fish or beef), may be found. While the potential for a reaction to these ingredients in medications exists, adverse events are rare, possibly because the amount of allergenic protein does not reach the threshold to cause a response. For more current information about potential allergens in medications and other medical products, package inserts and other references should be consulted, along with the clinician, pharmacist, as well as other members of the healthcare team, including dentists and anesthesia providers.

Vaccinations

While most vaccinations are safe for people with food allergies, some do contain food products, such as egg protein (e.g., yellow fever, some rabies vaccines), so some precautions may be warranted (Abrams et al., 2024) and should be discussed with an allergy provider. In addition, any "severe reaction (e.g., anaphylaxis) to a previous dose or vaccine component" is described as a contraindication by the (CDC, 2024).

Kelso (2022) recently underscored the safety of influenza vaccines for patients with egg allergies, agreeing with the American Academy of Pediatrics and other organizations that no special steps need to be taken for patients for flu shots in patients with egg allergies, but avoidance may be a personal preference, so there are egg free-influenza vaccine options available. Caution is warranted, however, for the yellow fever vaccine, which includes an allergy-testing protocol to ensure that the vaccine can be safely administered. Kelso (2022) also warns of the need to evaluate patients with a gelatin allergy more closely with allergy testing, or to provide a gelatin-free alternative. This warning is also relevant for patients with alpha-gal syndrome, with some reports of reactions to vaccines containing gelatin. Since this information may change, the reader is referred to the American Academy of (AAP), the Centers for Disease Control and Prevention (CDC) and other reliable sources of information for the most current ingredients such as the FDA-approved vaccine package insert for updated guidance.

Labeling for Allergens in Non-food Products

Nurses can also remind patients and families to remember to check non-food items to determine if there is a risk of allergen exposure. Families should be advised that allergens may also be hiding in unsuspecting items beyond medications, such as in cosmetics, pet foods, lotions, craft supplies, face paint, toothpaste, soaps, and gelatin (Bahna, 2023; Kids with Food Allergy, 2021).

Preventing Cross-Contact

Patients and caregivers should be counseled to avoid cross-contact with their allergen. Cross-contact occurs when a food comes in contact with another food and the allergenic proteins are transferred, as might occur when a spoon with milk on it is used in another safe food item. Cross-contact can occur when utensils are used for different food items. Other examples would be spreading hummus, wiping the knife, and then using the knife to spread butter, or using utensils on a grill with butter and then handling a dairy-free item. The food item is no longer safe since the allergen is now incorporated. Cross-contact is differentiated from cross-contamination, which infers the transfer of bacteria or viruses, but the latter term is often used incorrectly in this context.

Cross-contact can occur in the home, in restaurants, and in any setting where food is prepared or served. Some patients may have a severe reaction to trace amounts of the allergen from cross-contact, whereas others may have to ingest a larger amount of allergen to reach a threshold that induces a reaction. Some families will eliminate allergens from the home, but this is not always possible nor advisable when others live in the same household and do not avoid the allergen. In the home setting, cleaning plates, glasses, serving ware, and utensils with soap and water should be sufficient to remove allergens, and dishwashers will also be effective. While cooking foods at high temperatures is effective to destroy microorganisms, this process does not affect allergens, so effective cleaning is important.

Nurses can teach the patient and caregiver to have separate, clean cooking surfaces, such as cutting boards, serving platters, and pots and pans. They can advise patients to avoid shared serving utensils (such as ice cream scoopers, serving spoons, spatulas, measuring cups, pizza cutters, etc.) by adopting a different color for allergy-free foods. This practice can help keep allergens separate and prevent the transfer of allergenic proteins to safe foods. Preparing allergen-free foods first, and then handling other food items, can be helpful in preventing transfer of allergenic proteins. Any potential spill, splatter, or boiling over, for example, can spread an allergen, so care with food preparation is required, and warrants cooking or baking items separately. When grilling foods, care must be taken to remove any allergens from the grill surface and use of aluminum foil or pans can keep items allergen-free.

When serving meals, the person with allergies might be served (or serve themselves) first to avoid any inadvertent cross-contact. Depending on the age of the person with food allergies, careful observation and supervision is needed during meal and snack times to avert exposures. Care must be exercised in storing and handling allergenic foods, and areas where food is served should be cleaned thoroughly after every meal.

Storing products that contain food allergens carefully and preventing cross-contact is essential. Allergens can be segregated in separate drawers, shelves, or cabinets. Color-coded containers can be used for young children to alert them of allergens and also of safe foods. Some parents create a snack drawer of safe treats for the child with allergies that is separated from other foods. Of course, other foods should not come into contact with allergen-free food to minimize exposure. Other tips for avoiding cross-contact are available on our Resources Page via links to the Food Allergy Research and Education organization website and the Food Allergy & Anaphylaxis Connection Team website. Cross-contact is also discussed in the chapter "Food Allergy Management in Early Childhood Settings" on school age and the chapter "Food Allergy Management in Adolescents and Young Adults" on adolescent and young adults.

Managing Food Allergies Outside the Home

With foresight and understanding of potential risks, eating outside the home can be safely managed in most cases. Eating at restaurants and managing the school environment are important topics addressed here and in chapters "Food Allergy Management in Early Childhood Settings" and "Food Allergy Management in Adolescents and Young Adults". Eating outside the home, whether at a family holiday meal, a school function, a catered event at work, or at a restaurant, necessitates the same care and knowledge to be exercised every time food or drinks are consumed. The safe practices outlined here apply to any setting, from the local coffee shop or fast-food vendor to the potluck dinner or the fine dining establishment.

The person with allergies or their caregiver needs to verify that ingredients in any menu item are allergy-safe by asking questions about food preparation, segregation of allergens, and any special procedures put in place to ensure food for the person with allergies is safe from cross-contact and does not contain the allergen. Some common strategies to avoid allergens include avoiding unsafe situations by careful restaurant selection or skipping high-risk buffets and providing alternative meals, reviewing restaurant or gathering menus to ensure availability of safe food items, escalating discussions to the home or restaurant chef to ascertain ingredients and preparation practices, and ensuring communication about the severity of the allergy. For example, clarifications can include asking if French fries are cooked in the same oil as mozzarella sticks, if inquiring about dairy cross-contact, or if a frying pan is used for both fish and vegetables for a fish allergy. In addition, dining in restaurants on "off" hours to ensure adequate attention to allergy avoidance and calling ahead to discuss allergy protocols are some steps that can be taken to avoid risk of exposure. No restaurant meal or any meal prepared by someone else can be assumed to be safe without communicating and verifying safety precautions.

Using the acronym SNACK is a helpful way to think about eating out safely and can be adapted for any place where food is served.

- S: Share your concerns. Be open about food allergies and your safety needs even before you make a reservation. Start a conversation with the restaurant/venue in advance, and review menu items. Use allergy translation cards when needed.
- N: Never be without your epi. Be sure to always carry your epinephrine device so you are prepared for reactions and emergencies.
- A: Ask questions. Ask the cook/chef/manager questions about labels, ingredients in menu items, food preparation and presentation, allergy awareness, and allergy protocols.
- C: Cross-contact and cleaning. Cross-contact avoidance should be clearly understood and area cleaned if needed.
- K: Keep it simple. Keep food choices simple to avoid your allergens and consider bringing your own meal or snack if unsure about safety (Developed by J. Howard-Ruben, 2026).

Restaurant Dining

The American Academy of Allergy Asthma and Immunology (AAAAI) convened a work group on food allergy in restaurants and provided recommendations for both the restaurant industry and for people with food allergies around communication, knowledge, and safe practices for the industry and preparedness for patients and families (Carter et al., 2020). For example, restaurants should ask about allergies, offer training on food allergies regularly, ensure safe cleaning methods, and foster safe practices for food preparation and service. The latter would include preparing food for people with allergies in a special area, with color-coded equipment and by using technology and other communication tools to convey allergy information

Table 1 Summary of considerations for counseling food-allergic patrons on dining safely in restaurants

Communication	Consider notifying the restaurant in advance about the food allergy
	Involving the manager in the order may be helpful
	Consider requesting that the table surface is cleaned with soap and water or commercial wipes
	Consider providing written instructions about allergy for restaurant staff, such as a "chef card" or "allergy card" (www.foodallergy.org)
	Communicate with restaurant staff that trace amounts of allergen can cause a reaction
	Notify co-diners of food allergy
Knowledge	Nut-allergic patients should understand that certain food establishments more commonly serve nuts, such as Asian restaurants, bakeries, and ice cream shops
	Seafood-allergic patients should consider avoiding or take extra care when obtaining food from seafood restaurants
	Cross-contact is common in buffets where effective cleaning is difficult
	Simple dishes with clearly identified ingredients are safer than dishes with mixed ingredients
	Allergic ingredients may not always be visible
	If a mistake is made, patients should attempt to keep the dish at the table until a new dish without allergen is delivered
	When possible, patients should avoid sharing plates with other co-diners
Preparedness	Patients should consider dining at off-peak hours
	Developing a written anaphylaxis emergency care plan is helpful for patients in times of emergency
	Two epinephrine autoinjectors should be prescribed in case anaphylaxis occurs

Note. Used with permission from: Carter et al. (2020)

(p. 72). Key points for counseling patients and families are provided in the following table and can be adapted into a teaching plan for patient education (Table 1).

Traveling with Food Allergies

Traveling away from home, without the usual resources available, requires special attention to risk mitigation plans. Being prepared for traveling requires planning ahead for contingencies and always being prepared for food-induced emergencies. A travel checklist to use when planning a trip is available from Equal Eats (Fig. 2).

If patients and families do not speak the language of the country, or if they are unable to read labels, a major safety barrier exists. Using pictures of allergens and translated allergy cards or apps can assist with communication. A recent scoping review on traveling with food allergies emphasized the need to plan ahead, be prepared for managing food choices and allergic reactions, as well as to assess and plan for access to emergency health services. The authors also recommend using Google translate, carrying emergency action plans, and learning how to say epinephrine in the language of the travel country in case of an emergency (Bjelac et al., 2023).

EQUAL EATS

Travel Checklist

Be prepared and travel safely with dietary restrictions

WHEN BOOKING		
	Research airline policies	NOTES:
	Research accommodation's food options	
	Organize travel insurance	

ONE MONTH TO GO		
	Check and renew your/your child's medication	NOTES:
	Request doctor's letter (if required by airline)	
	Update emergency care/action plan	
	Order dietary translation cards	
	Gather local emergency #'s and hospital addresses	

ONE WEEK TO GO			
	Contact airline	**BUY SUPPLIES**	
	Ensure you have all medication		Antibacterial wipes
	Research restaurants and contact		Medication
NOTES:			Safe snacks
			Other:

ON THE DAY		ON THE PLANE	
	Talk to ground staff at airport		Tell crew about your restrictions
	Eat well before your flight/trip		Tell passengers around you
PACK IN CARRY-ON-LUGGAGE:			Make medication easily accessible
	Emergency medication	**WIPE DOWN:**	
	Emergency care/action plan		Armrest and headrest
	Doctor's note (for medication)		Tray table
	Safe snacks & antibacterial wipes		Seatbelt

AT THE DESTINATION		
	Visit local supermarket to stock up on safe food	NOTES:
	Show dietary card to resort chef or restaurants	
	Purchase safe food for return trip home	

www.equaleats.com

Fig. 2 Travel checklist. (Used with permission from: Food Allergy Travel Planning Checklist. n.d.. By Equal Eats. Accessed on February 22, 2026 at https://cdn.shopify.com/s/files/1/0258/9582/9613/files/Equal_Eats_Travel_Checklist_2026.pdf?v=1771753848)

FARE and other sources offer allergy chef cards or translation cards in English, Chinese, Dutch, French, German, Italian, Japanese, Portuguese, Spanish and Swedish, and more which can be used for travel and for use when there is a language issue. For example, Equal Eats offers multiple allergy translation cards available in a plastic card format in 52 languages that can be ordered for delivery or by instant download. The cards include both text and pictures, and cards for 700 allergens and other conditions (such as celiac) are available. An application is available for iOS and Android phones that allows the user to have access to unlimited languages with a paid subscription. See the Resources Page at the end of the book for websites related to allergen cards and apps.

For air travel, Bjelac et al. emphasize the need to carry multiple epinephrine devices and to carry on safe food, since availability of neither can be guaranteed by airlines. While epinephrine is required to be present on the plane, it may not be, and there are limitations to its use. Food service on the plane may be limited, and allergens may be present, so bringing safe foods available to eat during the trip is a prudent step. Some recommendations endorsed include preboarding to wipe the seating area and tray table. Allergic Living recently published a two-part (domestic and international) Airlines & Allergies Guide (Allergic Living, 2025) for accommodation information, policies, and emergency protocols on domestic airlines and international airlines (also see Resources Page for website).

Other Routes of Exposure to Allergens

Most allergic reactions are caused by eating the culprit food, but allergic reactions can also occur after other exposures, so they are briefly reviewed here to present a complete picture of exposure risk.

Skin Exposure

The literature suggests that the risk of anaphylaxis with skin exposure to a food allergen is minimal without oral ingestion (Golden et al., 2024), but there are a handful of case reports documenting such reactions (Foong et al., 2020; Jiang et al., 2024; Liccardi et al., 2004; Tan et al., 2001). While the skin serves as a barrier, there are situations where a reaction could result from skin exposure, particularly when the skin barrier is not intact, such as in eczema (Sicherer, 2022). More commonly, skin exposure, such as a kiss on the forehead by someone who recently consumed the specific allergen, or a small spill, may trigger a local skin reaction such as hives or redness. However, for infants and toddlers who may touch items with food residue and place objects or their hands in their mouth frequently, caution is advised (Wang et al., 2024).

Perry et al. (2004) conducted a study exploring removal of Ara h 1, a peanut protein, from tabletops and hands in a school setting. Various cleaning methods were compared using commercially available cleaning products, water, and dishwashing liquid. Only the dishwashing liquid left small amounts of allergen on the tabletops. A subsequent small study of book covers, tables, and toys found similar results, suggesting that allergens are easily removed with regular cleaning. However, porous and fabric-like materials were not assessed (Watson et al., 2015). Research in this area is very limited.

Hand cleaning, with water, hand sanitizer, commercial wipes and liquid soap in the Perry (2004) study, left "below detectable levels" for the commercial wipes and soap, but residual Ara h 1 at relatively high concentrations for water and antibacterial hand sanitizer. Commercial wipes and soap are more effective. Alcohol gel, foam, or spray may sanitize hands, but it does not remove the allergen to prevent contact exposures (Sicherer, 2022).

Exposure to Food Allergens in Saliva

Exposure to saliva from shared utensils, straws, or cups should also be avoided, as this can cause local and systemic reactions (Bahna, 2023; Maloney et al., 2006). Little is known about the clinical significance of these exposures, but at least one small study (Maloney) looked at peanut butter and its presence in saliva, where Ara h 1 protein was detectable within 5 min and then, for most, was undetectable at 60 min. A strategy of waiting for 60 min and then brushing teeth seemed to be most effective compared to other options (e.g., chewing gum, rinsing mouth). However, this information was based on a very small sample, which only included peanut butter and no other allergens. Exposure to allergens through saliva also can occur through intimate contact. See chapter "Food Allergy Management in Adolescents and Young Adults" for more information on this topic.

Exposure to Food Allergens from Inhalation

Reactions, and even sensitization, to food allergens can result from inhalation (Ramirez Jr & Bahna, 2009; Wang et al., 2024). For example, cooking, such as boiling milk or steam from frying an egg or fish, or work settings such as bakeries, flour mills, poultry farms, and seafood processing facilities, can disperse airborne food proteins. Wheat flour, seafood, soy, peanut, egg, and milk are noted in such cases, although a wide variety of foods have been implicated. These reactions may trigger symptoms similar to environmental allergies such as rhinitis, itchy eyes and nose, and respiratory symptoms like cough, wheezing or asthma, and rarely, anaphylaxis.

Occupational Exposure to Food Allergens

Occupational exposure to allergens can also cause allergic reactions, a scenario which may occur in industries where continuous allergen exposure is prevalent, and the routes of exposure may vary (Jeebhay & Baatjies, 2022). For example, the diagnosis of Baker's asthma and other respiratory conditions, as well as contact dermatitis, have been associated with exposure to food allergens. Anaphylaxis has also been correlated to airborne and contact exposure to allergens. An anaphylaxis registry identified 27 people with anaphylaxis associated with food handling, and included farmers and workers involved in preparing or handling food (Worm et al., 2024). Multiple food culprits were identified.

Passive Transfer of Food Allergens

Multiple routes of food allergen transfer have been posited, including transmission via placenta, breast milk, saliva, and blood products, although the clinical implications are not yet clear (Bahna, 2023). Saliva, as noted above, and semen are also implicated as conduits of food allergens and are discussed elsewhere see chapter "Food Allergy Management in Adolescents and Young Adults". Although not a route of exposure, transmission of food-specific IgE antibodies and atopic traits can happen through transplant (Bahna, 2023).

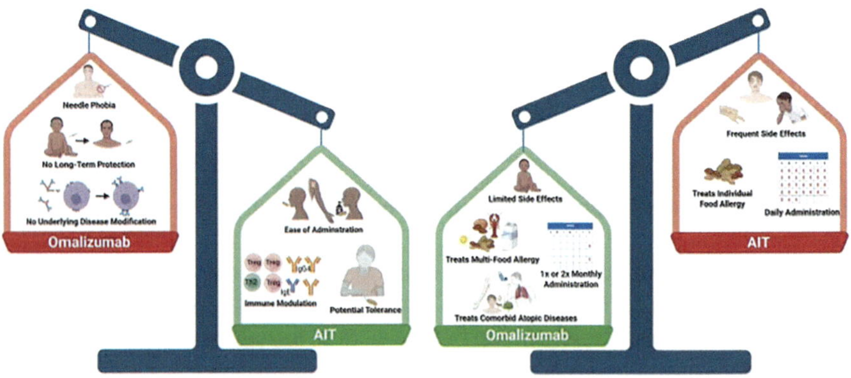

Fig. 3 Comparing the pros and cons of omalizumab and allergen-specific immunotherapy (AIT). There are many factors to consider when comparing the two types of therapies, including administration routes and frequency, long-term immune modulation, side effects, and comorbid allergic conditions. The left panel shows potential advantages of AIT (green) compared to omalizumab (red). The right panel shows advantages of omalizumab (green) compared to AIT (red). Note. Created in Biorender. Published under CC BY 4.0 https://creativecommons.org/licenses/by/4.0/. By Kulis et al. 2025

Moving Beyond Avoidance: Food Allergy Treatments

Over the last several years, food allergy management has moved beyond strict avoidance as the only treatment option. Many patients will still opt to continue avoiding their allergen and may choose not to pursue immunotherapy or biologic treatments. Some may be of an age where studies of effectiveness of therapies are limited, although future studies may determine the relative benefit of immunotherapy in adolescents and for adults.

Two treatments have been approved in the US recently for food allergy: Peanut Arachis Hypogaea (Palforzia) and Omalizumab (Xolair). The first treatment for a food allergy, Palforzia, a peanut oral immunotherapy (OIT), was approved by the United States Food and Drug Administration in 2020, but has now been discontinued by the manufacturer. Four years later, Xolair was approved for the indication of food allergies.

These treatments represent two major categories of therapeutics for food allergy: allergen-specific therapy (e.g., oral immunotherapy) and anti-IgE therapy (e.g., omalizumab as in Xolair). The treatment approach of allergen-specific immunotherapies (AIT) comprises oral immunotherapy (OIT), sublingual immunotherapy (SLIT), and epicutaneous immunotherapy (EPIT), while anti-IgE therapies are monoclonal antibodies that work by blocking IgE from binding to its receptor FcεRI. The two options are not a panacea, and they are certainly not perfect nor right for all patients, but they are a step forward in the treatment of food allergy. The following schematic helps to compare and contrast these two approaches to therapy (Fig. 3) (Kulis et al., 2025).

Allergen-Specific Immunotherapy

Conceptually, allergen-specific immunotherapy (AIT) is similar to aeroallergen or venom allergy desensitization via injections, and has not been standardized. The difference is that this exposure occurs via either oral (OIT) (e.g., the allergen in a powder or food form in precisely measured and prescribed amounts in office-based products and standardized protocols) or skin exposure (e.g., "peanut patch") and the doses are administered on a regular basis, such as daily ingestion or regular patch use. Other delivery methods have also been explored, such as epicutaneous therapy (EPIT) and sublingual immunotherapy (SLIT). Subcutaneous immunotherapy (SCIT) has not been explored extensively due to severe adverse outcomes and will not be presented here.

Oral Immunotherapy (OIT)

Oral immunotherapy (OIT) for confirmed IgE-mediated food allergy has emerged as an alternative to strict avoidance, but significant commitment and potential risks are involved, and this treatment cannot be considered as a cure for food allergies.

Patients and families must be fully informed of the risks and benefits, as well as the expected treatment outcomes, through a shared decision-making process. The *Consensus Report from the Food Allergy Research & Education (FARE) 2019 Oral Immunotherapy for Food Allergy Summit* (Pepper et al., 2020) provides guidance on the use of OIT in clinical practice, recommending that the treatment should be conducted by expert allergy staff under the supervision of board-certified or eligible allergists/immunologists with experience in food challenges, and with qualified staff and appropriate treatment facilities and access to emergency treatments and facilities.

OIT has been extensively studied for peanut allergy and researched to varying degrees for other allergens. Outcomes for OIT vary, with various terms coined, such as "free eating" (e.g., a restriction-free diet) or "bite-proof" (e.g., protective against most instances of cross-contact or accidental ingestion) (Inamdar & Mandal, 2022).

Oral immunotherapy treatments consist of the introduction of small amounts of an allergen which increases over time, aimed at decreasing the clinical reactivity threshold while also modulating the immune system (Bartha & Rodríguez Del Río, 2023, p. 239). Given continued consumption of the allergen, desensitization may be achieved. This increases the threshold amount of allergen that might elicit a reaction, providing protection from accidental ingestion. Sustained unresponsiveness is another term that is used, which is similar to the concept of remission, suggesting that even if the food is not eaten regularly, the patient will not react (McHenry et al., 2024). Whether the durability of this decrease in clinical reactivity will persist long-term, and under what conditions, remains to be seen with longer studies.

The optimal age for OIT seems to be in very young children when a "therapeutic window of opportunity" presents (Jones et al., 2022), where a post hoc analysis revealed greater remission rates in younger age groups (71% in children under 24 months, declining to 19% in those over age 3 to age 4). Some evidence suggests that immunotherapy earlier in life is more effective and safer (Bartha et al., 2024).

FDA-Approved Allergen-Specific Immunotherapy (Palforzia)

In 2020, Palforzia [Peanut Arachis Hypogaea (PTAH), peanut allergen powder, previously AR101], a form of daily oral immunotherapy (OIT) was the first OIT approved by the FDA for patients aged 1 to 17 years diagnosed with IgE-mediated peanut allergy to protect patients from a severe reaction due to accidental exposure to peanut (Aimmune Therapeutics, 2024; Lee et al., 2023). The treatment could be continued after age 17 for maintenance if started prior to age 17 years. However, Palforzia was discontinued by the manufacturer voluntarily (not due to safety issues) in July 2026. The drug provided peanut protein antigens in the form of capsules or sachets of defatted peanut protein powder that were added to food (Du Toit et al., 2023; Aimmune Therapeutics, 2024). Note that the treatment included a Black Box Warning for anaphylaxis due to a risk of severe reactions with the therapy (Aimmune Therapeutics, 2024).

Research Supporting Peanut OIT

Early studies (Vickery et al., 2017; Soller et al., 2019) provided some evidence for this treatment to desensitize the immune system to peanut. Pivotal studies provided additional evidence including the Peanut Allergy Oral Immunotherapy Study of AR101 for Desensitization in Children and Adults (PALISADE) clinical trial for children aged 4–17 years (The PALISADE Group of Clinical Investigators, 2018) and the Peanut Oral Immunotherapy Study of Early Intervention for Desensitization (POSEIDON) for children aged 1 < 4 years of age (Du Toit et al., 2023).

The PALISADE clinical trial included a double-blind placebo-controlled food challenge at the start and at the end of the trial. Inclusion criteria included patients with a peanut allergy age 4 to 55 years who reacted to ≤100 mg of peanut protein (The PALISADE Group of Clinical Investigators, 2018). The patients were randomized to the treatment group receiving AR101 peanut OIT or the placebo OIT group. The primary endpoint was one single dose of 600 mg or more of peanut protein in those aged 4 to 17 years without dose-limiting symptoms (The PALISADE Group of Clinical Investigators, 2018). The study included 551 participants originally with 496 aged 4–17 years and spanned 52 weeks. Results showed that 67.2% (250/372) of the participants in the treatment group met the end point vs. 4% (5/124) in the placebo group (The PALISADE Group of Clinical Investigators, 2018). Many participants did have mild to moderate symptoms (e.g., gastrointestinal symptoms like abdominal pain, nausea, vomiting; skin and mucosal symptoms; respiratory symptoms) and some instances of anaphylaxis were noted during the trial. 4.3% in the treatment group and 0.8% of the placebo group had severe symptoms (The PALISADE Group of Clinical Investigators, 2018).

The POSEIDON Phase III study was a randomized, double-blind, placebo-controlled clinical trial at multiple sites in the United States and Europe (Du Toit et al., 2023). Inclusion criteria included patients aged 1 to <4 years that reacted to >3 mg and ≤ 300 mg of peanut protein in one dose. Of 146 patients randomized to either the treatment group or placebo to determine statistical significance, 83 (84.7%) of the treatment group and 45 (93.8%) of the placebo group completed the trial (Du Toit et al., 2023). Attrition was due to either withdrawal of consent ($n = 5$, 5.1%) or adverse events ($n = 5$, 5.1%) (Du Toit et al., 2023). The primary end point was patients that could tolerate ≥600 mg of peanut protein without dose-limiting symptoms. Furthermore, the secondary endpoint was those patients that could tolerate 300 mg, 1000 mg, and additional endpoint of 2000 mg of peanut protein. Results showed that 73.5% (72) of the treatment group tolerated 600 mg single dose vs. 6.3% (3) of the placebo group (Du Toit et al., 2023). The dosing included an initial dose escalation of 0.5 mg up to 6 mg daily dose, updosing by incrementally titrating up to 300 mg daily dose, and maintenance of 300 mg daily dose (Du Toit et al., 2023). Most treatment-related adverse events reported were mild or moderate gastrointestinal and respiratory symptoms, although 2% experienced severe adverse events in the updosing period of the active treatment arm (Du Toit et al., 2023).

Other long-term studies on peanut OIT include the 3-year POISED study of 120 peanut allergic patients treated with peanut flour (treatment) or oat flour (placebo) aged 7–55 years post OIT who either continued maintenance or discontinued OIT

(Chinthrajah et al., 2019). The study found that 35% (21) of treatment group tolerated 4000 mg peanut protein while only 4% (1) of the placebo group could tolerate the same, and study authors noted that over time if participants stopped ingesting peanut or decreased the maintenance dose, this increased the risk of allergic reactions (Chinthrajah et al., 2019). Adverse events were mostly mild and were described as gastrointestinal or skin-related, but epinephrine use was reported in the treatment arm in years 1 and 2 of the study (Chinthrajah et al., 2019).

Additionally, the IMPACT study looked at patients 12 months to less than 4 years on long-term peanut OIT or placebo OIT for 134 weeks and then discontinuation for 26 weeks. At 134 weeks, the study found that 71% (68/96) of the treatment group vs. 2% (1) of the placebo group were desensitized to peanut protein on challenge of 5000 mg. After avoidance for 26 weeks, 21% (20/96) of the peanut OIT group were in remission vs. 2% (1/50) of the placebo group (Jones et al., 2022). The authors noted that most participants in the treatment arm experienced a dose-related reaction, but none were considered serious. However, epinephrine use to ameliorate symptoms was reported for 21 participants over the build-up and maintenance phases.

Overall, peanut allergen powder has been shown to increase tolerance to peanut protein and reduce the risk of severe reactions from accidental exposures in multiple clinical trials. Key studies, including PALISADE, POSEIDON, POISED, and IMPACT, demonstrated that a majority of children receiving this immunotherapy could tolerate higher doses of peanut protein compared to placebo, with the strongest results seen in younger children (Du Toit et al., 2023; Jeimy et al., 2024). While most adverse effects were mild to moderate gastrointestinal or respiratory symptoms, some participants experienced severe reactions, including anaphylaxis, highlighting the need for careful monitoring. Overall, this therapy offers an important treatment option that desensitizes the immune system to peanuts, but new peanut powder products will need to be evaluated in the future. In concept, the treatment has the potential to be disease modifying for some younger patients but typically requires continued maintenance dosing in most cases to sustain protection (Jeimy et al., 2024).

Food Oral Immunotherapy

Although only one form of OIT has been historically FDA-approved, many allergy providers offer OIT for most or all allergens, while others may limit the allergens that they consider treatable with OIT, which is consistent with variability in international guidelines. The intent of food OIT is desensitization early on and remission, or sustained unresponsiveness, over the longer term.

With this form of OIT, the general strategy is for the patient to take a prescribed very small "dose" of regular food purchased at a grocery store. The beginning dose is below the threshold for clinical reactivity for each patient. Daily doses at home commence with this low dose and continue to be gradually increased over time in a build-up phase. These increases occur after several weeks at a specific dose with supervised appointments for updosing (increasing the daily dose). Eventually, a maintenance dose is reached that is intended to offer protection from accidental allergen ingestion and also can curtail the severity of any reactions (Anagnostou et al., 2024). The maintenance dose then continues with daily dosing over an extended time period.

Food OIT is not presently considered a cure, and has multiple risks of adverse events, including anaphylaxis, eosinophilic esophagitis, as well as other symptoms, such as hives, oropharyngeal pruritus, and stomach pain (McHenry et al., 2024). Perrett (2022) lists asthma, concurrent illness, physical activity after dosing, menses, dosing on an empty stomach, pollen allergy, and irregular dosing as factors that can contribute to a higher risk of reaction. Patients participating in OIT in the office setting should be counseled as to the relative efficacy based on the available evidence, but also need to understand the potential side effects, adverse outcomes, and limitations. Bégin et al. (2020) offer ethical guidelines for patient-centered OIT, with recommendations and guidance for safe provision, patient selection, allergens that can be treated, likely clinical outcomes, patient-centered care, and more.

Successful OIT includes adherence to a specific dosing regimen, activity restrictions, and considerable commitment by the patient and family, so it may not be the right choice for everyone. For example, for children active in sports, scheduling quiet time with little activity may be challenging. On the other hand, in a highly motivated family, these obstacles may be overcome with planning and coordination of schedules.

Nurses often play an important role in managing patients undergoing OIT by being involved in teaching as well as answering questions about symptoms or dose modifications.

Russell et al. (2022) provide good insights into the multiple roles of the nurse in OIT treatment. For example, the authors suggest that general educational topics for OIT patients and families can include the following:

- Situations that may require holding or adjusting dose.
- Precision in dose measurement.
- Food intake prior to dosing.
- Appropriate foods to choose for mixing in dose.
- Regular scheduling of dose and rest/observation periods.
- Avoidance of activities that may affect body temperature around dosing.
- Alcohol timing restrictions.
- Factors that can contribute to reactions.
- Emergency preparedness for anaphylaxis.
- Management of asthma (Russell et al., 2022, p. 83).

Epicutaneous Immunotherapy

Immunotherapy delivered via the epicutaneous route is exemplified by the product Viaskin, also known as the "peanut patch." The patch contains micrograms (μg) of peanut allergen, applied via an adhesive device on the back between the scapulae

(Fleischer et al., 2020). Included in the device is a condensation chamber which collects water from the skin and combines it with peanut protein in powder form. The protein is absorbed by the skin and carried by Langerhans cells and the lymph system to lymph nodes where the allergic response is quelled by the immune system (DBV-Technologies, 2025). While the patch is not yet approved by the FDA, studies have pointed to both efficacy and safety for this approach to desensitization for peanut allergy.

The PEPITES study was a 12-month Phase 3 double-blind placebo-controlled clinical trial of children 4–11 years of age evaluating the feasibility and efficacy of epicutaneous treatment with Viaskin Peanut 250 μg patch vs. placebo. Results showed that 35.3% of the treatment group vs. 13.6% of the placebo group responded to treatment but the primary end point was not met (Fleischer et al., 2019, 2020). In addition, the PEOPLE (PEPITES open-label extension) study found long-term benefit with additional treatment (Fleischer et al., 2020). The REALISE trial (Pongracic et al., 2022) and its extension trial (Pongracic et al., 2025) explored adherence and safety of the patch in children aged 4–11. Safety in this patient population was confirmed, and long-term follow up also supported a favorable safety profile, with local skin reactions cited that decreased over time, and a low number of treatment-related anaphylaxis events reported (4.1%).

Greenhawt et al. (2025) also found in the EPITOPE trial that the patch could be used in children aged 1–3 and demonstrated desensitization with 67% meeting the primary end point vs. 33.5% in the placebo group.

The same manufacturer has also produced a milk skin patch for clinical trial evaluation. Safety and efficacy of the Viaskin milk dermal patch was reported in a study with participants aged 2–17 using three different μg doses: 150, 300 and 500. While safety was established, the milk patch treatment compared to placebo was statistically significant only for the children in the 2–11 age group. The group in this age category who received a 300-μg dose went on to have the highest level of double-blind food challenge proven desensitization, with most adverse effects classified as mild (97%) or moderate (63%) (Petroni et al., 2024).

To date, these EPIT studies point to a treatment effect on clinical reactivity. Overall, safety and efficacy data are promising, but more studies will confirm the durability of the response and will help to refine dosing and age groups likely to benefit. While local reactions have been common in studies thus far, the gastrointestinal symptoms associated with forms of OIT seem less prominent. Also, since little allergenic protein enters the bloodstream, anaphylaxis may be less likely to occur.

FDA approval of the Viaskin patches has not occurred at this time, so availability has been limited to clinical trials. The FDA required further studies to explore more about patch adhesion and duration of application. Should this approach to EPIT be approved, an advantage is that it does not require a rest period or any limitation on physical activities, so it would offer a patient-friendly treatment option for peanut, milk, and possibly other allergies.

Patches are one approach to EPIT, but others are being investigated, some in preclinical studies using a mouse model. Coated (with allergenic protein) microneedles, allergen application to skin that has been stripped by tape, and microperforation are some of the approaches under investigation (Hervé et al., 2023).

Sublingual Immunotherapy

Like non-proprietary or office-based OIT, sublingual immunotherapy (SLIT) for food allergies is not FDA-approved, but is being conducted in some settings, so will be only briefly discussed here. SLIT aims to desensitize patients with food allergies by using real food in liquid form or prepared solutions of diluted liquid allergen extract (Windom et al., 2024).

Some of the allergies treated with SLIT include kiwi, peanut, hazelnut, milk and peach. One form of SLIT involves holding the extract under the tongue for a period of time and then swallowing. Patients are observed for a specific period of time in the build-up phase, and preparation for any severe reaction or anaphylaxis is needed, but over the long-term, dosing is done at home. Unlike OIT, restrictions on activity and diet are not necessary (Chagarlamudi et al., 2024).

One of the earliest SLIT studies was a double-blind placebo-controlled trial in children with peanut allergy that resulted in some clinical desensitization as well as changes in immune response as measured by SPT, IgE and IgG4 testing (Kim et al., 2011). Fleischer et al. (2013, 2020) reported a randomized controlled trial using SLIT and showed patients in the treatment arm gained some level of desensitization, yet these participants experienced allergic symptoms during an initial challenge. The study raised questions about the length of time necessary to achieve clinically meaningful desensitization. A recent study of peanut SLIT in 1–11-year-old children over 48 months yielded evidence of desensitization, with itchy mouth the most common symptom (Kim et al., 2023). Those interested in the nursing care associated with SLIT are referred to a paper by Williams et al. (2025) which reports on their center's experience using real-food SLIT, including a reaction flow chart, instructions, dosing protocols, a list of supplies, a personalized action plan, and informed consent forms.

IgE-Mediated Therapies

Omalizumab, an Anti-IgE Monoclonal Antibody

Omalizumab (Xolair®) is an anti IgE monoclonal antibody that binds to IgE and reduces the severity of allergic reactions. Omalizumab is administered by subcutaneous injection every 2 or 4 weeks. Dosing schedule is calculated based on weight in kilograms and pretreatment serum total IgE level (IU/mL). Omalizumab has been used for over 20 years for allergic asthma, chronic urticaria, and chronic rhinosinusitis with nasal polyps (Genentech, 2024); therefore, there is a significant amount of data about its safe use. Marking a major milestone in active treatment of food allergies, the FDA-approved omalizumab in 2024 for patients 1 year and over with IgE-mediated food allergy as a treatment to help reduce allergic reactions with accidental exposure to one or more foods. Omalizumab treatment currently should be prescribed along with allergen avoidance (US FDA, 2024a, b; Genentech, 2024). It is important to note that omalizumab is not an emergency medication for anaphylaxis;

therefore, patients on omalizumab should be instructed to carry epinephrine for potential allergic reactions.

After years of setbacks, a trial, Omalizumab as Monotherapy and as Adjunct to Multi-Allergen Oral Immunotherapy (OUtMATCH), was conducted by the National Institute of Allergy and Infectious Disease in collaboration with an industry partner and successfully generated rigorous data that was used in the application for its use in treating food allergies (Anagnostou et al., 2024). The OUtMATCH study consisted of three stages to provide evidence for the use of omalizumab as a stand-alone therapy for patients with multiple food allergies. Stage 1 of the OUtMATCH clinical trial consisted of 180 patients who were between 1 and 55 years of age, allergic to peanut and two other study allergens (cashew, milk, egg, walnut, wheat, and hazelnut), randomized to either the omalizumab group or placebo for 16–20 weeks (Wood et al., 2024). Results of this phase of the study showed that 67% of the omalizumab group could tolerate the endpoint of 600 mg or more of a single dose of peanut (2.5 peanuts) vs. only 7% of the placebo group (Wood et al., 2024; Groetch et al., 2022). The percentage of patients who could tolerate a single dose of 1000 mg or more was 41% for cashew, 67% for egg, and 66% for milk (Wood et al., 2024). Some patients (14%) failed the trial and could not tolerate even 30 mg of peanut due to reactions (Wood et al., 2024).

In Stage 2, 117 participants from stage 1 were given omalizumab for 8 weeks and then randomized to either: (1) multi-allergen OIT with omalizumab for 8 weeks and then continued multi-allergen OIT with placebo for 44 weeks; or (2) placebo OIT with omalizumab for 8 weeks and then continued placebo OIT and omalizumab for 44 weeks (Wood et al., 2024). All patients who reacted to the lowest initial dose or could not reach maintenance were removed from the study. The results from Stage 2 showed 36% of the omalizumab group vs. 19% of the OIT group met the endpoint criteria of tolerance of greater than or equal to 2000 mg of all three study allergens (Wood et al., 2024). Adverse events were significantly higher for the OIT group.

An open-label extension of omalizumab for 24 weeks included 60 patients from Stage 1 who then entered Stage 3, which consisted of three groups: those that could eat the food after stopping omalizumab, those that needed rescue OIT (meaning they could not tolerate the allergen, but then were provided OIT treatment for that allergen) for 52 weeks, and those that needed to avoid the food (Dantzer et al., 2025). At the 12-month follow up, initial data show long-term success with omalizumab as 61–70% of patients were able to reintroduce milk, wheat, and egg into the diet and 38–56% were able to reintroduce peanuts and tree nuts (Danzter et al., 2025).

Overall, preliminary studies suggest that omalizumab appears to be superior to oral immunotherapy (OIT) for patients with multiple food allergies, especially with an extended course of omalizumab (Wood et al., 2025), but consumption of allergens reduced over time during long-term study after discontinuation of omalizumab. Many of the participants in the OIT group dropped out due to allergic reactions and side effects even after receiving omalizumab for a few weeks initially (Wood et al., 2025). The continued follow up of participants over time will produce more data on the long-term efficacy of omalizumab as a monotherapy for those with food allergies, and nurses interested in this therapy should follow the quickly evolving studies. Omalizumab is administered by subcutaneous injection via a prefilled syringe or auto-injector every 2 or 4 weeks, with the dosage based on total serum IgE test prior to treatment initiation and body weight in kilograms. Due to the viscosity of the drug solution, injection may take as long as 15 seconds. It is generally recommended that initial treatments (first three doses due to higher risk of anaphylaxis) should be administered in a healthcare setting. Following this initial treatment period, some patients and caregivers may be deemed appropriate for self-administration. Instructions for use, including choosing sites for injection, placement of multiple injections, and taking the device out of the refrigerator 30-45 minutes before injection are reviewed on the manufacturer web site (https://www.gene.com/download/pdf/xolair_prescribing.pdf)

Using a Shared Decision-Making Approach

Many providers are still working to understand the benefits and risks of these treatment options, as well as how to use shared decision-making to weigh these options with patients and their families. Shared decision-making engages both patients and providers in a process to help work through the pros and cons of a treatment decision to help discover what aligns most with the patient and family's goals and values. Shared decision-making by the patient, family and health care team is essential to help patients choose the treatment course that is best for them (Anagnostou, 2024), especially when there are so many variables to consider and no clear path (yet) to a cure.

Mack et al. (2024) outline that given the complexity of decisions about treatment for food allergies, using a shared decision-making process can be valuable to help clarify the potential benefits and harms as well as to incorporate the patient and family perspectives. Shared decision-making tools are available to help families discern whether treatment options should be considered (American College of Allergy, Asthma and Immunotherapy, n.d.; Greenhawt et al., 2020).

Future of Food Allergy Management

The advancement of food allergy science has accelerated at a rapid pace, with the transition from a passive avoidance and anaphylaxis precaution paradigm to one where interventions to prevent or treat food allergies are becoming mainstream. Allergen immunotherapy for foods, beyond oral immunotherapy, continues to be an area of intense research. Additional immunotherapy and biologic therapies are on the horizon, and vaccines, microbial therapies and genetic therapies are under consideration with varying degrees of research progress. Use of machine learning and data science may offer future options for food allergy treatment in conjunction with data analytics and personalized medicine.

Various biologic therapies, including anti-IL-33 etokimab, anti-IgE monoclonal antibody ligelizumab, IL-4 and IL-13 blocker dupilumab, anti-TSP tezepelumab, antialarmins, and Bruton's tyrosine kinase inhibitor, are among many candidates for food allergy treatment warranting further research and which could potentially be therapies at some point in the future (Sindher et al., 2025).

Since the gut and its microbial environment play a role in food allergy development, ongoing research exploring manipulation of the microbiome appears to be promising, and may someday include treatments with probiotics, prebiotics, and even fecal microbiota transplantation (Bartha et al., 2024).

The proliferation of potential treatment options is exciting and hopefully will lead to more effective treatments. This hope is tempered, however, by treatment burden, high cost, and the need for robust evidence of safety and efficacy. On balance, there are many reasons to be optimistic about current and future treatments for food allergy, as well as for new science that helps us understand how to prevent it from developing in the first place.

Conclusion

As treatment options for food allergies continue to expand, the role of nurses remains pivotal in helping patients and families understand the complex landscape of food allergy care. Beyond navigating emerging therapies, families must still continue to have a strong foundation of knowledge in allergen avoidance. In order to manage their everyday life with food allergies, they need to be confident about accurately interpreting allergen labeling and precautionary allergen labeling (PAL), recognizing hidden allergens in medications and non-food items, and preventing inadvertent exposures and cross-contact in their daily environment. Nurses are also key to empowering families to self-advocate when dining out and traveling and providing advice on how to stay vigilant. By combining education on traditional management strategies with guidance on new and promising therapies such as omalizumab (Xolair), oral immunotherapy (OIT), epicutaneous patch therapy, and sublingual immunotherapy, nurses and allergy providers help families make informed decisions that align with their goals and comfort levels. Through guidance on current best practices and awareness of future possibilities, nurses enhance patient safety, confidence, and quality of life as the field of food allergy care continues to advance.

References

Abrams, E. M., Zafack, J. G., Jensen, C., Bettinger, J. A., Top, K. A., Hildebrand, K. J., & Tunis, M. C. (2024). Vaccination and egg allergy: Considerations for family physicians. *Canadian family physician Medecin de famille canadien, 70*(1), 10–12. https://doi.org/10.46747/cfp.700110-x

Aimmune Therapeutics. (2024). PALFORZIA [Peanut (*Arachis hypogaea*) allergen powder-dnfp]: Highlights of prescribing information. https://www.fda.gov/media/134838/download?attachment

Allergic Living (2025). Allergic Living's Airlines and Allergies Guide. Retrieved on June 22, 2026 from https://www.allergicliving.com/2025/07/11/allergic-livings-airlines-allergies-guide-domestic/

Allergen Disclosure In Non-Food Articles Act (ADINA), H.R. 3821, 119th Cong. (2025).

American College of Allergy, Asthma, & Immunology (n.d.). *Peanut allergy treatment shared-decision-making tool*. https://acaai.org/resource/should-my-child-try-peanut-allergy-treatment/. Accessed on 28 Aug 2025.

Anagnostou, A. (2024). Shared decision-making in food allergy: Navigating an exciting era. *Annals of Allergy, Asthma & Immunology: Official Publication of the American College of Allergy, Asthma, & Immunology, 132*(3), 313–320. https://doi.org/10.1016/j.anai.2023.09.004

Anagnostou, A., Mack, D. P., Johannes, S., Shaker, M., Abrams, E. M., DeSanto, K., & Greenhawt, M. (2024). The safety and efficacy of baked egg and Milk dietary advancement therapy: A systematic review and meta-analysis. *The Journal of Allergy and Clinical Immunology. In Practice, 12*(9), 2468–2480. https://doi.org/10.1016/j.jaip.2024.06.016

Bahna, S. L. (2023). New insights in hidden food allergies. *Journal of Food Allergy, 5*(1), 19–24. https://doi.org/10.2500/jfa.2023.5.230003

Baker, M. G., & Sampson, H. A. (2018). Phenotypes and endotypes of food allergy: A path to better understanding the pathogenesis and prognosis of food allergy. *Annals of Allergy, Asthma & Immunology: Official Publication of the American College of Allergy, Asthma, & Immunology, 120*(3), 245–253. https://doi.org/10.1016/j.anai.2018.01.027. Redirecting.

Bartha, I., & Rodríguez Del Río, P. (2023). Clinical outcomes of efficacy in food allergen immunotherapy trials. *Current Opinion in Allergy and Clinical Immunology, 23*(3), 239–245. https://doi.org/10.1097/ACI.0000000000000905

Bartha, I., Almulhem, N., & Santos, A. F. (2024). Feast for thought: A comprehensive review of food allergy 2021–2023. *The Journal of Allergy and Clinical Immunology, 153*(3), 576–594. https://doi.org/10.1016/j.jaci.2023.11.918

Bégin, P., Chan, E. S., Kim, H., et al. (2020). CSACI guidelines for the ethical, evidence-based and patient-oriented clinical practice of oral immunotherapy in IgE-mediated food allergy. *Allergy, Asthma and Clinical Immunology, 16*(20). https://doi.org/10.1186/s13223-020-0413-7

Bjelac, J., Abrams, E. M., & Iglesia, E. G. A. (2023). Food allergies on vacation – There and back again. *Annals of Allergy, Asthma, & Immunology, 130*(4), 438–443. https://doi.org/10.1016/j.anai.2023.01.008

Carter, C. A., Pistiner, M., Wang, J., & Sharma, H. P. (2020). Food allergy in restaurants work group report. *The Journal of Allergy and Clinical Immunology. In Practice, 8*(1), 70–74. https://doi.org/10.1016/j.jaip.2019.09.013

Centers for Disease Control and Prevention. (CDC). (2024). *Vaccines and immunizations. Contraindications and precautions*. https://www.cdc.gov/vaccines/hcp/imz-best-practices/contraindications-precautions.html. Accessed on 27 Aug 2025.

Chagarlamudi, H., Smith, H. G., & Kim, E. H. (2024). A review of sublingual immunotherapy for treatment of peanut allergy. *Journal of Food Allergy, 7*(1), 14–20. https://doi.org/10.2500/jfa.2025.7.250007

Chang, F., Eng, L., & Chang, C. (2023). Food allergy labeling laws: International guidelines for residents and travelers. *Clinical Reviews in Allergy & Immunology, 65*(2), 148–165. https://doi.org/10.1007/s12016-023-08960-6

Chinthrajah, R. S., Purington, N., Andorf, S., Long, A., O'Laughlin, K. L., Lyu, S. C., Manohar, M., Boyd, S. D., Tibshirani, R., Maecker, H., Plaut, M., Mukai, K., Tsai, M., Desai, M., Galli, S. J., & Nadeau, K. C. (2019). Sustained outcomes in oral immunotherapy for peanut allergy (POISED study): A large, randomised, double-blind, placebo-controlled, phase 2 study. *The Lancet (British Edition), 394*(10207), 1437–1449. https://doi.org/10.1016/S0140-6736(19)31793-3

Dantzer, J., Virkud, Y., Wang, J., Sicherer, S., Groetch, M., Shreffler, W., Pyle, D., Kim, E., Keet, C., Kulis, M., Mudd, K., Sindher, S., Long, A., Scurlock, A., Jones, S., Leung, D., Lanser, B., Vickery, B., Ezhuthachan, I., & Wood, R. (2025). Introduction of allergenic foods after treatment with omalizumab. *Journal of Allergy and Clinical Immunology, 155*(2), AB445–AB445. https://doi.org/10.1016/j.jaci.2024.12.1024

Du Toit, G., Brown, K. R., Vereda, A., Irani, A.-M., Tilles, S., Ratnayake, A., Jones, S. M., & Vickery, B. P. (2023). Oral immunotherapy for peanut allergy in children 1 to less than 4 years of age. *NEJM Evidence, 2*(11), EVIDoa2300145. https://doi.org/10.1056/EVIDoa2300145

DBV-Technologies. (2025). *DBV aims to unlock the powerful immune properties of the skin*. Accessed 12.19.25 at https://dbv-technologies.com/our-science/viaskin-platform/

Equal Eats. (n.d.-a). *Allergy translation cards*. https://equaleats.com. Accessed on 27 Aug 2025. Food Allergy Cards | Translation Cards in 52 Languages—Equal Eats.

Equal Eats. (n.d.-b). *Food allergy travel planning checklist—Equal eats*. https://equaleats.com/blogs/news/food-allergy-travel-planning-checklist. Accessed on 28 Aug 2025.

FAACT. How to prevent cross-contact and accidental environmental exposure (n.d.). Avoiding Cross-Contact Allergen Contamination | FAACT. https://www.foodallergyawareness.org/foodallergy-and-anaphylaxis/cross-contact/. Accessed on 26 Aug 2025.

Fleischer, D. M., Burks, A. W., Vickery, B. P., Scurlock, A. M., Wood, R. A., Jones, S. M., Sicherer, S. H., Liu, A. H., Stablein, D., Henning, A. K., Mayer, L., Lindblad, R., Plaut, M., Sampson, H. A. (2013). Consortium of Food Allergy Research (CoFAR). Sublingual immunotherapy for peanut allergy: a randomized, double-blind, placebo-controlled multicenter trial. *J Allergy Clin Immunol, 131*(1):119–127.e1-7. https://doi.org/10.1016/j.jaci.2012.11.011. PMID: 23265698; PMCID: PMC3550002.

Fleischer, D. M., Greenhawt, M., Sussman, G., Bégin, P., Nowak-Wegrzyn, A., Petroni, D., Beyer, K., Brown-Whitehorn, T., Hebert, J., Hourihane, J. O., Campbell, D. E., Leonard, S., Chinthrajah, R. S., Pongracic, J. A., Jones, S. M., Lange, L., Chong, H., Green, T, D., Wood, R., Cheema, A., Prescott, S. L., Smith, P., Yang, W., Chan, E. S., Byrne, A., Assa'ad, A., Bird, J. A., Kim, E. H., Schneider, L., Davis, C, M., Lanser, B. J., Lambert, R., Shreffler, W. (2019). Effect of epicutaneous immunotherapy vs placebo on reaction to peanut protein ingestion among children with peanut allergy: the pepites randomized clinical trial. *JAMA, 321*(10), 946–955. https://doi.org/10.1001/jama.2019.1113. PMID: 30794314; PMCID: PMC6439674.

Fleischer, D. M., Shreffler, W. G., Campbell, D. E., Green, T. D., Anvari, S., Assa'ad, A., Bégin, P., Beyer, K., Bird, J. A., Brown-Whitehorn, T., Byrne, A., Chan, E. S., Cheema, A., Chinthrajah, S., Chong, H. J., Davis, C. M., Ford, L. S., Gagnon, R., Greenhawt, M., Hourihane, J. O., & Sampson, H. A. (2020). Long-term, open-label extension study of the efficacy and safety of epicutaneous immunotherapy for peanut allergy in children: PEOPLE 3-year results. *The Journal of Allergy and Clinical Immunology, 146*(4), 863–874. https://doi.org/10.1016/j.jaci.2020.06.028

Food Allergy Research & Education. (2020). *How to avoid cross-contact*. https://www.foodallergy.org/sites/default/files/2020-11/FARE_AvoidCrossContact-110920.pdf. Accessed on 27 Aug 2025.

Food Allergy Research & Education. (2025). *Update to FDA guidance for food allergen labeling*. https://www.foodallergy.org/fare-blog/update-fda-guidance-food-allergen-labeling. Accessed on 27 Aug 2025.

Food Allergy Research & Education. (n.d.). *Food allergy chef cards*. https://www.foodallergy.org/resources/food-allergy-chef-cards. Accessed on 27 Aug 2025.

Foong, R. X., Turner, P. J., & Fox, A. T. (2020). Fatal anaphylaxis due to transcutaneous allergen exposure: An exceptional case. *The Journal of Allergy and Clinical Immunology. In Practice, 8*(1), 332–333. https://doi.org/10.1016/j.jaip.2019.09.023

Gallagher, A., Cronin, C., Heng, T. A., McKiernan, A., Tobin, C., Flores, L., McGinley, A. M., Loughnane, C., Velasco, R., O'B. Hourihane, J., & Trujillo, J. (2024). Dietary advancement therapy using milk and egg ladders among children with a history of anaphylaxis. *The Journal of Allergy and Clinical Immunology: In Practice, 12*(8), 2135–2143. https://doi.org/10.1016/j.jaip.2024.04.057

Genentech. (2024). *XOLAIR: Highlights of prescribing information*. Retrieved from https://www.accessdata.fda.gov/drugsatfda_docs/label/2024/103976s5245lbl.pdf

Gene.com (2024). Xolair prescribing. Retrieved June 22, 2026 from https://www.gene.com/download/pdf/xolair_prescribing.pdf

Golden, D. B. K., Wang, J., Waserman, S., Akin, C., Campbell, R. L., Ellis, A. K., Greenhawt, M., Lang, D. M., Ledford, D. K., Lieberman, J., Oppenheimer, J., Shaker, M. S., Wallace, D. V., Abrams, E. M., Bernstein, J. A., Chu, D. K., Horner, C. C., Rank, M. A., Stukus, D. R., Collaborators, & Wang, J. (2024). Anaphylaxis: A 2023 practice parameter update. *Annals of Allergy, Asthma & Immunology: Official Publication of the American College of Allergy, Asthma, & Immunology, Annals of Allergy, Asthma & Immunology, 132*(2), 124–176. https://doi.org/10.1016/j.anai.2023.09.015

Greenhawt, M., Shaker, M., Winders, T., Bukstein, D. A., Davis, R. S., Oppenheimer, J., Fleischer, D. M., Kim, E., Chan, E. S., Stukus, D. R., & Matlock, D. (2020). Development and acceptability of a shared decision-making tool for commercial peanut allergy therapies. *Annals of Allergy, Asthma & Immunology: Official Publication of the American College of Allergy, Asthma, & Immunology, 125*(1), 90–96. https://doi.org/10.1016/j.anai.2020.01.030

Greenhawt, M., Albright, D., Anvari, S., Arends, N., Arkwright, P. D., Bégin, P., Blümchen, K., Brown-Whitehorn, T., Cassell, H., Chan, E. S., Ciaccio, C. E., Deschildre, A., Divaret-Chauveau, A., Dorris, S., Dorsey, M., Du Toit, G., Eiwegger, T., Erlewyn-Lajeunesse, M., Fleischer, D. M., Ford, L. S., & Burks, A. W. (2025). Efficacy and safety of epicutaneous immunotherapy in Peanut-allergic toddlers: Open-label extension to EPITOPE. *The Journal of Allergy and Clinical Immunology. In Practice, 13*(5), 1176–1187.e7. https://doi.org/10.1016/j.jaip.2025.02.004

Groetch, M., Mudd, K., Woch, M., Schaible, A., Gray, B. E., Bird, J. A., Jones, S., Kim, E. H., Lanser, B. J., Poyser, J., Rogers, N., Babineau, D. C., Spergel, A. R., Shreffler, W., Sicherer, S., Spergel, J., Vickery, B. P., Chinthrajah, R. S., & Wood, R. (2022). Retail food equivalents for post-OIT dosing in the OUtMATCH clinical trial. *The Journal of Allergy and Clinical Immunology in Practice (Cambridge, MA), 11*(2), 572–580.e2. https://doi.org/10.1016/j.jaip.2022.10.022

Ham, J. H., Suh, S. M., Cha, J. E., Ahn, K., Sohn, M. G., & Kim, H. Y. (2025). Global perspectives on allergen labeling: Harmonization of regulations and practices. *Allergy, Asthma & Immunology Research, 17*(3), 288–303. https://doi.org/10.4168/aair.2025.17.3.288

Hervé, P. L., Dioszeghy, V., Matthews, K., Bee, K. J., Campbell, D. E., & Sampson, H. A. (2023). Recent advances in epicutaneous immunotherapy and potential applications in food allergy. *Frontiers in Allergy, 4*, 1290003. https://doi.org/10.3389/falgy.2023.1290003

Inamdar, S. R., & Mandal, B. (2022). Approaches to maintenance dosing during oral immunotherapy. *Journal of Food Allergy, 4*(2), 98–101. https://doi.org/10.2500/jfa.2022.4.220030

Jeebhay, M. F., & Baatjies, R. (2022). Occupational inhalant allergy in food handling occupations. *Current Opinion in Allergy and Clinical Immunology, 22*(2), 64–72. https://doi.org/10.1097/ACI.0000000000000804

Jeimy, S., Yu, N., Chan, E. S., & Cook, V. (2024). Oral immunotherapy for treatment of food allergy in infants and preschoolers. *CMAJ: Canadian Medical Association journal = journal de l'Association medicale canadienne, 196*(23), E790–E791. https://doi.org/10.1503/cmaj.231478

Jiang, N. N., Xiang, L., Huang, H. J., & Hou, X. L. (2024). Unusual anaphylaxis induced by food allergen inhalation or skin contact. *Asia Pacific Allergy, 14*(2), 93–96. https://doi.org/10.5415/apallergy.0000000000000118

Jones, S. M., Kim, E. H., Nadeau, K. C., Nowak-Wegrzyn, A., Wood, R. A., Sampson, H. A., Scurlock, A. M., Chinthrajah, S., Wang, J., Pesek, R. D., Sindher, S. B., Kulis, M., Johnson, J., Maloney, J. M., Chapman, M. D., & Sicherer, S. H. (2006). Peanut allergen exposure through saliva: Assessment and interventions to reduce exposure. *The Journal of Allergy and Clinical Immunology, 118*(3), 719–724. https://doi.org/10.1016/j.jaci.2006.05.017

Jones, S. M., Kim, E. H., Nadeau, K. C., Nowak-Wegrzyn, A., Wood, R. A., Sampson, H. A., Scurlock, A. M., Chinthrajah, S., Wang, J., Pesek, R. D., Sindher, S. B., Kulis, M., Johnson, J., Spain, K., Babineau, D. C., Chin, H., Laurienzo-Panza, J., Yan, R., Larson, D., Qin, T., & Immune Tolerance Network. (2022). Efficacy and safety of oral immunotherapy in children aged 1–3 years with peanut allergy (The Immune Tolerance Network IMPACT trial): A randomised placebo-controlled study. *Lancet (London, England), 399*(10322), 359–371. https://doi.org/10.1016/S0140-6736(21)02390-4

Kelso, J. M. (2014). Potential food allergens in medications. *The Journal of Allergy and Clinical Immunology, 133*(6), 1509–1520. https://doi.org/10.1016/j.jaci.2014.03.011

Kelso, J. M. (2022). The adverse reactions to vaccines practice parameter 10 years on-what have we learned? *Annals of Allergy, Asthma & Immunology: Official Publication of the American College of Allergy, Asthma, & Immunology, 129*(1), 35–39. https://doi.org/10.1016/j.anai.2022.01.026

Kids with Food Allergy. (2021). *Potential food allergens in preschool and school activities*. https://www.kidswithfoodallergies.org/wp-content/uploads/2022/12/potential-food-allergens-in-preschool-daycare-activities-crafts.pdf. Accessed on 18 Dec 2025.

Kids With Food Allergies (2026). Living with Food Allergies. Retrieved on June 22, 2026 at https://kidswithfoodallergies.org/living-with-food-allergies/

Kim, E. H., Keet, C. A., Virkud, Y. V., Chin, S., Ye, P., Penumarti, A., Smeekens, J., Guo, R., Yue, X., Li, Q., Kosorok, M. R., Kulis, M. D., & Burks, A. W. (2023). Open-label study of the efficacy, safety, and durability of peanut sublingual immunotherapy in peanut-allergic children. *The Journal of Allergy and Clinical Immunology, 151*(6), 1558–1565.e6. https://doi.org/10.1016/j.jaci.2023.01.036

Kim, E. H., Bird, J. A., Kulis, M., Laubach, S., Pons, L., Shreffler, W., Steele, P., Kamilaris, J., Vickery, B., & Burks, A. W. (2011). Sublingual immunotherapy for peanut allergy: Clinical and immunologic evidence of desensitization. *Journal of Allergy and Clinical Immunology, 127(3)*, 640–646.e1. https://doi.org/10.1016/j.jaci.2010.12.1083. Epub 2011 Feb 1. PMID: 21281959; PMCID: PMC3052379.

Kulis, M. D., Humphrey, J. R., Krempski, J. W., Kim, E. H., & Smeekens, J. M. (2025). Anti-IgE therapy versus allergen-specific immunotherapy for food allergy: Weighing the pros and cons. *Frontiers in Immunology, 16*, 1617153. https://doi.org/10.3389/fimmu.2025.1617153

Lambert, R., Grimshaw, K. E. C., Ellis, B., Jaitly, J., & Roberts, G. (2017). Evidence that eating baked egg or milk influences egg or milk allergy resolution: A systematic review. *Clinical and Experimental Allergy: Journal of the British Society for Allergy and Clinical Immunology, 47*(6), 829–837. https://doi.org/10.1111/cea.12940

Lee, T., Edwards-Salmon, S., & Vickery, B. P. (2023). Current and future treatments for peanut allergy. *Clinical and Experimental Allergy, 53*(1), 10–24. https://doi.org/10.1111/cea.14244

Lee, E. C. K., Trogen, B., Brady, K., Ford, L. S., & Wang, J. (2024). The natural history and risk factors for the development of food allergies in children and adults. *Current Allergy and Asthma Reports, 24*(3), 121–131. https://doi.org/10.1007/s11882-024-01131-3

Liccardi, G., De Falco, F., Gilder, J. A., D'Amato, M., & D'Amato, G. (2004). Severe systemic allergic reaction induced by accidental skin contact with cow milk in a 16-year-old boy. A case report. *Journal of Investigational Allergology & Clinical Immunology, 14*(2), 168–171.

Mack, D. P., Greenhawt, M., & Anagnostou, A. (2023). Are there hidden dangers associated with milk and egg dietary advancement therapy? *The Journal of Allergy and Clinical Immunology: In Practice, 11*(4), 1056–1062. https://doi.org/10.1016/j.jaip.2022.12.015

Mack, D. P., Greenhawt, M., Bukstein, D. A., Golden, D. B. K., Settipane, R. A., & Davis, R. S. (2024). Decisions with patients, not for patients: Shared decision-making in allergy and immunology. *The Journal of Allergy and Clinical Immunology. In Practice, 12*(10), 2625–2633. https://doi.org/10.1016/j.jaip.2024.05.046

Maloney, J. M., Chapman, M. D., & Sicherer, S. H. (2006). Peanut allergen exposure through saliva: Assessment and interventions to reduce exposure. *The Journal of Allergy and Clinical Immunology, 118*(3), 719–724. https://doi.org/10.1016/j.jaci.2006.05.017

McHenry, M., Bégin, P., Chan, E. S., et al. (2024). Food oral immunotherapy. *Allergy, Asthma and Clinical Immunology, 20*(Suppl 3), 82. https://doi.org/10.1186/s13223-025-00948-5

Pepper, A. N., et al. (2020). Consensus report from the Food Allergy Research & Education (FARE) 2019 Oral Immunotherapy for Food Allergy Summit. *Journal of Allergy and Clinical Immunology, 146*(2), 244–249. https://doi.org/10.1016/j.jaci.2020.05.027

Perrett, K. P., Sindher, S. B., Begin, P., Shanks, J., & Elizur, A. (2022). Advances, practical implementation, and unmet needs regarding Oral immunotherapy for food allergy. *The Journal of Allergy and Clinical Immunology. In Practice, 10*(1), 19–33. https://doi.org/10.1016/j.jaip.2021.10.070

Perry, T. T., Conover-Walker, M. K., Pomés, A., Chapman, M. D., & Wood, R. A. (2004). Distribution of peanut allergen in the environment. *The Journal of Allergy and Clinical Immunology, 113*(5), 973–976. https://doi.org/10.1016/j.jaci.2004.02.035

Petroni, D., Bégin, P., Bird, J. A., Brown-Whitehorn, T., Chong, H. J., Fleischer, D. M., Gagnon, R., Jones, S. M., Leonard, S., Makhija, M. M., Oriel, R. C., Shreffler, W. G., Sindher, S. B., Sussman, G. L., Yang, W. H., Bee, K. J., Bois, T., Campbell, D. E., Green, T. D., & Wood, R. A. (2024). Varying doses of epicutaneous immunotherapy with viaskin milk vs placebo in children with cow's milk allergy: A randomized clinical trial. *JAMA Pediatrics, 178*(4), 345. https://doi.org/10.1001/jamapediatrics.2023.6630

Pongracic, J. A., Gagnon, R., Sussman, G., Siri, D., Oriel, R. C., Brown-Whitehorn, T. F., Green, T. D., Campbell, D. E., Anvari, S., Berger, W. E., Bird, J. A., Chan, E. S., Cheema, A., Chinthrajah, R. S., Chong, H. J., Dowling, P. J., Fineman, S. M., Fleischer, D. M., Gonzalez-Reyes, E., Kim, E. H., & Bégin, P. (2022). Safety of epicutaneous immunotherapy in peanut-allergic children: REALISE randomized clinical trial results. *The Journal of Allergy and Clinical Immunology. In Practice, 10*(7), 1864–1873.e10. https://doi.org/10.1016/j.jaip.2021.11.017

Pongracic, J. A., Gagnon, R., Sussman, G., Siri, D., Oriel, R. C., Brown-Whitehorn, T. F., Anvari, S., Berger, W. E., Bird, J. A., Chan, E. S., Chinthrajah, R. S., Chong, H. J., Fineman, S. M., Fleischer, D. M., Gonzalez-Reyes, E., Kim, E. H., Lanser, B. J., MacGinnitie, A., Mehta, H., Petroni, D., & Bégin, P. (2025). Long-term safety of epicutaneous immunotherapy in peanut-allergic children: An open-label active treatment (REALISE study). *The Journal of Allergy and Clinical Immunology. In Practice, 13*(5), 1190–1200.e3. https://doi.org/10.1016/j.jaip.2025.02.024

Ramirez, D. A., Jr., & Bahna, S. L. (2009). Food hypersensitivity by inhalation. *Clinical and Molecular Allergy: CMA, 7*, 4. https://doi.org/10.1186/1476-7961-7-4

Russell, A. F., Cooke, A. J. T., Kagan, O., & Stieb, E. S. (2022). Multifaceted role of the registered nurse on an oral immunotherapy clinical team. *Journal of Food Allergy, 4*(2), 78–85. https://doi.org/10.2500/jfa.2022.4.220014

Sicherer, S. (2022). *The complete guide to Food allergies in adults and children*. Johns Hopkins University Press.

Sicherer, S. H., & Sampson, H. A. (2018). Food allergy: A review and update on epidemiology, pathogenesis, diagnosis, prevention, and management. *The Journal of Allergy and Clinical Immunology, 141*(1), 41–58. https://doi.org/10.1016/j.jaci.2017.11.003

Sindher, S. B., O'Rourke, E., Tan, W., Chin, A. R., & Chinthrajah, R. S. (2025). Emerging role of novel Therapeutics. *Immunology and Allergy Clinics of North America, 45*(3), 419–427. https://doi.org/10.1016/j.iac.2025.04.008

Soller, L., Abrams, E. M., Carr, S., Kapur, S., Rex, G. A., Leo, S., Lidman, P. G., Yeung, J., Vander Leek, T. K., McHenry, M., Wong, T., Cook, V. E., Hildebrand, K. J., Gerstner, T. V., Mak, R., Lee, N. J., Cameron, S. B., & Chan, E. S. (2019). First real-world safety analysis of preschool peanut oral immunotherapy. *The Journal of Allergy and Clinical Immunology: In Practice, 7*(8), 2759–2767.e5. https://doi.org/10.1016/j.jaip.2019.04.010

Tan, B. M., Sher, M. R., Good, R. A., & Bahna, S. L. (2001). Severe food allergies by skin contact. *Annals of Allergy, Asthma & Immunology: Official Publication of the American College of Allergy, Asthma, & Immunology, 86*(5), 583–586. https://doi.org/10.1016/S1081-1206(10)62908-0

The PALISADE Group of Clinical Investigators. (2018). AR101 oral immunotherapy for Peanut allergy. *New England Journal of Medicine, 379*(21), 1991–2001. https://doi.org/10.1056/NEJMoa1812856

U.S. Food & Drug Administration. (2024a). *FDA approves first medication to help reduce allergic reactions to multiple foods after accidental exposure*. Retrieved on August 10, 2025, https://www.fda.gov/news-events/press-announcements/fda-approves-first-medication-help-reduce-allergic-reactions-multiple-foods-after-accidental

U.S. Food & Drug Administration. (2024b). *The FASTER act: Sesame is the ninth major food allergen*. Retrieved on August 27, 2025. https://www.fda.gov/food/food-allergies/faster-act-sesame-ninth-major-food-allergen

U.S. Food & Drug Administration. (2025). *Questions and answers regarding food allergens guidance for industry: Questions and answers regarding food allergen labeling* (Edition 5) | FDA. https://www.fda.gov/regulatory-information/search-fda-guidance-documents/guidance-industry-questions-and-answers-regarding-food-allergen-labeling-edition-5. Accessed on 27 Aug 2025.

Vickery BP, Berglund JP, Burk CM, Fine JP, Kim EH, Kim JI, Keet CA, Kulis M, Orgel KG, Guo R, Steele PH, Virkud YV, Ye P, Wright BL, Wood RA, Burks AW. Early oral immunotherapy in peanut-allergic preschool children is safe and highly effective. J Allergy Clin Immunol. 2017 Jan;139(1):173-181.e8. doi: 10.1016/j.jaci.2016.05.027. Epub 2016 Aug 10.

Wang, J., Lieberman, J. A., Wallace, D. V., Waserman, S., & Golden, D. B. K. (2024). Anaphylaxis in practice: A guide to the 2023 practice parameter update. *The Journal of Allergy and Clinical Immunology. In Practice, 12*(9), 2325–2336. https://doi.org/10.1016/j.jaip.2024.06.036

Watson, W. T., Woodrow, A., & Stadnyk, A. W. (2015). Removal of peanut allergen Ara h 1 from common hospital surfaces, toys and books using standard cleaning methods. *Allergy, Asthma & Clinical Immunology, 11*, 4. https://doi.org/10.1186/s13223-015-0069

Windom, R. R., Seitz, S., Ly, J. B., Dunn, N., Fergeson, J., & Windom, H. H. (2024). Food sublingual immunotherapy: Safety and simplicity of a real food updosing protocol. *The Journal of Allergy and Clinical Immunology: In Practice, 12*(9), 2447–2453.e1. https://doi.org/10.1016/j.jaip.2024.05.007

Williams, B. A., Baaske, A., Soller, L., Erdle, S. C., Wong, T., Mak, R., Schroeder, N. D., & Chan, E. S. (2025). The use of grocery-sourced real-food solutions in sublingual immunotherapy for food allergies. *Annals of Allergy, Asthma & Immunology, 135*(1), 79–86.e9. https://doi.org/10.1016/j.anai.2025.03.001. Epub 2025 Mar 8. PMID: 40064397.

Wood, R. A., Togias, A., Sicherer, S. H., Shreffler, W. G., Kim, E. H., Jones, S. M., Leung, D. Y. M., Vickery, B. P., Bird, J. A., Spergel, J. M., Iqbal, A., Olsson, J., Ligueros-Saylan, M., Uddin, A., Calatroni, A., Huckabee, C. M., Rogers, N. H., Yovetich, N., Dantzer, J., & Chinthrajah, R. S. (2024). Omalizumab for the treatment of multiple food allergies. *New England Journal of Medicine, 390*(10), 889–899. https://doi.org/10.1056/nejmoa2312382

Wood, R., Jones, S., Dantzer, J., Sicherer, S., Wang, J., Shreffler, W., Pyle, D., Kim, E., Keet, C., Kulis, M., Sindher, S., Long, A., Scurlock, A., Leung, D., Lanser, B., Bird, J. A., Parrish, C., Vickery, B., Ezhuthachan, I., & Chinthrajah, R. S. (2025). Treatment of multi-food allergy with omalizumab compared to omalizumab-facilitated multi-allergen OIT. *Journal of Allergy and Clinical Immunology, 155*(2), AB444–AB444. https://doi.org/10.1016/j.jaci.2024.12.1022

Worm, M., Höfer, V., Dölle-Bierke, S., Bilo, M. B., Hartmann, K., Sabouraud-Leclerc, D., & Treudler, R. (2024). Occupational anaphylaxis-data from the anaphylaxis registry. *Allergy, 79*(3), 702–710. https://doi.org/10.1111/all.15974

Disparities in Food Allergy

Josie Howard-Ruben and Melinda Fitzgerald

Introduction

Health disparities are the result of multiple forces, including broad economic policies, political influences, structural racism, and social norms, all of which can, in turn, impact the social determinants of health (WHO, Social Determinants of Health, 2025). Social determinants of health comprise factors related to education, health care, community resources, financial stability, and safe communities. The Centers for Disease Control and Prevention has adapted the World Health Organization's definition of social determinants of health (SDOH), described as "non-medical factors that affect health outcomes" and "include the conditions in which people are born, grow, work, live, and age" as well as other factors that are present in an individual's life in the larger environment (Healthy People 2030, n.d.) which may contribute to health-related outcomes (see Fig. 1) (CDC, 2024). Housing, education, work opportunities, the economy, and other societal systems can lead to disparities that have a powerful impact on healthcare inequities (Davis et al., 2021), and in turn on the challenges of living with food allergies.

Economic stability impacts socioeconomic status (SES), a factor that has broad implications for other SDOH. If an individual or family has a low SES, their ability to access health care, live in safe areas, engage with community resources, and easily obtain the kind of food they need close to home may be limited. Food allergy affects people across the socioeconomic spectrum, so identifying issues associated

J. Howard-Ruben (✉)
Rush University College of Nursing, Chicago, IL, USA
e-mail: josie_howard-ruben@rush.edu

M. Fitzgerald
Mobile Care Chicago, Chicago, IL, USA
e-mail: mfitzgerald@mobilecarefoundation.org

J. Doucette, J. Howard-Ruben (eds.), *Comprehensive Food Allergy Management for Nurses*, https://doi.org/10.1007/978-3-032-28647-5_5

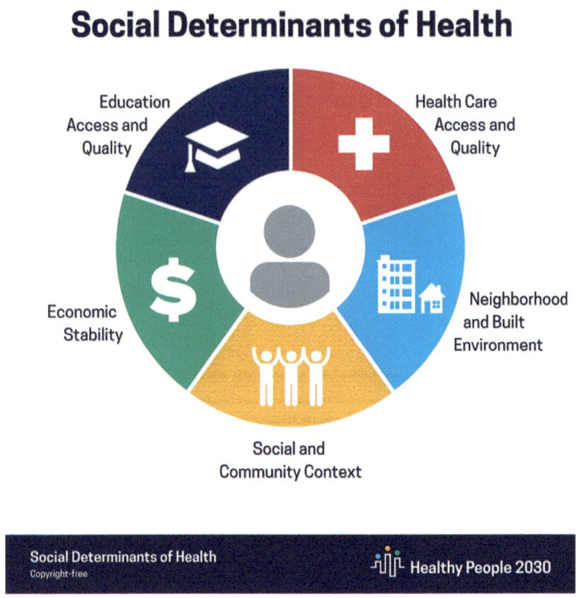

Fig. 1 Social determinants of health. (Used with permission from: Healthy People 2030, U.S. Department of Health and Human Services, Office of Disease Prevention and Health Promotion. Public Domain. Retrieved August 15, 2025, from https://health.gov/healthypeople/objectives-and-data/social-determinants-health)

with SDOH and addressing them with a multipronged approach can help improve health outcomes in the population of patients and families coping with food allergies.

Expanding on the socioeconomic factors that contribute to food allergy disparities, the SDOH Health Care Access and Quality model considers these factors and their salience at the patient, provider, community and policy level (Perry et al., 2024). At the patient level, health literacy, insurance coverage, educational attainment, and income are identified as factors. At the provider level, provider and clinical trial diversity, cultural competence, quality and availability of specialty care are considered. Walkability, safe food options, housing, air quality, environmental exposures, and green space are important community level needs. Finally, policies at every level, from local health code regulations to institutional policies, to regulatory policies, all must be steeped in an understanding of allergic disease.

While everyone experiencing IgE-mediated food allergy must confront healthcare challenges and the impact of this condition on everyday life, for those impacted by SDOH, including not only economic challenges, but lack of educational opportunities, lack of access to basic and specialty care, food insecurity and unequal resources in the community and neighborhood, the challenges become even more difficult. Protudjer et al. (2025) assert that SDOH are significant factors affecting the capacity to handle life with food allergies, and can result in delayed diagnosis, barriers to specialty care, insufficient patient and family education for food allergy management, and inadequate access to safe foods. Furthermore, the authors note that health-promoting behaviors such as allergen avoidance through accessing safe food, accurate and timely diagnosis, access to emergency medications and services, availability of clinical trials to evaluate newer therapies, the latest treatment options, and other self-care strategies, may not be accessible to some people due to these disparities, so optimal health with food allergies is compromised (Protudjer et al., 2025). For example, people with food allergy who are without access to specialty care do not receive an accurate diagnosis, may not have access to emergency epinephrine, and may be more likely to access emergency care to manage allergic reactions (Tepler et al., 2022).

A survey of members of the American College of Allergy, Asthma and Immunology confirmed many of these challenges and found that 68% of member respondents believed that racial disparities negatively affect care of people with skin of color with food allergy and atopic dermatitis (Corbett et al., 2023). Among the issues identified by more than half of the respondents were lack of access to a specialist who takes Medicaid, lack of awareness of symptoms and conditions, inadequate or no insurance coverage, and costs associated with treatment, all of which encompass problems rooted in SDOH.

Managing a diagnosis of food allergy requires coordination of many aspects of daily living that fall under the umbrella of the SDOH and requires access to an array of resources, both in the healthcare system and in the community environment. Udemgba et al. (2023) presented a broad perspective and framework for both the current barriers and proposed interventions to address health disparities across multiple allergic diseases, including food allergy. An overview of inequities and proposed interventions, some of which are discussed later in this chapter, is provided as shown in Fig. 2. Not all of these factors can be addressed by clinicians, but nurses can make a difference by providing resources to address SDOH and food allergy disparities.

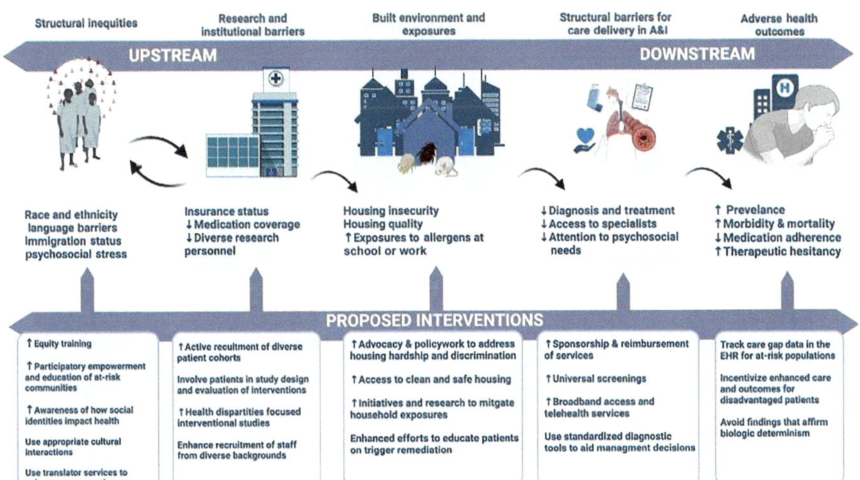

Fig. 2 Framework for upstream and downstream effects of health disparities in allergic and immunologic diseases. Upstream factors of structural inequity, barriers to research, and the built environment effects on adverse outcomes and barriers to care in allergy-immunology are shown. Proposed interventions and examples of future research needs are described. A&I, Allergy & Immunology; EHR, electronic health record. (Created using Biorender.com). (Used with permission from: Udemgba et al. (2023))

How Healthcare Disparities Can Impact People with a Food Allergy Diagnosis

Consistent with these models, the concept of "food allergy disparities" is an emerging idea that encompasses a variety of these factors that broadly align with SDOH (Leeds & Nowak-Wegrzyn, 2022). The authors summarized the factors impacting disparities in food allergy and note that these are understudied in this population (see Figs. 2 and 3).

The following US-based scenarios illustrate some of the challenges faced by people with food allergy disparities underscoring the impact of SDOH on food allergy management.

Scenario 1

A mother with a 6-year-old daughter, recent newcomer to America, learned of the daughter's shellfish allergy after a severe reaction during a family celebration. The family faces multiple challenges in managing her condition: limited English proficiency, unfamiliarity with the US healthcare system, and a lack of culturally responsive care. Though she obtained an epinephrine auto-injector at the pharmacy, the instructions were not available in her first language, and no interpreter was available.

At school, the student's allergy was not documented because mom struggled to understand enrollment paperwork. At home, family members often question the legitimacy of the allergy, citing cultural norms around food and health beliefs. These challenges leave the student vulnerable to accidental exposure.

This scenario highlights the critical need for language services, translated medical materials, and cultural competence among providers to ensure safety and understanding for newcomer families navigating food allergy care.

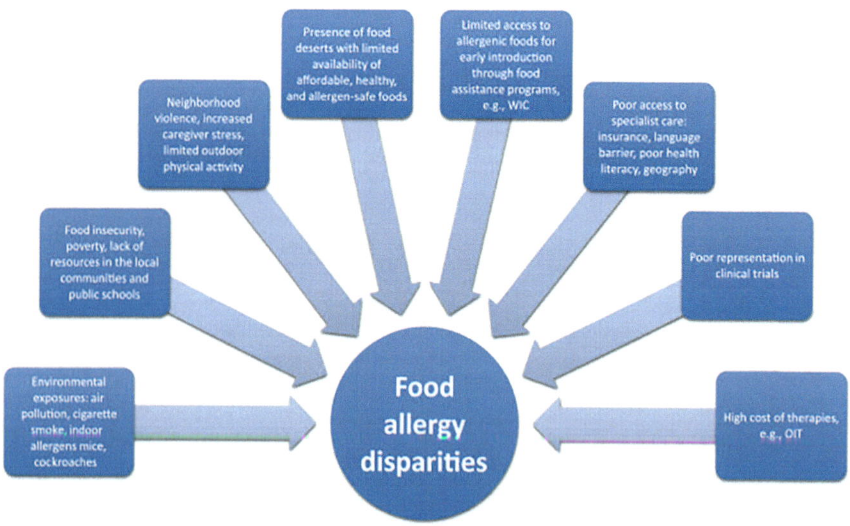

Fig. 3 Food allergy disparities. (Used with permission from: Defining socioeconomic and racial disparities in food allergy: The time is now. By Leeds & Nowak-Wegrzyn (2022))

Scenario 2

A family living in a low-income neighborhood includes a 7-year-old child who has a life-threatening peanut allergy. Despite the caregiver's proactive efforts, including preparing allergen-free meals and informing the school staff about the allergy, the child's school lacks the infrastructure to support children with food allergies. The cafeteria continues to serve peanut products due to budget limitations. The lack of safe food options for the student, as well as cross-contact concerns, are both real safety issues. In addition, the staff members are not trained in food allergy safety and have not had epinephrine device training. Compounding the problem, the school nurse works part-time at the site and is not immediately available for emergencies.

One afternoon, the student ate a snack from a classmate, unaware that it contained a peanut warning. A delayed response by staff, and their unfamiliarity with administration of an epinephrine auto-injector, led to a 911 call and a frightening trip to the emergency room.

This experience underscores the disparities faced by families in low-income communities: under-resourced schools, inconsistent staff training, and lack of systemic support can all result in preventable health emergencies.

Scenario 3

A young adult living in a rural community has allergies to eggs and soy that have persisted since diagnosis in childhood. Following a job loss, they lost their private health insurance and now rely solely on emergency departments for care. Specialty allergy care is only available in a large city several hours away, and regular visits to an allergist have been deferred due to the cost and limited availability of an allergist. Their prescription for an epinephrine device has expired, and the cost to replace it would be more than they can afford. They continue to carry an expired device, aware of the risks, and know that they need to explore other options, but are not sure where to start. Insurance coverage options are confusing, and the COBRA offered after job termination was too expensive to purchase. Egg- and soy-free products add to the cost of food, and the young adult uses available resources to purchase safe food. Without insurance, consistent healthcare access, routine follow-up, or consistent support, the young adult's ability to manage food allergies is compromised.

This clinical scenario reflects the consequences of systemic barriers faced by the uninsured and the urgent need for policy changes that increase access to specialty care, allergy-safe foods, and affordable medications, including safety net options during times of crisis.

AAAAI Position Statement on Health Disparities in Food Allergy

Acknowledging the need to focus on health disparities, the American Academy of Allergy, Asthma & Immunology issued a position statement on addressing health disparities in food allergy, citing that all facets of food allergy care, from prevention to diagnosis to management can be adversely affected (AAAAI, 2025).

The statement suggests that gaps in access to food allergy prevention may be impacted by social and cultural practices, such as differing breastfeeding practices and the timing of food introduction. Access to timely diagnosis is also not universal, and variability in healthcare insurance coverage (e.g., Medicaid) may limit the access to allergy specialists and the care and education provided in these settings, according to the position statement. In addition, access to emergency epinephrine might also be threatened by limited access to health care specialists or prescriptions. The high cost of food allergy treatments is a barrier for many patients, but when patients experience SDOH or inadequate healthcare, access to epinephrine or other therapies may be out of reach.

Treatment plans may require significant financial resources, an unrealistic time commitment, such as when patients or caregivers hold several jobs or do not have flexible work hours, and access to reliable transportation. Participation in clinical trials may not be realistic when researchers are not readily or geographically available, when time or financial resources are limited, or when a lack of trust in the research process exists.

Failure to enroll representative minority populations in clinical trials adversely impacts their acceptance and practicality in different populations (Maldonado-Puebla et al., 2024). Notably, Smith and Kim (2021) point out the underrepresentation of Black children in a series of oral immunotherapy (OIT) trials and underscores the challenge of the time-intensive appointment structure for implementation of OIT, a requirement which may not be feasible when parents are working at a job with little flexibility, as may be the case with low-income families.

The AAAAI position statement on health disparities also notes the prevalence of food insecurity, reporting that 1 in 5 children with food allergy (FA) may be at risk of food insecurity (2025). All or some of these factors can adversely impact the mental health burden of food allergies and quality of life, and taken together, the impact can be significant. The position statement authors identified many opportunities for improvement in food allergy care in patients experiencing these disparities, including some allergists not accepting Medicaid, inadequate participation in clinical trials, and lack of access to care.

Table 1 highlights key points from this AAAAI position statement, reflecting the gaps in care and possible solutions that the allergy care community can implement. Improvements in Medicaid coverage acceptance in the allergy care community and more equitable treatment and care access are highlighted.

Access to Allergy Specialty Care

Due to the lack of board-certified allergists, access to allergy specialists is already limited. Exacerbating this shortage is the fact that many allergists do not accept Medicaid, which provides healthcare coverage for many children in the US. Additionally, barriers to care are not limited to the number of available specialists, but also due to underrepresentation of diversity of culture and ethnicity in practicing allergists.

Table 1 Gaps, unmet needs, and proposed action steps to address health disparities in FA

Gaps and unmet needs	Proposed action steps to address health disparities in FA
Poor acceptance of Medicaid populations in our practices	Increase Medicaid participation from all allergists
Lack of understanding of the relative importance of FA compared with other diagnoses and life constraints in ethnically and racially minoritized groups	Conduct focus groups within ethnically and racially minoritized groups to better understand how they value FA and what is culturally appropriate in different populations
Limited participation by ethnically and racially minoritized populations in FA research to allow better generalization of findings	Increase participation of ethnically and racially minoritized populations in research and support further research in the area of health disparities in FA to obtain more robust data
Prevalence rate estimates of FA in ethnically and racially minoritized populations are currently limited by indirect assessment	Use better and more accurate diagnostic methods in studies assessing prevalence Raise awareness of the probability that health disparities likely exist in FA
Barriers to accessing care, especially access to specialist care	Diversify the workforce within the allergy and immunology specialty Expand advocacy efforts alongside an increased push for policy changes that ensure all food-allergic individuals have access to needed resources Incorporate educational initiatives and alternate health care modalities for providing care

Note. Printed with permission from Addressing Health Disparities in Food allergy: A Position Statement of the AAAAI Prior Authorization Task Force. In the American Academy of Allergy, Asthma & Immunology (2025, p. 58).

Compounding the workforce issue are geographic barriers, which can impact both people living in rural areas, as well as those in locations not served by an allergist. The state of Alaska, as an example, has only 9 board-certified allergists, New Mexico has 22, and Wyoming has 1 (ABMS, 2024). Federal policies may also impact rural healthcare, as hospitals are forced to close, and finding specialty care may require traveling long distances and reliable transportation may not be available.

Food Allergy in the Context of Food Insecurity

Food insecurity suggests that access to a healthy and nutritious food supply in socially acceptable ways is uncertain (NASEM, 2006, p.43), and represents a serious problem for those with specific dietary product needs. A survey of US households found that about 10.5% of households (13.8 million) reported low (6.6%) or very low (3.9%) levels of food security (Coleman-Jensen, 2021). Food insecurity leads to multiple adverse outcomes, including poor nutritional status, hunger, and adverse psychological effects. In children, adverse effects include physical, mental, and developmental issues, including poor school performance. Feeding

America (Dewey et al., 2025) lists many examples of people and groups who may face food insecurity and hunger, ranging from children to seniors, to those living in various geographic locations, and many others, such as low-income households, newcomers to America, and those with disabilities, but people all across America are affected (p. 2).

In patients with food allergies, allergen avoidance is still the standard of care, so specific products are often needed, such as products made on dedicated manufacturing lines, or egg- or nut-free items, or bread products free of sesame flour. In addition, foods appropriate for early introduction of allergens may be difficult to obtain, resulting in a missed opportunity for primary prevention of food allergies. People with food allergies are susceptible to the problem of food insecurity, as allergen-free foods safe for a specific individual may not be readily available, may be challenging to obtain, requiring special ordering or visiting several stores, and may cost more.

In an update to Gupta et al. (2013) findings about the economic burden of food allergy (originally reported at over $24 billion), a recent report (Warren et al., 2025) using a Markov economic modeling approach, projected an "annual societal cost" impact in the US for food allergies of $370.8 billion (p.1675), with $22,234 cost per year patient estimated. The primary contributor in the updated estimates was indirect costs incurred by patients and/or their caregivers. In the projection scenarios, costs were higher for children and adolescents than for adults. However, in a more conservative model, not considering indirect costs, the "annual societal cost" was projected to be $39.6 billion. The individual annual costs for each patient were projected to be $2375 (p. 1676, Fig. 2 in supplementary materials), which included nearly $400 annually for allergy-safe foods and $468 for direct medical costs, as well as other direct and indirect costs (Warren et al., 2025). Regardless of the analytic approach, the economic burden of food allergy is significant, particularly for those with food insecurity.

Access to foods within the community where people reside has been described as geographic food access (Eldin et al., 2025). Food deserts, where availability of healthy foods may be limited, are often a feature of low-income communities and may impact patients with food allergies (Ogbogu et al., 2021). The USDA has moved away from the term food desert to the phrasing "low-income, low-access" (LILA) (Jones et al., 2024). In many of these LILA locations, in urban areas, groceries stores may be a mile or more away from home, and in rural areas, the distance can be 10 miles or more. Though this topic appears to be understudied, one could assume that allergen-friendly foods are also less available in these locations.

Unfortunately, food insecurity is not always assessed in patients with food allergy, as noted in a small survey ($n = 59$) conducted by the Food Insecurity Work Group of the American Academy of Allergy Asthma & Immunology (AAAAI) and a committee of the Center for Food Allergy and Asthma (Shroba et al., 2022). About 75% of the respondents reported that they did not routinely screen patients for food insecurity, and nearly as many did not know if their patients with food allergy had experienced food insecurity recently. Lack of knowledge, unfamiliarity with resources, and comfort level were the most frequent barriers reported (Shroba). Eldin et al. (2025) investigated food insecurity in the pediatric allergy population

For each of the following statements, please tell me which one is "often true," "sometimes true" or "never true" for the past 12 months, that is since last [name of current month].

1) We (I) worried whether our food would run out before we (I) got money to buy more

Often true Sometimes true Never true

2) The food that we (I) bought just didn't last and we (I) didn't have money to get more

Often true Sometimes true Never true

Please answer question 3 only if you have a child with a documented food allergy.

3) We (I) worried that my child's allergen-free food(s) would run out before we (I) had money to buy more.

Often true Sometimes true Never true

Fig. 4 Hunger Vital Sign Questionnaire. (Used with permission from Eldin et al., 2025. The original tool includes the first two questions and no fee or license is required to use the original Hunger Vital Sign™ Hager et al. (2010))

using the Hunger Vital Sign Questionnaire (Hager et al., 2010), with an additional question added about allergen-free foods for those with diagnosed food allergies (see Fig. 4). The authors reported that in pediatric patients with food allergies, about 1 in 5 families reported food insecurity. They noted that adding a food insecurity ICD-10 code (Z59.41 ICD-10) would allow the health care team to identify, track and intervene for cases of food insecurity.

Overall, recommendations to address food insecurity include screening patients, recording the ICD-10 code, and providing informational resources about food banks, other local programs, and privately funded pantries. All these interventions can be implemented by nurses, in collaboration with nutritionists and other members of the healthcare team. On a more comprehensive systems level, Jones et al. (2024) call for a "cross-sector partnership" to address food insecurity in food allergy which includes every facet of the healthcare system, as well as policy makers, researchers, and funding and advocacy groups (p. 365).

Access to Medications

The cost of medications for patients with food allergies varies by country and insurance coverage (when available). For example, without insurance coverage, two epinephrine autoinjectors (EAIs) can cost anywhere from $600–800 in the US. While there are many variables governing what a specific patient will be required to pay for epinephrine devices or other therapies, insurance coverage and patient benefit programs can help defray these costs, but the patient responsibility is often still substantial.

Not only can a lack of health insurance coverage or limited prescription coverage contribute to a lack of equity in prescription access, but other barriers, such as so-called "pharmacy deserts" in underserved communities, higher prices, disparate prescribing practices, and limited access to specialists, all may affect the ability to obtain needed medications (Essien et al., 2021).

A newer concept called "pharmacoequity" refers to ensuring that all people are able to access the prescription drugs required to manage their health issues, regardless of their ethnicity, race, resources or socioeconomic status (Essien et al., 2021). Lack of pharmacoequity is driven by larger system failures and requires complex solutions. Pharmacoequity is not specific to food allergy but is relevant due to the high cost of medications.

Leveraging Alternative Healthcare Delivery Models

Some proposed alternative delivery models have emerged in food allergy care, including telehealth and mobile health clinics. One solution proposed is to implement telehealth services in "tele-allergy" visits (Waibel & Perry, 2022). However, this option does not apply to the many diagnostic tests required in food allergy management, including lab draws, skin prick tests, and oral food challenges. Another potential model is the deployment of mobile health clinics for food allergy care. An integrative review of the literature reflecting mobile health clinics for primary care explored the populations who use these clinics, how they used them, and chronic disease health outcomes (Coaston et al., 2022). Though food allergies were not mentioned in the review, asthma featured prominently, and outcomes related to emergency room utilization, hospitalization and disease management improved.

For example, favorable outcomes for children with asthma using a mobile clinic (Breathmobile) have been reported (Morphew et al., 2017), so mobile clinics could be a feasible option for some aspects of food allergy diagnosis and management and might be explored in prospective trials or demonstration projects. Another program features an asthma mobile unit, which provides families with comprehensive care that goes beyond respiratory health by incorporating assessments for food allergies, which are often closely linked to asthma management. During visits, families receive education on identifying cross-reactivity between common allergens, understanding food labels to prevent accidental exposures, and proper administration of an epinephrine auto-injector in case of emergencies. The clinical team also collaborates with parents and schools to develop individualized action plans, ensuring that children are safe, supported, and able to fully participate in school activities while effectively managing both their asthma and food allergies (Allergy & Asthma Network, 2024). Telehealth and food allergy (Allergy & Asthma Network, 2025) is also being explored in clinical settings to address the shortage of allergists (also see chapter "Advancing Food Allergy Care: The Role of the Certified Allergy Nurse Educator"), partly due to changes in practice during the COVID-19 epidemic, but literature is sparse in this area to date.

Conclusion

Many solutions to disparities impacting food allergies have been proposed in recent years, including calls for more complete epidemiologic data, increased access to specialty care, more diversity in food allergy providers, more affordable and accessible treatments, solutions for food insecurity, and more participation in clinical trials by those experiencing health disparities.

Recently, with the intent to explore solutions related to "daily life, diagnosis, prevention, and daily treatment," Northwestern's Center for Food Allergy and Asthma Research (CFAAR) engaged interest holders and experts in a Summit for Advancing Equity in Food Allergy (Yang et al., 2025, p. 2292). Among the improvement opportunities identified were strengthening public preparedness, community collaboration, provider and allergy care access, policy reform, and research innovation (Yang et al., 2025). This work is foundational to the development of broad-based initiatives across multiple systems to overcome barriers in food allergy care.

Nurses can participate in addressing social determinants of health and food allergy disparities by drawing from organizational, governmental, and community resources available to help patients manage their food allergies more effectively. Table 2 outlines nursing interventions that can address these social determinants and drivers of health disparities in food allergies.

Table 2 How nurses can help to address social determinants of health and food allergy disparities

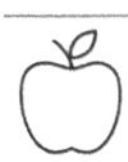	Implement recommended guidelines for primary prevention of food allergies Screen for social determinants of health, using tools such as the free social needs screening tool https://www.aafp.org/dam/AAFP/documents/patient_care/everyone_project/patient-short-print.pdf Screen patients for food insecurity using validated tools like the Hunger Vital Signs tool, a validated 2 question tool or PRAPARE® (Protocol for Responding to And Assessing Patients' Assets, Risks, and Experiences), available in more than 25 languages https://prapare.org/the-prapare-screening-tool/ Educate about resources to help families access safe foods, such as food benefits (e.g., supplemental nutrition assistance program [SNAP] and special supplemental nutrition program for women, infants, and children [WIC]), food pantries Explore securing safe food https://www.securingsafefood.org/ a US-based nonprofit focused on food insecurity and safe food for people with food allergies Provide resources such as local charities and food pantries, vouchers or gift cards for groceries or local farmers markets, Feeding America https://www.feedingamerica.org/find-your-local-foodbank USDA hunger hotline https://www.usa.gov/emergency-food-assistance 1-866-348-6479 or (1-877-842-6273 for Spanish) Refer to nutritionist when available Explore culturally appropriate food options

(continued)

Table 2 (continued)

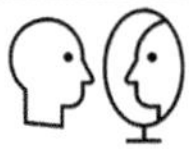	Conduct assessment of social and emotional stress Provide referrals for social and emotional support Refer to online and in-person food allergy support groups Promote self-care behaviors to help reduce anxiety
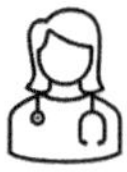	Assess access to a community health clinic for primary care Explore care sites, such as school-based clinics, mobile care, telehealth, federally qualified health centers (FHQC) Refer to health navigators if available Foster awareness of available clinical trials in the community Enlist benefit specialists or insurance navigators to assist with medical insurance enrollment Inform about patient assistance programs managed by pharmaceutical companies and others
	Screen for indoor and outdoor allergens in the home Provide interventions to reduce exposures to environmental allergens Engage with daycare, childcare and educational settings to provide evidence-based guidance on care of the child with food allergy Advocate for healthy communities, green space, playgrounds and enhanced safety
	Assess for implicit bias and language barriers Utilize available translation services Assess literacy with screening tools Create educational programs considering health literacy Employ health literacy toolkits such as Agency for Healthcare Research and Quality (AHRQ) Health Literacy Universal Precautions Toolkit https://www.ahrq.gov/sites/default/files/publications2/files/health-literacy-universal-precautions-toolkit-3rd-edition.pdf Collaborate with community health workers

Note. Table developed by Josie Howard-Ruben and Melinda Fitzgerald adapted from content in Leeds & Nowak-Wegrzyn (2022), Healthy People (2030), Perry et al. (2024), and Feeding America (2025)

Acknowledgments Dr. Fitzgerald wishes to acknowledge the invaluable contributions of Matt Siemer at Mobile Care Clinic in Chicago, Illinois, whose dedication and service have significantly advanced community-centered care and the mission of this work.

Conflict of Interest The authors declare no conflict of interest.

References

Allergy & Asthma Network. (2024). *Planning for school with food allergies*. Allergy & Asthma Network https://allergyasthmanetwork.org/food-allergies/planning-for-school-with-food-allergies/

American Academy of Allergy, Asthma & Immunology. (2025). Addressing health disparities in food allergy: A position statement of the AAAAI prior authorization task force. *The Journal of Allergy and Clinical Immunology, 155*(1), 53–61. https://doi.org/10.1016/j.jaci.2024.10.008

American Board of Medical Specialties (ABMS). (2024). *Board certification report 2023–2024*. Retrieved on January 24, 2026, from https://www.abms.org/wp-content/uploads/2024/11/2023_24_ABMSCertReport_FNLPosting11_1.pdf

Asthma & Allergy Network (2025, October 9). *How telemedicine improves access to allergy care*. Accessed on December 16, 2025. https://allergyasthmanetwork.org/podcast/telehealth-for-food-allergies/

Centers for Disease Control and Prevention. Public Health Professionals Gateway. (2024, May 15). *Social determinants of health*. Accessed on August 15, 2025. https://www.cdc.gov/public-health-gateway/php/about/social-determinants-of-health.html

Coaston, A., Lee, S. J., Johnson, J., Hardy-Peterson, M., Weiss, S., & Stephens, C. (2022). Mobile medical clinics in the United States post-affordable care act: An integrative review. *Population Health Management, 25*(2), 264–279. https://doi.org/10.1089/pop.2021.0289

Coleman-Jensen, A., Rabbitt, M. P., & Gregory, C. A. (2021). *Household food security in the United States in 2020*. Economic Research Service; US Department of Agriculture Economic Research Report No. ERR-298. Retrieved on August 1, 2024, from https://www.ers.usda.gov/publications/pub-details/?pubid=102075

Corbett, M., Allen, A., Bobo, N., Foggs, M. B., Fonacier, L. S., Gupta, R., Kowalsky, R., Martinez, E., Begolka, W. S., Zachary, C., & Blaiss, M. S. (2023). Proposed solutions by the American College of Allergy, Asthma, and Immunology and advocacy experts to address racial disparities in atopic dermatitis and food allergy. *Annals of Allergy, Asthma & Immunology, 130*(3), 392–396.e2. https://doi.org/10.1016/j.anai.2022.12.017

Davis, C. M., Apter, A. J., Casillas, A., Foggs, M. B., Louisias, M., Morris, E. C., Nanda, A., Nelson, M. R., Ogbogu, P. U., Walker-McGill, C. L., Wang, J., & Perry, T. T. (2021). Health disparities in allergic and immunologic conditions in racial and ethnic underserved populations: A work group report of the AAAAI committee on the underserved. *The Journal of Allergy and Clinical Immunology, 147*(5), 1579–1593. https://doi.org/10.1016/j.jaci.2021.02.034

Dewey, A., Hilvers, J., Dawes, S., Harris, V., Hake, M., and Engelhard, E. (2025). Map the meal gap: a report of local food insecurity and food costs in the United States in 2023. *Feeding America National Organization*. https://www.feedingamerica.org/research/map-the-meal-gap/overall-executive-summary

Eldin, M., Campbell, S., Lee, M., Nowak-Wegrzyn, A., & Varshney, P. (2025). Food insecurity screening in the allergy/immunology clinic: A work group report of the AAAAI adverse reactions to foods committee. *The Journal of Allergy and Clinical Immunology in Practice (Cambridge, MA), 13*(5), 1050–1056.e2. https://doi.org/10.1016/j.jaip.2025.02.011

Essien, U. R., Dusetzina, S. B., & Gellad, W. F. (2021). A policy prescription for reducing health disparities—Achieving pharmacoequity. *JAMA, 326*(18), 1793–1794. https://doi.org/10.1001/jama.2021.17764

Feeding America. (2025). *Food insecurity among the overall population in the United States*. Accessed on 30 Aug 2025, at https://map.feedingamerica.org

Gupta, R., Holdford, D., Bilaver, L., Dyer, A., Holl, J. L., & Meltzer, D. (2013). The economic impact of childhood food allergy in the United States. *JAMA Pediatrics, 167*(11), 1026–1031. https://doi.org/10.1001/jamapediatrics.2013.2376

Hager, E. R., Quigg, A. M., Black, M. M., Coleman, S. M., Heeren, T., Rose-Jacobs, R., Cook, J. T., Ettinger de Cuba, S. A., Casey, P. H., Chilton, M., Cutts, D. B., Meyers, A. F., & Frank, D. A. (2010). Development and validity of a 2-item screen to identify families at risk for food insecurity. *Pediatrics, 126*(1), 26–32. https://doi.org/10.1542/peds.2009-3146

Healthy People 2030, U.S. Department of Health and Human Services, Office of Disease Prevention and Health Promotion. (n.d.). Retrieved August 15, 2025, from https://health.gov/healthypeople/objectives-and-data/social-determinants-health

Jones, S. M., Anvari, S., Coleman, A., Pesek, R. D., Kloepfer, K. M., Perry, T. T., Jefferson, A. A., Doan, D., Andres, A., Doderer, M., Hilbun, A., Solomon, R., & Scurlock, A. M. (2024). Food insecurity and allergic diseases: A call to collective action. *The Journal of Allergy and Clinical Immunology, 153*(2), 359–367. https://doi.org/10.1016/j.jaci.2023.10.019

Leeds, S., & Nowak-Wegrzyn, A. (2022). Defining socioeconomic and racial disparities in food allergy: The time is now. *Annals of Allergy, Asthma & Immunology: Official Publication of the American College of Allergy, Asthma, & Immunology, 129*(4), 391–392. https://doi.org/10.1016/j.anai.2022.07.018. PMID: 36155692

Maldonado-Puebla, M., Akenroye, A., Busby, J., Cardet, J. C., & Louisias, M. (2024). Pharmacoequity in allergy-immunology: Disparities in access to medications for allergic diseases and proposed solutions in the United States and globally. *The Journal of Allergy and Clinical Immunology in Practice (Cambridge, MA), 12*(2), 272–280. https://doi.org/10.1016/j.jaip.2023.11.005

Morphew, T., Altamirano, W., Bassin, S. L., & Galant, S. P. (2017). The Breathmobile improves the asthma medication ratio and decreases emergency department utilization. *The American Journal of Managed Care, 23*(4), e120–e126.

National Academies of Sciences, Engineering, and Medicine. (2006). Food insecurity and hunger in the United States: An assessment of the measure. Panel to review the U.S. Department of Agriculture's Measurement of Food Insecurity and Hunger. In G. S. Wunderlich & J. L. Norwood (Eds.), *Committee on National Statistics, Division of Behavioral and Social Sciences and Education*. The National Academies Press. https://doi.org/10.17226/9502

Ogbogu, P. U., Capers, Q., 4th, & Apter, A. J. (2021). Disparities in asthma and allergy care: What can we do? *The Journal of Allergy and Clinical Immunology: In Practice, 9*(2), 663–669. https://doi.org/10.1016/j.jaip.2020.10.030

Perry, T. T., Grant, T. L., Dantzer, J. A., Udemgba, C., & Jefferson, A. A. (2024). Impact of socioeconomic factors on allergic diseases. *The Journal of Allergy and Clinical Immunology, 153*(2), 368–377. https://doi.org/10.1016/j.jaci.2023.10.025

Protudjer, J. L. P., Davis, C. M., Gupta, R. S., & Perry, T. T. (2025). Social determinants and quality of life in food allergy management and treatment. *The Journal of Allergy and Clinical Immunology: In Practice, 13*(4), 745–750. https://doi.org/10.1016/j.jaip.2025.02.016

Shroba, J., Das, R., Bilaver, L., Vincent, E., Brown, E., Polk, B., Ramos, A., Russell, A. F., Bird, J. A., Ciaccio, C. E., Lanser, B. J., Mudd, K., Sood, A., Vickery, B. P., & Gupta, R. (2022). Food insecurity in the food allergic population: A work group report of the AAAAI adverse reactions to foods committee. *The Journal of Allergy and Clinical Immunology: In Practice, 10*(1), 81–90. https://doi.org/10.1016/j.jaip.2021.10.058

Smith, H. G., & Kim, E. H. (2021). Increasing diversity in peanut oral immunotherapy research and accessibility. *The Journal of Allergy and Clinical Immunology: In Practice, 9*(5), 2132–2133. https://doi.org/10.1016/j.jaip.2021.02.010

Tepler, E., Wong, K. H., & Soffer, G. K. (2022). Health disparities in pediatric food allergy. *Annals of Allergy, Asthma & Immunology: Official Publication of the American College of Allergy, Asthma, & Immunology, 129*(4), 417–423. https://doi.org/10.1016/j.anai.2022.04.022

Udemgba, C., Sarkaria, S. K., Gleeson, P., Bryant-Stephens, T., Ogbogu, P. U., Khoury, P., & Apter, A. J. (2023). New considerations of health disparities within allergy and immunology. *The Journal of Allergy and Clinical Immunology, 151*(2), 314–323. https://doi.org/10.1016/j.jaci.2022.11.004

Waibel, K. H., & Perry, T. T. (2022). Telehealth and allergy services in rural and regional locations that lack specialty services. *The Journal of Allergy and Clinical Immunology: In Practice, 10*(10), 2507–2513.e1. https://doi.org/10.1016/j.jaip.2022.06.025

Warren, C., Whittington, M. D., Bilaver, L., Kratochvil, D., Liu, R., Seetasith, A., ... Gupta, R. (2025). Estimating the societal economic burden of food allergy in the United States. *Journal of Medical Economics, 28*(1), 1669–1681. https://doi.org/10.1080/13696998.2025.2563462

World Health Organization. (2025). Social determinants of health. https://www.who.int/news-room/fact-sheets/detail/social-determinants-of-health

Yang, M. S., Warren, C. M., Engel, M. L., Samady, W., Sansweet, S. R., Kanaley, M. K., Folger, E. V. W., Shankar, S., Gupta, R. S., & Bilaver, L. A. (2025). Strategic directions for advancing equity in food allergy: Takeaways from CFAAR's summit for advancing equity in food allergy. *The Journal of Allergy and Clinical Immunology: In Practice, 13*(9), 2290–2297. https://doi.org/10.1016/j.jaip.2025.05.024

Early Introduction of Food Allergens

Kristen Bowersox, Laura Biazon, and Julianne Doucette

Introduction

In previous chapters, we have established that the prevalence of food allergies has notably increased since the 1990s, imposing a significant burden not only on patients, caregivers, and schools, but also on the healthcare system. The financial impact of food allergies on American families is substantial; the most up-to-date cost analysis estimated the United States (US) spent $24.8 billion in 2011, which equates to $35.8 billion in 2025 dollars (Gupta et al., 2013; U.S. Bureau of Labor Statistics, n.d.). Most of this burden is experienced by family opportunity costs such as leaving work outside the home to homeschool, or to switch careers to jobs with more flexibility to care for the child with food allergies. Beyond the financial burdens, the psychological distress, fear, and anxiety experienced by these families is significant. One study found 36.6% of children with food allergies report being bullied as a result of their condition (Schepel et al., 2025), and there are many other psychosocial issues associated with food allergies.

However, imagine a future where food allergies could be prevented for many individuals. The recent shift in focus from managing food allergies and allergic reactions to preventing them by helping to develop tolerance during infancy is a promising development. Preventing food allergy before it starts is a primary

K. Bowersox (✉)
Nationwide Children's Hospital, Columbus, OH, USA
e-mail: Kristen.Bowersox1@nationwidechildrens.org

L. Biazon
University of Virginia, Charlottesville, VA, USA
e-mail: Lib3gq@virginia.edu

J. Doucette
College of Nursing, Rush University, Chicago, IL, USA
e-mail: Julianne_Doucette@rush.edu

J. Doucette, J. Howard-Ruben (eds.), *Comprehensive Food Allergy Management for Nurses*, https://doi.org/10.1007/978-3-032-28647-5_6

prevention strategy, and there is even emerging evidence that if an infant develops a food allergy, early oral immunotherapy (OIT) may be an approach to induce tolerance or even remission (Jones et al., 2022). In contrast to previous recommendations, which advised delaying introduction of potential food allergens, early introduction of allergens may prove to be effective in alleviating the burden of food allergies for future generations.

> An ounce of prevention is worth a pound of cure.
> —Benjamin Franklin

History of Food Allergy Management and Food Introduction Recommendations

Cases of allergic reactions to foods were described in ancient Greek and Chinese literature, but the mechanism of food allergies was not established until the past century. Studies by Prausnitz in the 1920s established the immunologic basis of allergic reactions, and with the discovery of IgE in 1967, the process of Type I (immediate) hypersensitivity reactions became understood (Bahna, 2024). RAST and ImmunoCap testing became more widely available in the 1970s, increasing public awareness of food allergies (Bahna, 2024). As parents and clinicians hoped to decrease the risk of children developing allergic sensitivities to foods, they looked to professional medical organizations to provide recommendations for the introduction of potential food allergens.

Originally, a randomized controlled trial (RCT) in 1989 showed that maternal avoidance of allergens in the diet combined with delayed introduction of allergens in the infant's diet may reduce the development of food allergy (Conway et al., 2024; Zeiger et al., 1989). This set the stage for recommendations to avoid allergens in both the mother and infant for many years. Later, the maternal avoidance of allergens was dropped from recommendations, noting that infant weight gain suffered, and the correlation between avoidance of allergens and the development of food allergy was not strong (Conway et al., 2024). In 2000, the American Academy of Pediatrics (AAP) released its first position statement on food allergies, recommending avoidance of cow's milk until 12 months, eggs until 24 months, and peanuts, tree nuts, fish, and seafood until 3 years of age in a child's diet (Abrams & Becker, 2015). The American College of Allergy, Asthma, and Immunology (ACAAI) supported these recommendations in their consensus statement in 2006 (Fiocchi, 2006). However, the data supporting these recommendations was limited and based mostly on expert opinion, and as pediatric clinicians followed the guidelines in subsequent years, the prevalence of food allergy continued to increase at alarming rates. According to CDC data, the prevalence of reported food allergy in children under age 18 in the USA increased 18% between 1997 and 2007 (Branum & Lukacs, 2008), *see* Fig. 1. Similarly, the number of annual hospital discharges of children under 18 years old with a diagnosis related to food allergy more than doubled when comparing 2001–2003 with 2004–2006 (Branum & Lukacs, 2008), *see* Fig. 2.

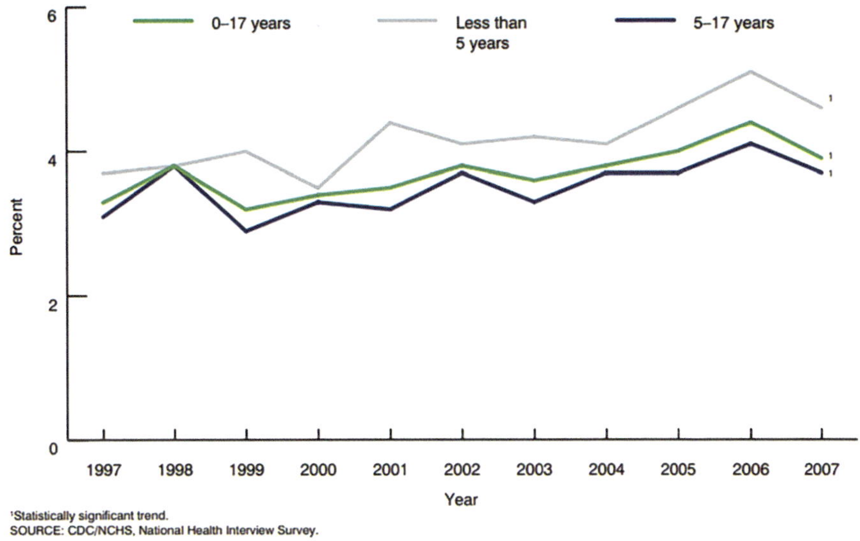

Fig. 1 *Food allergy in children under 18 years in the USA, 1997–2007. From:* Percentage of children under age 18 years who had a reported food or digestive allergy in the past 12 months, by age group: USA, 1997–2007. (Used with permission from: NCHS Data Brief (Branum & Lukacs, 2008). Open Access. https://www.cdc.gov/nchs/data/databriefs/db10.pdf)

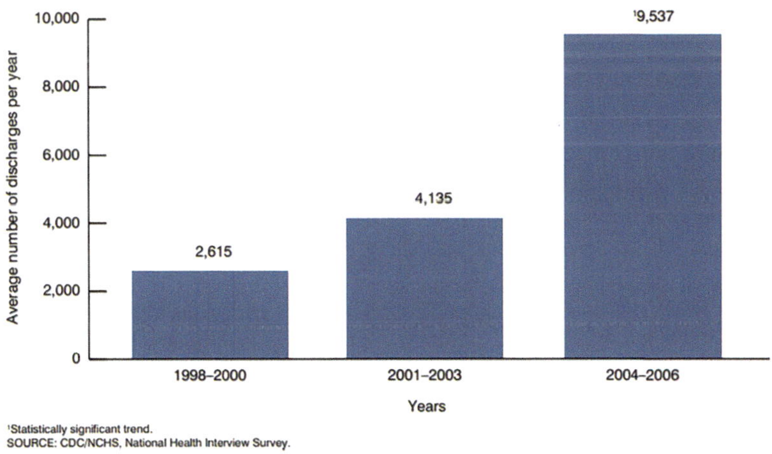

Fig. 2 Hospital discharges per year among children under 18 years, 1998–2006. *From:* Average number of hospital discharges per year among children under 18 years with any diagnosis related to food allergy: USA, 1998–2006. (Used with permission from: NCHS Data Brief (Branum & Lukacs, 2008). Open Access. https://www.cdc.gov/nchs/data/databriefs/db10.pdf)

These trends led to a revision by the AAP in 2008 with a new clinical report recommending that potential food allergens should *not* be delayed beyond 4–6 months (Greer, 2008). Similarly, in 2010, the National Institute of Allergy and Infectious Diseases (NIAID) guidelines recommended "Introduction of solid foods should not be delayed beyond 4 to 6 months of age. Potentially allergenic foods may be introduced at this time as well" (Boyce et al., 2011). NIAID also specified that mothers should not avoid potential food allergens in their diets during pregnancy or lactation, as this strategy is not shown to lower the rate of food allergies in children (Boyce et al., 2011). However, there was still insufficient data at the time to definitively show that early introduction would prevent allergy.

Around the same time, researchers in the United Kingdom (UK) began noticing an interesting trend in peanut allergy: Jewish children living in the UK had 10-times greater rates of peanut allergy than Jewish children living in Israel (Du Toit et al., 2008). Since the two groups shared a common genetic ancestry, the researchers hypothesized that an environmental factor was causing the difference. Upon further investigation, researchers found that, in contrast to children in the UK whose caregivers followed the guidelines to avoid peanut exposure until 36 months old, the children in Israel were regularly fed peanut-containing foods starting at 8 months old (Du Toit et al., 2008). Thus, the study suggested, "These findings raise the question of whether early introduction of peanut during infancy, rather than avoidance, will prevent the development of peanut allergy" (Du Toit et al., 2008). Smaller studies in 2011 and 2012 suggested a pattern that early introduction of baked milk and baked egg, respectively, accelerated the tolerance of unbaked forms of these foods into allergic children's diets compared with strict avoidance (Kim et al., 2011; Leonard et al., 2012).

These studies were foundational to the LEAP study, published in 2015. This study focused on a high-risk group of infants who already had a diagnosis of severe eczema and/or egg allergy aged 4–11 months and randomized them to two groups: one that began consumption of peanut protein between 4 and 11 months and continued consumption throughout the study, and one group that avoided peanut protein for the first 5 years (Du Toit et al., 2015). The infants who consumed safe peanut products early in infancy had an overall 81% reduction in the development of peanut allergy upon follow-up at age 5 years (Du Toit et al., 2015). This was a pivotal study setting off a cascade of changes to guidelines and recommendations globally, including in the USA and Europe. The science for early introduction is clear for peanut protein, but what have studies shown for other common food allergens? And how have food allergy guidelines changed recently?

Many clinical trials related to early introduction have been conducted in the last 15 years; however, there is still work to be done to verify the benefits of early introduction for a broader population (de Silva et al., 2020).

Review of Early Introduction Studies Beyond LEAP

Other studies beyond LEAP have helped inform current clinical guidelines and are briefly discussed here. Early introduction of allergens is emerging as a potential secondary prevention option in the management of food allergy, at least for some allergens, but studies are ongoing.

Peanut Early Introduction Studies

LEAP-On Study (Persistence of Oral Tolerance to Peanut): (Du Toit et al., 2015)

A follow-up to the original LEAP trial, the LEAP-On (Du Toit et al., 2015) involved 556 high-risk participants from the LEAP cohort, who were assessed for peanut allergy at 72 months of age after 12 months of peanut avoidance. The results demonstrated that early introduction of peanuts in high-risk infants led to a sustained reduction in peanut allergy prevalence, even after a long period of abstinence (Du Toit et al., 2015).

Immune Tolerance Network Peanut OIT in Toddlers (IMPACT): (Jones et al., 2022)

IMPACT was a USA-based RCT involving 146 peanut-allergic toddlers aged 12–48 months (Jones et al., 2022). The study evaluated the effects of early peanut oral immunotherapy (OIT) lasting approximately 2.5 years on desensitization and remission. Children consumed gradually increasing doses of peanut protein with a goal maintenance dose of up to 2000 mg/day. In the peanut OIT group, 71% of children could tolerate a 5000 mg peanut challenge, compared with only 2% in the placebo group. Then they avoided peanuts for 6 months, and 21% of treated children achieved sustained unresponsiveness (remission) versus 2% in the placebo group. Children under age 2 years had the highest remission rates, suggesting a stronger benefit with earlier intervention (Jones et al., 2022).

The IMPACT trial is the most definitive study to date showing that very early peanut OIT not only induces desensitization, but also may help infants, toddlers, or children allergic to peanuts achieve remission. Rates of sustained unresponsiveness were highest in the youngest participants.

Egg Early Introduction Studies

The Solids Timing for Allergy Research (STAR): (Palmer et al., 2013)

This clinical trial included 86 high-risk infants with eczema randomized to receive pasteurized raw whole-egg powder in one arm of the study or placebo (rice powder) at 4 months of age. At 8 months of age, both groups were given a cooked egg challenge. At 1-year of age, there was a non-significant trend toward a lower rate of egg allergy in the early introduction group vs. whole cooked egg at age 8 months. However, the trial ended early due to 31% of infants in the early egg group having reactions (Palmer et al., 2013).

Beating Egg Allergy Trial (BEAT): (Tan et al., 2017)

The BEAT study was a randomized clinical trial of 319 infants with at least 1 first-degree relative with allergic disease. Daily freeze-dried whole raw egg powder (from 4–6 months) was compared to a daily dose of placebo (rice powder) on IgE sensitization to egg white, based on skin prick testing (SPT) responses of 3 mm or greater at 12 months and symptoms of clinical egg allergy. Within the first week of the study, 10% of infants reacted to the raw egg powder, but early introduction of egg was associated with a reduction of egg sensitization at 12 months of age (Tan et al., 2017).

Starting Time for Egg Protein (STEP): (Palmer et al., 2017)
Conducted in Australia, this RCT compared 820 infants with a family history of allergic disease to investigate the effects of early pasteurized raw egg powder (from 4–6 months) vs. placebo on egg allergy development. Results showed no significant difference in egg allergy prevalence between the early introduction and control groups. However, there was a non-significant trend toward a reduced risk of egg allergy in the 4–6-month-old group compared to introduction at 10 months. A per-protocol analysis also found that significantly fewer children in the early introduction group had egg allergy at 12 months (Palmer et al., 2017).

Hen's Egg Allergy Prevention (HEAP): (Bellach et al., 2017)
This RCT examined the effects of early pasteurized raw egg introduction (from 4 to 6 months) on egg allergy development in 406 infants from the general population in Germany. Results showed no significant difference in egg allergy prevalence or sensitization between the early introduction and control groups (Bellach et al., 2017).

Prevention of Egg Allergy with Tiny Amount Intake (PETIT): (Natsume et al., 2017)
The PETIT RCT examined the effects of early, stepwise introduction of cooked egg powder on egg allergy development in 147 infants in Japan. The intervention group consumed 50 mg of heated egg per day from 6–9 months of age and then increased consumption to 250 mg per day until 12 months of age, while the control group received a placebo. The study found that heated egg powder at age 6 months significantly reduced the risk of egg allergy by 78% compared with avoidance until age 12 months (Natsume et al., 2017). The PETIT study is perhaps the most successful egg RCT and the only one that used cooked egg powder.

***Note on Evidence for Egg Allergy Prevention**
Although most early egg trials by themselves did not yield significant results (likely due to using raw forms of egg), five systematic reviews, one meta-analysis, and one RCT support targeted early cooked egg introduction in infants (Al-Saud & Sigurdardóttir, 2018; de Silva et al., 2020; Fleischer et al., 2021; Ierodiakonou et al., 2016; Matsumoto et al., 2018; Obbagy et al., 2019; Perkin et al., 2019).

Milk Study

Strategy for Prevention of Milk Allergy by Daily Ingestion of Infant Formula in Early Infancy (SPADE): (Sakihara et al., 2021)

The SPADE RCT, conducted in Japan, examined the effects of early introduction of cow's milk formula (10 ml daily starting at 1–2 months) on cow's milk allergy (CMA) development in 312 "low-risk" infants. Results showed a significant reduction in milk allergy prevalence in the early introduction group. Only 0.8% of the early introduction group developed a milk allergy compared with 6.8% of the control group (Sakihara et al., 2021).

Multiple Food Studies

Enquiring About Tolerance (EAT Study): (Perkin et al., 2016)

The EAT RCT studied 1303 exclusively breastfed infants from the general population, comparing early introduction of six allergenic foods (peanut, cow's milk, cooked egg, sesame, whitefish, and wheat) beginning at 3 months compared to standard introduction of solids at 6 months. Notably, this study demonstrated the safety of early introduction as results in this arm of the study did not show any increased risk of food allergy development. Early introduction did not impact breastfeeding, and there were no cases of anaphylaxis in the early introduction group. The per-protocol analysis revealed a significant reduction in food allergy (particularly egg and peanut) prevalence in the early introduction group. However, the intention-to-treat analysis did not show a significant difference between the two groups. Researchers thought this was likely due to the difficulty of following protocols for many foods at once, as many families had difficulties with incorporating and maintaining 6 foods (Perkin et al., 2016).

Preventing Atopic Dermatitis and Allergies in Children (PreventADALL): (Skjerven et al., 2022)

The PreventADALL study, a multicenter, cluster-randomized trial involving 2397 infants from a general population, examined the effects of early food introduction (small amounts of peanut, milk, wheat, and egg from 3 months multiple times per week) and/or skin emollients on food allergy and atopic dermatitis development. Results showed that early food introduction combined with eczema treatment was associated with a reduced risk of food allergy at age 3 years, while skin emollients alone did not significantly affect food allergy development. Smaller doses of food allergens may be sufficient to build tolerance, but more studies are needed (Skjerven et al., 2022).

The Cow's Milk Early Exposure Trial (COMEET): (Lachover-Roth et al., 2023)

COMEET was an Israeli interventional study that found babies receiving early cow's milk formula followed by cessation of formula and then exclusive breastfeeding after the first few days of life were the most at risk of developing cow's milk allergy (CMA). Those infants that continued to receive some cow's milk over time during the first 2 months of life even if breastfed developed CMA less often (Lachover-Roth et al., 2023).

Systematic Review and Meta-analysis (Scarpone et al., 2023)

A systematic review and meta-analysis examined 23 early introduction studies and concluded introduction of allergens before 1 year reduced the development of food allergy; however, it was noted that the studies had a high rate of attrition. The authors concluded further studies on early introduction of multiple foods in a manner acceptable to infants and parents is needed (Scarpone et al., 2023).

Review of Food Allergy Guidelines and Consensus Statements

As mentioned earlier in this chapter, the *2010 NIAID Guidelines for the Diagnosis and Management of Food Allergy* (NIAID Sponsored Expert Panel, 2010) were the first major U.S. effort to standardize food allergy care. Authors stressed that diagnosis was based on history plus testing, not just positive skin or IgE results, and the oral food challenge was emphasized as the gold standard. Management centered on strict allergen avoidance, emergency readiness with epinephrine, and nutritional support. At the time, the guidance on infant feeding was cautious: Early allergen introduction was not expressly recommended, but delaying beyond 4–6 months was not advised either. The authors concluded there was not enough evidence to support deliberately delaying allergen introduction as was recommended by experts in the past.

The *2017 NIAID Addendum Guidelines* were developed in direct response to the LEAP trial. Du Toit et al. (2015) used peanut SPT to prescreen infants, excluding those with a wheal >4 mm to minimize risk during oral food challenges. This prescreening strategy was adopted into the NIAID Addendum Guidelines, which recommend that high-risk infants (those with severe eczema, egg allergy, or both) undergo SPT before peanut introduction. Infants with a wheal ≥8 mm were considered likely allergic and referred to a specialist, while those with 3–7 mm required an in-office oral challenge. If cleared, peanut should be introduced between 4 and 6 months in high-risk infants, and around 6 months in those with mild to moderate eczema (Togias et al., 2017).

Unlike the U.S. risk-based approach, countries like Australia and the UK recommend universal early peanut introduction without screening. Australia's EarlyNuts study showed a dramatic increase in early peanut introduction after their 2016 guideline update—from 28% in 2007–2011 to 78% by 2018–2019 (Soriano et al., 2021). In contrast, USA uptake of the NIAID guidelines was disappointing. Multiple surveys reported poor physician awareness and low implementation rates

(Chang et al., 2020; Gupta et al., 2020; Saini et al., 2021a, b; Sandhu et al., 2021), with many pediatricians uncomfortable conducting oral challenges. Additionally, a national survey found that nearly half of new U.S. parents preferred to delay peanut introduction until after 11 months, reflecting poor public awareness and uptake (Greenhawt et al., 2018).

2021 North American Consensus Guidelines

The most current organizational recommendations regarding primary prevention of food allergies through nutrition come from the publication of a consensus document from the American Academy of Allergy, Asthma, and Immunology (AAAAI); American College of Allergy, Asthma, and Immunology (ACAAI); and the Canadian Society for Allergy and Clinical Immunology (CSACI) (Fleischer et al., 2021). The authors acknowledge there is sufficient evidence to include egg as a target food for early introduction alongside peanut. They also recommend that all infants be introduced to peanut and egg beginning around 6 months of life, irrespective of relative risk and that screening is "not required." They pointed out that implementation of early allergen introduction in the USA and Canada lags behind other developed countries like Australia with strong public health infrastructures. Additionally, screening high-risk infants likely leads to delays in early introduction causing them to miss a critical window of opportunity. Finally, they recommend, "Recruiting more implementation science researchers into the field, devoting more research funding to implementation, incorporating best practices from other successful countries, and other strategies are needed" (Fleischer et al., 2021, p. 18).

European Guidelines

In 2021, the European Academy of Allergy and Clinical Immunology (EAACI) updated the 2014 guidelines with recommendations to introduce cooked egg to all infants and infant-safe peanut in populations with high prevalence rates without routine pre-screening during routine complementary feeding during infancy (Halken et al., 2021). The update to the guidelines suggested that 4–6 months of age was the ideal time to introduce these allergens to prevent the development of food allergy. Overall, the updated guidelines suggest that families feed infants typical foods consumed by their community around 4–6 months of age when the infant is developmentally ready and not avoid feeding allergenic foods. Furthermore, updates to the guidelines included the recommendation that infants avoid exposure to cow's milk formula during the first week after birth to avoid early sensitization (Halken et al., 2021). See Fig. 3 for a summary of all food allergy research and guidelines.

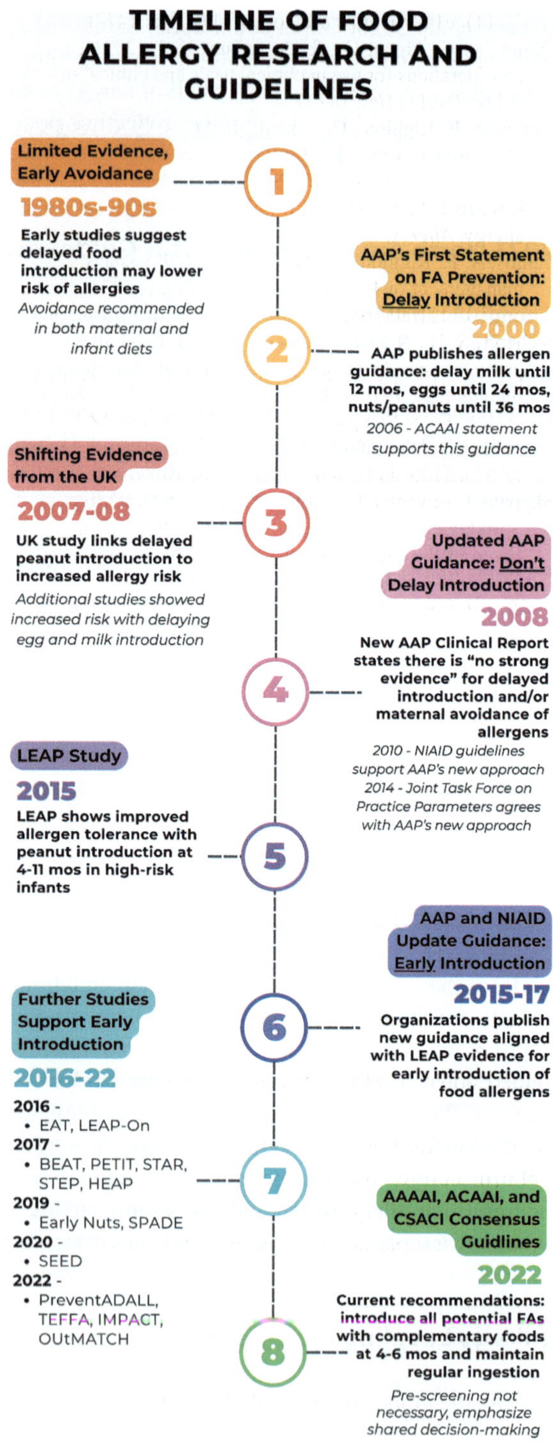

Fig. 3 Summary timeline of Food Allergy Research and Guidelines from 1980 to present. *Note.* Source: Timeline created by Kristen Bowersox, APRN. (Content adapted from Abrams and Becker (2015), Bellach et al. (2017), Conway et al. (2024), Du Toit et al. (2008, 2015), Lachover-Roth et al. (2023), Palmer et al. (2013, 2017), Perkin et al. (2016), Tan et al. (2017), and Sakihara et al. (2021))

Universal Implementation

The 2021 North American Consensus Guidelines (Fleisher et al., 2021) give a strong recommendation for universal implementation of egg and peanut early introduction based on the available literature, a cost analysis, and the national guidelines of other countries. The cost analysis indicates that compared to other policies, universal introduction cost less, prevented more cases of food allergy, and produced better long-term quality of life for patients (Fleischer et al., 2021). It is noteworthy, however, that the EAACI guidelines apply caution to the generalizability of the evidence to all countries and are careful to say the early introduction recommendations apply to countries where peanut allergy prevalence is currently high.

Risk Stratification and Prescreening

As mentioned, the North American Consensus Guidelines state that pre-screening infants is "not required" and recent Canadian Guidelines take it a step further and say prescreening is "not recommended" (Chan et al., 2024). Fleischer et al. (2021) cite the Australian Early Nuts Study, which recommends a non-screening approach that has been demonstrated to be safe and highly effective in supporting adherence to early introduction guidelines. However, risk stratification remains important in order to focus on infants and families with the highest risk. Fleischer et al. (2021) define the highest risk infants as having severe eczema and infants with mild-moderate eczema and/or parent history of atopic disease as being at some increased risk of developing food allergy. Besides the *2017 NIAID Addendum Guidelines,* no major guideline from developed countries recommends a pre-screening approach. Ultimately, pre-screening approaches may lead to a delay in early introduction for the infants that need it the most.

Early and Often

Newer guidelines emphasize the need to continue a food on a regular basis once it is introduced into the diet. For example, in 2023 the Australasian Society of Clinical Immunology and Allergy recommended to "continue to give the foods to the child regularly (twice weekly), as part of a varied diet, to maintain tolerance. Trying a food and then not giving it regularly may result in food allergy development" (Australasian Society of Clinical Immunology and Allergy, 2023).

Helping to Make Early Introduction Practical for Families

The "Window of Opportunity" and Barriers to Early Introduction

A notable risk of not adhering to the early introduction guidelines is missing what Du Toit and team (2018, p. 33) have termed, "a window of opportunity"—the period of time during a child's first year of life within which to influence a tolerogenic response to potential food allergens. Du Toit suggests this window exists between 4 and 11 months of age, with specific response depending on the individual child's history of other food allergies, eczema, and/or additional risk factors. Roberts et al. (2023) narrow this window even further, suggesting a need for early peanut introduction by 6 months of age for the whole population, with even earlier intervention from 4 months of age in children with eczema. A 2021 study found that while less than 20% of infants with severe eczema under 6 months reacted to peanuts during an oral food challenge, that number grew to 50% at 8 months of age (Keet et al., 2021). Clearly, time is of the essence for introducing food allergens, particularly for infants with underlying risk factors. Nurses play an essential role in confronting informational and psychological barriers to early introduction of food allergens, thus increasing the number of children who are able to benefit from this window of opportunity.

In an analysis of parental feedback to the EAT trial, Voorheis (2019) found that infant food refusal, parental fears about reactions, and practical barriers were the most common reasons caregivers did not comply with early introduction recommendations, *see* Fig. 4. Voorheis also found that poor adherence was associated with

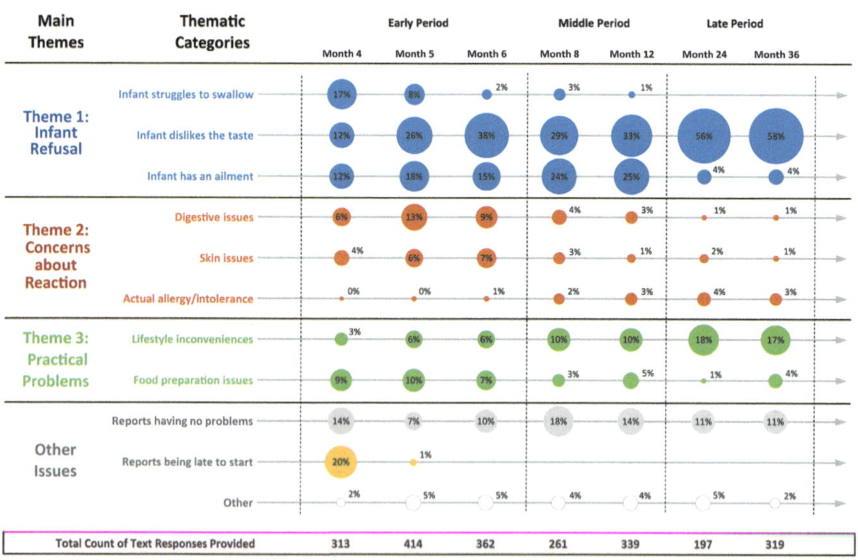

Fig. 4 Longitudinal bubble chart of caregiver responses to Enquiring About Tolerance (EAT). (Used with permission from: Paula Voorheis et al. Elsevier. Published under CC BY 4.0 https://creativecommons.org/licenses/by/4.0/)

older maternal age, non-white ethnicity, and lower maternal quality of life at enrollment, so increased attention to families with these risk factors is key. Regarding infant food refusal, repeated exposure to novel or disliked foods that occurs in a positive, supportive environment has been shown to promote the acceptance of and eventual preference for those foods (Voorheis, 2019). Practical barriers should be addressed in an individualized approach such as helping caregivers identify ways to offer foods in a desired consistency, presenting foods in a palatable way, and adopting a consistent routine for mealtimes (Voorheis, 2019). Companies have begun producing infant meals specifically containing food allergens and marketed to decrease allergy risk; these products may be useful to some families but may also be cost-prohibitive to others.

Patient education focusing on methods of safe infant feeding, the relatively low incidence of food allergy, and evidence that first-time reactions tend to be mild in infants compared to older age groups can help address parental fears (Biazon, 2022). Acknowledgement of the change in food introduction guidelines helps to assuage caregiver concern and confusion too. Additionally, if allergenic foods can be encouraged not only for their potential to prevent food allergies but also for their healthfulness to the developing child, decision-making may be positively influenced (Voorheis, 2019).

According to Tepler et al. (2022), common difficulties with early introduction cited by pediatricians include uncertainty about implementation of early introduction guideline recommendations, clinic time limitations, and pediatric office capability to conduct supervised oral challenges. Nursing staff informed about food allergy prevention and management can provide patient education to decrease these barriers. A written decision aid for early introduction could be a useful tool in this approach to shared decision-making between providers and families (Schroer et al., 2021), such as an algorithm below (see Fig. 5) or pediatric food allergy resources. It is essential for nurses to work closely with allergists to ensure that high-risk infants are seen promptly and do not miss the window of opportunity for preventing food allergies.

Shared Decision-Making

Although the North American Consensus authors advocate for a universal approach without pre-screening, they also support the use of shared decision-making regarding screening and in-office oral food challenges (Fleischer et al., 2021). For example, in the case of an infant with severe atopic dermatitis living in a rural setting without quick access to emergency services, perhaps the provider and caregivers will feel more comfortable screening. If screening is performed, the primary care provider (PCP) should refer to the NIAID-AG algorithm for appropriate follow-up, and avoid food panel testing due to poor positive predictive values of tests (Togias et al., 2017). If a caregiver of an infant with a sibling with food allergies is fearful of doing early introduction, perhaps that parent would be better supported with an

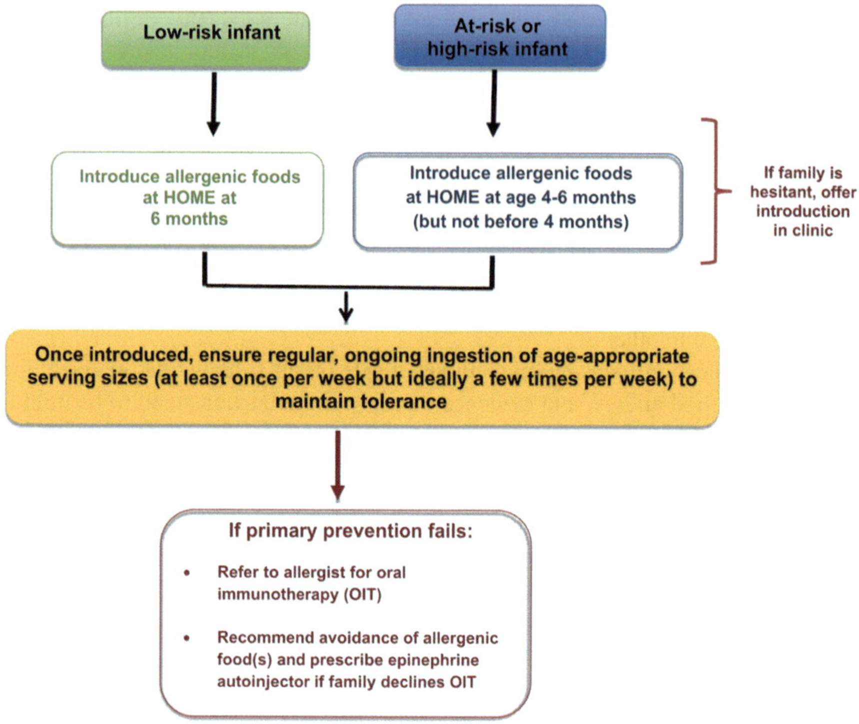

Fig. 5 Simplified algorithm for the primary prevention of food allergy. *Note.* Simplified algorithm for the primary prevention of food allergy. (Used with permission from: By Edmond S. Chan. In: Primary prevention of food allergy: beyond early introduction, https://doi.org/10.1186/s13223-024-00924-5, BMC, Part of Springer Nature, Published under CC BY 4.0 https://creativecommons.org/licenses/by/4.0/)

in-office oral food challenge or urgent (time is of the essence!) allergy referral. Virtual visits may be a convenient option to help reduce anxiety in caregivers when attempting early introduction for the first time at home. PCPs and nurses should individualize care, while remaining acutely aware of the potential harms of over-screening (poor positive predictive values, delay in infants who need it the most) and knowledgeable of the rationale behind current evidence-based guidelines.

Nursing Role in Educating Parents and Caregivers on Early Introduction

Nurses should start the conversation early, around the 1–2-month well-baby visit, before the baby is ready developmentally for complementary foods. Then, recommend introduction of safe peanut-based foods in the infant's diet around 4–6 months if the infant is ready for solid food (see Fig. 6).

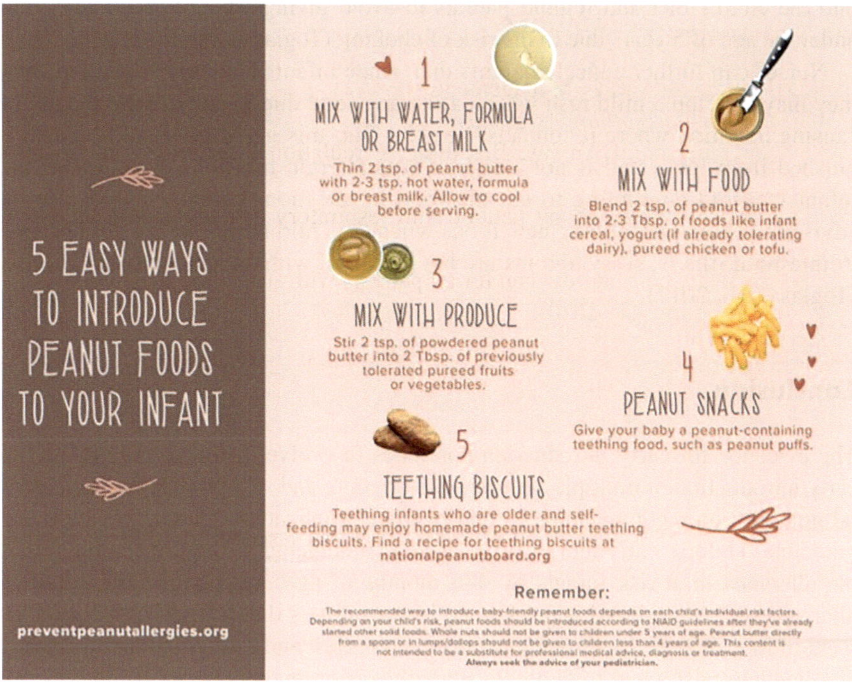
5 EASY WAYS
TO INTRODUCE
PEANUT FOODS
TO YOUR INFANT
preventpeanutallergies.org
1
MIX WITH WATER, FORMULA
OR BREAST MILK
Thin 2 tsp. of peanut butter with 2-3 tsp. hot water, formula or breast milk. Allow to cool before serving.
2
MIX WITH FOOD
Blend 2 tsp. of peanut butter into 2-3 Tbsp. of foods like infant cereal, yogurt (if already tolerating dairy), pureed chicken or tofu.
3
MIX WITH PRODUCE
Stir 2 tsp. of powdered peanut butter into 2 Tbsp. of previously tolerated pureed fruits or vegetables.
4
PEANUT SNACKS
Give your baby a peanut-containing teething food, such as peanut puffs.
5
TEETHING BISCUITS
Teething infants who are older and self-feeding may enjoy homemade peanut butter teething biscuits. Find a recipe for teething biscuits at
nationalpeanutboard.org
Remember:
The recommended way to introduce baby-friendly peanut foods depends on each child's individual risk factors. Depending on your child's risk, peanut foods should be introduced according to NIAID guidelines after they've already started other solid foods. Whole nuts should not be given to children under 5 years of age. Peanut butter directly from a spoon or in lumps/dollops should not be given to children less than 4 years of age. This content is not intended to be a substitute for professional medical advice, diagnosis or treatment.
Always seek the advice of your pediatrician.

Fig. 6 Five easy ways to introduce peanut foods to your infant. (Used with permission from: National Peanut Board. (2025). Five easy ways to introduce peanut foods to your infant retrieved from https://nationalpeanutboard.org/news/5-easy-ideas-to-introduce-peanut-to-infants/)

Instructions for Safe Peanut Introduction to Infants (National Peanut Board, 2025; Togias et al., 2017)

1. Mix 2 tsp of smooth peanut butter thinned with 2–3 tsp. of warmed breast milk, water, or formula (cool before feeding).
2. Blend 2 tsp of smooth peanut butter/peanut powder into 2–3 tbsp of infant cereal, fruit, applesauce, or yogurt (if not dairy allergic).
3. Mix 2 tsp of smooth peanut butter/peanut powder into 2 tbsp of any fruit or vegetable purees.
4. Once peanut is introduced into the diet safely, the allergen should be included in the infant's diet 3 times a week continually to prevent the development of food allergy and incorporating peanut into baked goods and sauces and/or provide teething biscuits with peanut protein into toddlerhood.

The Addendum Guidelines advise that the infant receive 2 grams of peanut protein in an age-appropriate food (approximately 2 teaspoons of peanut butter/powder) at any meal or snack three times a week. Parents and caregivers should be advised to avoid giving peanut butter in lumps or dollops on a spoon until after 4 years of age due to choking risks. Peanuts should not be the first food introduced into the child's diet and remind parents to avoid giving whole nuts to any child under the age of 5 years due to the risk of choking (Togias et al., 2017).

Nurses can further educate parents that, since infants have very sensitive skin, they may develop a mild rash when eating any food due to enzymes in the saliva causing irritation where it contacts the skin. But, this irritation should be distinguished from hives and is not a sign of true allergic reaction or reason for the infant to avoid continuing to eat the food in question. Parents should also be advised to avoid introducing new foods when the child is sick with a cold or gastrointestinal illness, so symptoms are not confused with an anaphylactic reaction (Togias et al., 2017).

Conclusion

The evidence for early introduction continues to evolve. Clinical trials related to early introduction of multiple allergens are ongoing and will provide further parental guidance on recommendations and practical application. Current research and guidelines endorse early introduction of all complementary foods, including possible allergens in at-risk infants by 4–6 months of age, and continued feeding of allergens once introduced and tolerated in the infant's diet to reduce the development of food allergy. As trusted educators, advocates, and care-coordinators, nurses are uniquely positioned to facilitate shared decision-making, support food allergy guidelines, and assist families to overcome barriers to prevent food allergy. Whether virtually guiding an anxious mother with a food allergy through her baby's first peanut introduction, debunking myths about anaphylaxis, or partnering with a patient scheduler to accelerate infant allergy referrals, nurses are well-positioned to ensure caregivers of infants receive comprehensive food allergy prevention education as the science evolves. The resources page at the end of the book includes websites containing information on early introduction of other allergens.

References

Abrams, E. M., & Becker, A. B. (2015). Food introduction and allergy prevention in infants. *CMAJ: Canadian Medical Association Journal = Journal de l'Association Medicale Canadienne, 187*(17), 1297–1301. https://doi.org/10.1503/cmaj.150364

Al-Saud, B., & Sigurdardóttir, S. T. (2018). Early introduction of egg and the development of egg allergy in children: A systematic review and meta-analysis. *International Archives of Allergy and Immunology, 177*(4), 350–359. https://doi.org/10.1159/000492131

Australasian Society of Clinical Immunology and Allergy. (2023). *ASCIA fast facts: Infant feeding and allergy prevention*. https://www.allergy.org.au/images/pc/ff/ASCIA_PC_FAST_FACTS_Infant_feeding_allergy_prevention_2023.pdf

Bahna, S. L. (2024). History of food allergy and where we are today. *The World Allergy Organization Journal, 17*(5), 100912. https://doi.org/10.1016/j.waojou.2024.100912

Bellach, J., Schwarz, V., Ahrens, B., Trendelenburg, V., Aksünger, Ö., Kalb, B., et al. (2017). Randomized placebo-controlled trial of hen's egg consumption for primary prevention in infants. *Journal of Allergy and Clinical Immunology, 139*(5), 1591–1599.

Biazon, L. (2022). *Integration of early introduction guidelines for the primary prevention of food allergy into infant well child checks within a pediatric primary care setting*. University of Virginia. https://doi.org/10.18130/h2dj-qs32

Boyce, J. A., Assa'ad, A., Burks, A. W., Jones, S. M., Sampson, H. A., Wood, R. A., Plaut, M., Cooper, S. F., Fenton, M. J., Arshad, S. H., Bahna, S. L., Beck, L. A., Byrd-Bredbenner, C., Camargo, C. A., Jr, Eichenfield, L., Furuta, G. T., Hanifin, J. M., Jones, C., Kraft, M., Levy, B. D., … Schwaninger, J. M. (2011). Guidelines for the diagnosis and management of food allergy in the United States: summary of the NIAID-sponsored expert panel report. *Nutrition research (New York, N.Y.), 31*(1), 61–75. https://doi.org/10.1016/j.nutres.2011.01.001

Branum, A. M., & Lukacs, S. L. (2008). Food allergy among U.S. children: Trends in prevalence and hospitalizations. *NCHS Data Brief, 10*, 1–8. Hyattsville, National Center for Health Statistics.

Chan, E. S., Abrams, E. M., Mack, D. P., Protudjer, J. L. P., & Watson, W. (2024). Primaryprevention of food allergy: Beyond early introduction. *Allergy, Asthma & Clinical Immunology, 20*(Suppl 3), Article 71. https://doi.org/10.1186/s13223-024-00924-5

Chang, A., Cabana, M. D., LaFlam, T. N., Patel, S., & Okumura, M. (2020). Early peanut introduction and testing: A framework for general pediatrician beliefs and practices. *Pediatric Allergy, Immunology, and Pulmonology*. https://doi.org/10.1089/ped.2020.1190

Conway, A. E., Greenhawt, M., Abrams, E. M., & Shaker, M. S. (2024). Food allergy prevention through the decades: An ounce of humility is worth a pound of cure. *Journal of Food Allergy, 6*(1), 3–14. https://doi.org/10.2500/jfa.2024.6.230018

de Silva, D., Halken, S., Singh, C., Muraro, A., Angier, E., Arasi, S., Arshad, H., Beyer, K., Boyle, R., Du Toit, G., Eigenmann, P., Grimshaw, K., Hoest, A., Jones, C., Khaleva, E., Lack, G., Szajewska, H., Venter, C., Verhasselt, V., et al. (2020). Preventing food allergy in infancy and childhood: Systematic review of randomised controlled trials. *Pediatric Allergy and Immunology, 31*(7), 813–826. https://doi.org/10.1111/pai.13273

Du Toit, G., Katz, Y., Sasieni, P., Mesher, D., Maleki, S. J., Fisher, H. R., Fox, A. T., Turcanu, V., Amir, T., Zadik-Mnuhin, G., Cohen, A., Livne, I., & Lack, G. (2008). Early consumption of peanuts in infancy is associated with a low prevalence of peanut allergy. *The Journal of Allergy and Clinical Immunology, 122*(5), 984–991. https://doi.org/10.1016/j.jaci.2008.08.039

Du Toit, G., Roberts, G., Sayre, P. H., Bahnson, H. T., Radulovic, S., Santos, A. F., Brough, H. A., Phippard, D., Basting, M., Feeney, M., Turcanu, V., Sever, M. L., Gomez Lorenzo, M., Plaut, M., & Lack, G. (2015). Randomized trial of peanut consumption in infants at risk for peanut allergy. *New England Journal of Medicine, 372*(9), 803–813. https://doi.org/10.1056/nejmoa1414850

Du Toit, G., Sampson, H. A., Plaut, M., Burks, A. W., Akdis, C. A., & Lack, G. (2018). Food allergy: Update on prevention and tolerance. *The Journal of Allergy and Clinical Immunology, 141*(1), 30–40. https://doi.org/10.1016/j.jaci.2017.11.010

Fiocchi, A., Assa'ad, A., Bahna, S., Adverse Reactions to Foods Committee, & American College of Allergy, Asthma and Immunology. (2006). Food allergy and the introduction of solid foods to infants: A consensus document. Adverse Reactions to Foods Committee, American College of Allergy, Asthma and Immunology. *Annals of Allergy, Asthma & Immunology: Official Publication of the American College of Allergy, Asthma, & Immunology, 97*(1), 10–77. https://doi.org/10.1016/s1081-1206(10)61364-6

Fleischer, D. M., Chan, E. S., Venter, C., Spergel, J. M., Abrams, E. M., Stukus, D., et al. (2021). A consensus approach to the primary prevention of food allergy through nutrition: Guidance from the American Academy of Allergy, Asthma & Immunology; The American College of Allergy, Asthma & Immunology; and the Canadian Society for Allergy and Clinical Immunology. *Journal of Allergy and Clinical Immunology: In Practice, 9*(1), 22–43.e4. https://doi.org/10.1016/j.jaip.2020.11.002

Greenhawt, M., Chan, E. S., Fleischer, D. M., Hicks, A., Wilson, R., Shaker, M., Venter, C., & Stukus, D. (2018). Caregiver and expecting caregiver support for early peanut introduction guidelines. *Annals of Allergy, Asthma & Immunology: Official Publication of the American College of Allergy, Asthma, & Immunology, 120*(6), 620–625. https://doi.org/10.1016/j.anai.2018.03.001

Greer, F. R., Sicherer, S. H., Burks, A. W., American Academy of Pediatrics Committee on Nutrition, & American Academy of Pediatrics Section on Allergy and Immunology. (2008). Effects of early nutritional interventions on the development of atopic disease in infants and children: The role of maternal dietary restriction, breastfeeding, timing of introduction of complementary foods, and hydrolyzed formulas. *Pediatrics, 121*(1), 183–191. https://doi.org/10.1542/peds.2007-3022

Gupta, R. S., Warren, C. M., Smith, B., Blumenstock, J. A., Jiang, J., Davis, M. M., et al. (2013). The economic impact of childhood food allergy in the United States. *JAMA Pediatrics, 167*(11), 1026–1031. https://doi.org/10.1001/jamapediatrics.2013.2376

Gupta, R. S., Bilaver, L. A., Johnson, J. L., Hu, J. W., Jiang, J., Bozen, A., Martin, J., Reese, J., Cooper, S. F., Davis, M. M., Togias, A., & Arbes, S. J. (2020). Assessment of pediatrician awareness and implementation of the addendum guidelines for the prevention of peanut allergy in the United States. *JAMA Network Open, 3*(7), e2010511. https://doi.org/10.1001/jamanetworkopen.2020.10511

Halken, S., Muraro, A., de Silva, D., Khaleva, E., Angier, E., Arasi, S., Arshad, H., Bahnson, H. T., Beyer, K., Boyle, R., Du Toit, G., Ebisawa, M., Eigenmann, P., Grimshaw, K., Hoest, A., Jones, C., Lack, G., Nadeau, K., O'Mahony, L., et al. (2021). EAACI guideline: Preventing the development of food allergy in infants and young children (2020 update). *Pediatric Allergy and Immunology, 32*(5), 843–858. https://doi.org/10.1111/pai.13496

Ierodiakonou, D., Garcia-Larsen, V., Logan, A., Groome, A., Cunha, S., Chivinge, J., Robinson, Z., Geoghegan, N., Jarrold, K., Reeves, T., Tagiyeva-Milne, N., Nurmatov, U., Trivella, M., Leonardi-Bee, J., & Boyle, R. J. (2016). Timing of allergenic food introduction to the infant diet and risk of allergic or autoimmune disease a systematic review and meta-analysis. *JAMA-Journal of the American Medical Association, 316*(11), 1181–1192. https://doi.org/10.1001/jama.2016.12623

Jones, S. M., Kim, E. H., Nadeau, K. C., Nowak-Wegrzyn, A., Wood, R. A., Sampson, H. A., et al. (2022). Efficacy and safety of oral immunotherapy in children aged 1–3 years with peanut allergy (the Immune Tolerance Network IMPACT trial): A randomised placebo-controlled study. *The Lancet, 399*(10322), 359–371.

Keet, C., Pistiner, M., Plesa, M., Szelag, D., Shreffler, W., Wood, R., et al. (2021). Age and eczema severity, but not family history, are major risk factors for peanut allergy in infancy. *Journal of Allergy and Clinical Immunology, 147*(3), 984–991.

Kim, J. S., Nowak-Węgrzyn, A., Sicherer, S. H., Noone, S., Moshier, E. L., & Sampson, H. A. (2011). Dietary baked milk accelerates the resolution of cow's milk allergy in children. *The Journal of Allergy and Clinical Immunology, 128*(1), 125–131.e2. https://doi.org/10.1016/j.jaci.2011.04.036

Lachover-Roth, I., Cohen-Engler, A., Furman, Y., Shachar, I., Rosman, Y., Meir-Shafrir, K., et al. (2023). Early, continuing exposure to cow's milk formula and cow's milk allergy: The COMEET study, a single center, prospective interventional study. *Annals of Allergy, Asthma & Immunology, 130*(2), 233–239.

Leonard, S. A., Sampson, H. A., Sicherer, S. H., Noone, S., Moshier, E. L., Godbold, J., & Nowak-Węgrzyn, A. (2012). Dietary baked egg accelerates resolution of egg allergy in children. *The Journal of Allergy and Clinical Immunology, 130*(2), 473–80.e1. https://doi.org/10.1016/j.jaci.2012.06.006

Matsumoto, K., Mori, R., Miyazaki, C., Ohya, Y., & Saito, H. (2018). Are both early egg introduction and eczema treatment necessary for primary prevention of egg allergy? *The Journal of Allergy and Clinical Immunology, 141*(6), 1997–2001.e3. https://doi.org/10.1016/j.jaci.2018.02.033

National Peanut Board. (2025). *How to introduce peanut to babies early*. https://nationalpeanutboard.org/resources/videos/how-to-introduce-peanut-to-babies-early/

Natsume, O., Kabashima, S., Nakazato, J., Yamamoto-Hanada, K., Narita, M., Kondo, M., et al. (2017). Two-step egg introduction for prevention of egg allergy in high-risk infants with eczema (PETIT): A randomised, double-blind, placebo-controlled trial. *The Lancet, 389*(10066), 276–286.

NIAID-Sponsored Expert Panel. (2010). Guidelines for the diagnosis and management of food allergy in the United States: Report of the NIAID-sponsored expert panel. *The Journal of Allergy and Clinical Immunology, 126*(6 Suppl), S1–S58. https://doi.org/10.1016/j.jaci.2010.10.007

Obbagy, J. E., English, L. K., Wong, Y. P., Butte, N. F., Dewey, K. G., Fleischer, D. M., Fox, M. K., Greer, F. R., Krebs, N. F., Scanlon, K. S., & Stoody, E. E. (2019). Complementary feeding and food allergy, atopic dermatitis/eczema, asthma, and allergic rhinitis: A systematic review. *American Journal of Clinical Nutrition, 109*(1), 890S–934S. https://doi.org/10.1093/ajcn/nqy220

Palmer, D. J., Metcalfe, J., Makrides, M., Gold, M. S., Quinn, P., West, C. E., et al. (2013). Early regular egg exposure in infants with eczema: A randomized controlled trial. *Journal of Allergy and Clinical Immunology, 132*(2), 387–392.

Palmer, D. J., Sullivan, T. R., Gold, M. S., Prescott, S. L., & Makrides, M. (2017). Randomized controlled trial of early regular egg intake to prevent egg allergy. *Journal of Allergy and Clinical Immunology, 139*(5), 1600–1607.

Perkin, M. R., Logan, K., Marrs, T., Radulovic, S., Craven, J., Flohr, C., et al. (2016). Enquiring About Tolerance (EAT) study: Feasibility of an early allergenic food introduction regimen. *Journal of Allergy and Clinical Immunology, 137*(5), 1477–1486.

Perkin, M. R., Bahnson, H. T., Logan, K., Marrs, T., Radulovic, S., Knibb, R., Craven, J., Flohr, C., Mills, E. N., Versteeg, S. A., van Ree, R., Lack, G., & Enquiring About Tolerance (EAT) study team. (2019). Factors influencing adherence in a trial of early introduction of allergenic food. *The Journal of Allergy and Clinical Immunology, 144*(6), 1595–1605. https://doi.org/10.1016/j.jaci.2019.06.046

Roberts, G., Bahnson, H. T., Du Toit, G., O'Rourke, C., Sever, M. L., Brittain, E., Plaut, M., & Lack, G. (2023). Defining the window of opportunity and target populations to prevent peanut allergy. *The Journal of Allergy and Clinical Immunology, 151*(5), 1329–1336. https://doi.org/10.1016/j.jaci.2022.09.042

Saini, S. D., Hassan, M., & DeBiasi, A. (2021a). Implementation gaps in the NIAID peanut allergy prevention guidelines: A qualitative study of pediatric clinician perspectives. *The Journal of Allergy and Clinical Immunology: In Practice, 9*(4), 1706–1708. https://doi.org/10.1016/j.jaip.2020.11.043

Saini, S., Tran, C.-L., Huang, J., Seth, D., & Poowuttikul, P. (2021b). A quality improvement initiative to improve resident-physician practices regarding peanut introduction in infancy. *Journal of Allergy and Clinical Immunology, 147*(2), AB101. https://doi.org/10.1016/j.jaci.2020.12.377

Sakihara, T., Otsuji, K., Arakaki, Y., Hamada, K., Sugiura, S., & Ito, K. (2021). Randomized trial of early infant formula introduction to prevent cow's milk allergy. *Journal of Allergy and Clinical Immunology, 147*(1), 224. https://doi.org/10.1016/j.jaci.2020.08.021

Sandhu, S., Hanono, M., Rabin, C., Harriz, R., Nagarajan, S., & Vastardi, M.-A. (2021). Assessment of early peanut introduction guidelines among pediatricians in an inner-city hospital. *Journal of Allergy and Clinical Immunology, 147*(2), AB99. https://doi.org/10.1016/j.jaci.2020.12.372

Scarpone, R., Kimkool, P., Ierodiakonou, D., Leonardi-Bee, J., Garcia-Larsen, V., Perkin, M. R., & Boyle, R. J. (2023). Timing of allergenic food introduction and risk of immunoglobulin e-mediated food allergy: a systematic review and meta-analysis. *JAMA pediatrics, 177*(5), 489–497. https://doi.org/10.1001/jamapediatrics.2023.0142

Schepel, I. R., Humiston, T., D'Ambrosi, G., Dupuis, R., Monuteaux, M. C., Herbert, L. J., et al. (2025). Food allergy-related bullying: Risk factors and psychosocial functioning. *Pediatric Allergy and Immunology, 36*(4), e70081.

Schroer, B., Groetch, M., Mack, D. P., & Venter, C. (2021). Practical challenges and considerations for early introduction of potential food allergens for prevention of food allergy. *The Journal of Allergy and Clinical Immunology. In Practice, 9*(1), 44–56.e1. https://doi.org/10.1016/j.jaip.2020.10.031

Skjerven, H. O., Lie, A., Vettukattil, R., Rehbinder, E. M., LeBlanc, M., Asarnoj, A., et al. (2022). Early food intervention and skin emollients to prevent food allergy in young children (PreventADALL): A factorial, multicentre, cluster-randomised trial. *The Lancet, 399*(10344), 2398–2411.

Soriano, V., Peters, R., Ponsonby, A.-L., Perrett, K., Dharmage, S., Gurrin, L., & Koplin, J. (2021). Has the prevalence of peanut allergy changed following earlier introduction of peanut? The Earlynuts study. *Journal of Allergy and Clinical Immunology, 147*(2), AB236. https://doi.org/10.1016/j.jaci.2020.12.009

Tan, J. W., Tham, E. H., Panetta, J. M., et al. (2017). Beating Egg Allergy Trial (BEAT): Raw egg powder introduction. *Clinical & Experimental Allergy, 47*(8), 1029–1037. https://doi.org/10.1111/cea.12931

Tepler, E., Wong, K. H., & Soffer, G. K. (2022). Health disparities in pediatric food allergy. *Annals of Allergy, Asthma & Immunology: Official Publication of the American College of Allergy, Asthma, & Immunology, 129*(4), 417–423. https://doi.org/10.1016/j.anai.2022.04.022

Togias, A., Cooper, S. F., Acebal, M. L., Assa'ad, A., Baker, J. R., Beck, L. A., Block, J., Byrd-Bredbenner, C., Chan, E. S., Eichenfield, L. F., Fleischer, D. M., Fuchs, G. J., Furuta, G. T., Greenhawt, M. J., Gupta, R. S., Habich, M., Jones, S. M., Keaton, K., Muraro, A., et al. (2017). Addendum guidelines for the prevention of peanut allergy in the United States: Report of the National Institute of Allergy and Infectious Diseases-sponsored expert panel. *The Journal of Allergy and Clinical Immunology, 139*(1), 29–44. https://doi.org/10.1016/j.jaci.2016.10.010

U.S. Bureau of Labor Statistics. (n.d.). *CPI inflation calculator*. U.S. Department of Labor. Retrieved July 10, 2025, from https://www.bls.gov/data/inflation_calculator.htm

Voorheis, P., Bell, S., Cornelsen, L., Quaife, M., Logan, K., Marrs, T., Radulovic, S., Craven, J., Flohr, C., Lack, G., Perkin, M. R., & Enquiring About Tolerance (EAT) study team. (2019). Challenges experienced with early introduction and sustained consumption of allergenic foods in the Enquiring About Tolerance (EAT) study: A qualitative analysis. *The Journal of Allergy and Clinical Immunology, 144*(6), 1615–1623. https://doi.org/10.1016/j.jaci.2019.09.004

Zeiger, R. S., Heller, S., Mellon, M. H., et al. (1989). Effect of combined maternal and infant food-allergen avoidance on development of atopy in early infancy: A randomized study. *The Journal of Allergy and Clinical Immunology, 84*, 72–89.

Food Allergy Management in Early Childhood Settings

Laura Warnock Koo, Erin O'Grady, and Leslie Speer

Introduction

With the incidence of food allergies in children on the rise, it is imperative that early childhood settings, including daycares and primary/elementary schools, be equipped with the knowledge and skills to care for those with food allergies. Globally, food allergy affects approximately one in twelve children with an increasing prevalence (Tanno & Demoly, 2022). In the United States, food allergy affects an estimated 6%–8% of children, or about one in thirteen children (Gupta et al., 2018; Asthma and Allergy Foundation of America, Elijah-Alavi Foundation, 2022). Nurses are integral to educating families and facility staff on allowing these children to attend school in a safe and inclusive environment. Food allergy reactions are unpredictable, and about one in four students who have a severe reaction at school have no known history of food allergy (Centers for Disease Control and Prevention [CDC], 2013). Early recognition and prompt treatment is vital for a positive outcome during an allergic reaction. All staff, including teachers, administration staff, and kitchen workers, must be trained in preventing, recognizing, and treating allergic reactions so children can safely attend these settings (Waserman et al., 2021). Living with food allergies can potentially lead to a decreased quality of life especially if

L. W. Koo (✉)
University of Maryland School of Nursing, Baltimore, MD, USA
e-mail: lkoo@umaryland.edu

E. O'Grady
Food Allergy Nurses Association (FANA), Great Neck, NY, USA
e-mail: erin.th.ogrady@gmail.com

L. Speer
Monroe Carell Jr. Children's Hospital at Vanderbilt, Nashville, TN, USA
e-mail: leslie.m.speer@vumc.org

J. Doucette, J. Howard-Ruben (eds.), *Comprehensive Food Allergy Management for Nurses*, https://doi.org/10.1007/978-3-032-28647-5_7

participation in certain activities, such as school craft projects, is limited out of fear of reacting (Waserman et al., 2021). Nurses can help improve children's quality of life by advocating for safety in all settings. Many prevention strategies can help ensure children remain safe, and these will be discussed throughout this chapter. While school management strategies may vary by region, the basic principles of food allergy prevention and recognition for children from infancy through primary school remain the same. Nurses in school and childcare settings are key players who provide staff training for food allergy management and advocate for institutional policies related to exposure prevention, epinephrine access, and emergency management. Nurses should remain up to date with the latest best practices for the prevention, recognition, and management of allergic reactions and learn about the relevant policies in childcare and school settings.

Risk Prevention Strategies in Childcare and Schools

The standard of care for preventing a food-induced anaphylaxis or allergic reaction is avoiding the food allergen (Golden et al., 2024). Therefore, methods to prevent allergen exposure are the primary strategies to manage food allergies. In childcare and school settings where young children require adult supervision for their safety, the facility staff caring for these children are the key players who must prevent allergen exposure. Facility staff members may include teachers, childcare workers, aides, food service workers, administrators, nurses, maintenance staff, bus drivers, and other childcare/school personnel (Centers for Disease Control and Prevention CDC, 2013; Waserman et al., 2021). Significant strategies for reducing the risk of allergen exposure include annual staff education, institutional emergency preparedness, and institutional-based policies and guidelines (Santos et al., 2022). Yet, food allergy management practices, policies, and guidelines vary widely from one jurisdiction to another and from one school or childcare center to another (Asthma and Allergy Foundation of America, Elijah-Alavi Foundation, 2022; Santos et al., 2022; Food Allergy Canada, 2024).

The most common policies and guidelines for food allergy management in early childhood institutions include recognizing anaphylaxis, using individual and institutional emergency management plans, and facilitating the availability of epinephrine devices. Other policies or guidelines to prevent allergen exposure recommend staff training include topics such as safe handling of food, handwashing, surface cleaning, reading food labels, no food sharing, mealtime supervision, allergen-safe zones (tables or desks) for children who are unable to self-manage, reviewing classroom projects for allergens, planning for special events and off-site activities, teacher-parent communication, educating children and parents, and more (Table 1) (CDC, 2013; Waserman et al., 2021; Santos et al., 2022; National Allergy Council, 2023a, b; Food Allergy Management in Schools Advisory Panel [FAMS], 2024). Of note, the evidence does not support the use of allergen-free zones, such as "peanut-free tables," except in settings where children cannot self-manage avoidance of allergens, such as infants or toddlers (Waserman et al., 2021; Golden et al., 2024). Such food restrictions may induce a false sense of security, decrease vigilance, and increase the

Table 1 Strategies to prevent food allergen exposure and respond to food-induced anaphylaxis in early childhood settings

Location	Recommended strategies
Facility site-wide	Stock undesignated epinephrine Have quick access to epinephrine Allow students who are mature enough to self-carry epinephrine devices Train staff in the prevention, recognition, and treatment of allergic reactions to foods Use epinephrine only for suspected anaphylaxis, rather than for all types of allergic reactions Wash hands with soap and water before and after handling food Require up-to-date individual emergency care plans Implement site-wide protocols or universal emergency care plans for allergic reactions to food Do not prohibit specific foods site-wide Nurses should educate children, parents, and staff about food allergies
Classroom	Do not establish allergen-restricted zones, except in limited circumstances (infants, toddlers; physical or cognitive impairments) Prevent cross-contact of food allergens bystoring snacks or meals appropriately Avoid using food allergens in projects, crafts, snacks, celebrations Offer non-food prizes and gifts Avoid ordering food from restaurants; allergens may be present but not reported Help students read food labels to avoid ingesting allergens Support parents who provide allergen-safe snacks in case of unexpected circumstances Inform substitute teachers about children with special needs, including food allergies
Cafeteria	Do not establish allergen-restricted zones, except in limited circumstances (infants, toddlers; physical or cognitive impairments) Prevent cross-contact of food allergens through allergen-safe food preparation and serving and cleaning surfaces with recommended products such as soap and water or disinfectants Read all food labels for allergens and re check labels with each purchase Be prepared to share food and all ingredients in foods served; keep labels for at least 24 h after servicing; keep contact info for all vendors to request ingredient information Make reasonable meal accommodations per doctor's dietary orders Provide copies of menus in advance to parents for planning Do not permit sharing food or utensils Create procedures for identifying children with food allergies and maintaining privacy protections with parent and student cooperation. Report mistakes (cross-contact mishaps, ingredient list errors) immediately to administrators & parents

(continued)

Table 1 (continued)

Location	Recommended strategies
Transportation	Do not allow eating on buses except for those with special needs (e.g., diabetes)
Events (excursions, celebrations, before or after school activities)	Plan to ensure safety of those with food allergies on field trips and during events or extracurricular activities Prevent cross-contact of food allergens by packaging meals and snacks safely Identify special needs before trips or events; find out if location is safe for young children with food allergies Make sure events are consistent with food allergy policies
Physical education and recess	Plan to ensure safety of children with food allergies during physical education and recess

Note: All recommendations are subject to local laws, regulations, and institutional policies
Adapted from Refs. (CDC, 2013; FAMS, 2024; National Allergy Council, 2023a, b; Santos et al., 2022; Waserman et al., 2021)

risks of isolation or bullying (Waserman et al., 2021; Lawlis et al., 2017). Therefore, some policies or guidelines should be changed according to the current evidence.

Recognizing Anaphylaxis in Young Children

Anaphylaxis and allergic reactions can present in many different ways. All staff members at schools and other early childhood settings must be familiar with the various signs of an allergic reaction. In multiple countries, including Australia and the United States, guidelines recommend age-appropriate education for children to help raise awareness and manage anaphylaxis (National Allergy Council, 2023b; Keller & Stanislo, 2023). Symptoms during an allergic reaction can vary in type and severity with each response. Anaphylaxis is defined as a serious, systemic hypersensitivity reaction that is usually rapid in onset and may cause death. Severe anaphylaxis is characterized by potentially life-threatening compromise in respiration and/or circulation, and it may occur without typical skin features, circulatory shock, or compromised breathing being present (Golden et al., 2024).

Recognizing anaphylaxis in young children and infants can be challenging. Infants and young children are unable to communicate their symptoms effectively, and many signs of anaphylaxis in infants can be indistinguishable from normal infant behaviors. Significant symptoms to look for in this age group include sudden behavior changes such as inconsolable crying, withdrawal, irritability or clinging, pulling, scratching, fingers in mouth or ears, cough, throat clearing, and voice changes (Golden et al., 2024). Studies suggest infants experience skin symptoms more often during an allergic reaction compared to older children, though caregivers working with this young age group should also be aware of all possible symptoms of an allergic reaction (Golden et al., 2024). Because symptoms in this age group rely heavily on objective symptoms, high-quality training on recognition and prompt intervention is critical (Also see Table 1, chapter "Understanding the Diagnosis and Management of Food Allergy Part I: IgE-Mediated Food Allergy and Anaphylaxis" and Fig. 2, chapter "Food Allergy Management in the Hospital Setting").

If an allergic reaction is suspected, staff should immediately follow the child's emergency care plan if one is in place or general emergency policies for treating allergic reactions (Golden et al., 2024). While knowing which children have food allergies is helpful for risk prevention, caregivers should be knowledgeable about general emergency response policies for an allergic reaction in a child with no known history or no plan in place because one in four students who have a severe reaction at school have no known history of food allergy (CDC, 2013). Early recognition of an allergic reaction can be the difference between a swift recovery and a potentially fatal outcome.

Increased awareness about food allergies and allergic reactions for caregivers and students can lead to faster treatment and help create an environment where those with food allergies feel supported. Posters with age-appropriate pictures and descriptions of allergic reactions can aid in creating this environment. Posters, flyers, and interactive learning activities for families, caregivers, and facility staff are available online, many of which are printable and free. A collection of these resources can be found in the Resources Page at the end of the book. Nurses can also recommend additional online training resources for facility staff that provide education on recognizing and treating allergic reactions.

Emergency Response for Anaphylactic Reactions

It is estimated that a median of 10% (range 0%–29%) of reported cases of anaphylaxis in children of any severity occur at childcare centers or schools across studies in Spain, Japan, Australia, and the United States (Waserman et al., 2021). According to the Organisation for Economic Co-operation and Development (2023), an international organization that helps countries compare and set policies, the time spent in primary education varies. The United States and Australia have the highest average number of hours, about one-third of the child's waking hours, while Spain and Japan have lower average hours, spending around 20% less time in school. While the risk of anaphylaxis in schools is low, the amount of time a child spends in school is high (Hall & Nielsen, 2020). This makes it vital for schools and childcare centers to have a plan to handle food allergy reactions if they occur.

International practice guidelines developed by interest holders from Canada, the United States, Mexico, Japan, Ireland, Australia, and Italy report that institutional policies for treating allergic reactions in childcare centers and schools vary widely and often depend on local laws and policies in the respective countries. These practice guidelines for childcare and school staff recommend following individualized allergy emergency care plans, maintaining stock epinephrine, and implementing a general emergency response plan for children with no known history of food allergy (Waserman et al., 2021). Individualized allergy emergency care plans should be kept in a location that caregivers can easily access in an emergency but not visible to the public to protect patient privacy (Waserman et al., 2021).

Prompt epinephrine administration for severe reactions is the gold standard for food allergy reaction treatment and is most effective in preventing poor outcomes;

for patients without a history of food allergy, stock or undesignated epinephrine may be used for treatment if available. Epinephrine should be used when symptoms of anaphylaxis are present, and emergency medical services be notified immediately (Waserman et al., 2021). The international guidelines recommend against preemptively administering epinephrine when no symptoms are present. However, exceptions or special considerations should be given to situations involving impaired consciousness, explicit instructions from the child's signed allergy emergency care plan indicating otherwise, and based on local laws and policies (Waserman et al., 2021).

In the United States (US), guidelines outline the importance of preparing for food allergy emergencies, recommending the availability of open communication systems, quick access to emergency care plans and epinephrine, prompt use of epinephrine when needed, and immediate notification of emergency medical services (CDC, 2013; Sicherer et al., 2025). In addition, the guidelines recommend clear role identification for staff members in an emergency with simple and easy-to-follow instructions. This is especially important when the staff member delegated to administer the epinephrine device is not a licensed health professional (CDC, 2013).

International Perspectives on Management Guidelines in Early Childhood Settings

International food allergen regulations vary from country to country based on the prevalence of allergies to specific food allergens, legislative updates, and other factors. More than 80 countries, including organizations of country groups (such as the European Union), have regulations for food allergen labeling. Nationally recognized allergens range from a low of eight in many countries to 15 recognized allergens in the European Union and 16 allergens in South Korea (Food Allergy Research and Resource Program, University of Nebraska Lincoln, 2024). According to a scoping review of food allergy management in schools in Asian-Pacific countries, no studies mentioned food-induced anaphylaxis emergency management plans or school staff training programs (Lee, 2022). In contrast, in a scoping review of food-induced anaphylaxis management in schools in the United States, Canada, Australia, and Europe, twelve studies within 5 years were identified related to school training programs (Santos et al., 2022; Lee, 2022). The European Academy of Allergy and Immunology (EAAI) and Global Allergy and Asthma Excellence Network (GA^2LEN) taskforce, comprised of representatives from fourteen European countries or national societies, created action points for schools, clinicians, and families to consider for advocacy and implementation within local districts institutional policies (Muraro et al., 2010).

The United States, Canada, and Australia recognize the autonomy of states and territories to implement voluntary guidelines or best practices for managing food allergies in schools and early childhood settings within their jurisdictions (CDC, 2013; Santos et al., 2022; Food Allergy Canada, 2024). This means there is great variability in mandatory versus recommended state or local requirements of these early childhood institutions for food allergy and anaphylaxis management (Asthma and Allergy Foundation of America, Elijah-Alavi Foundation, 2022; Santos et al., 2022; Food Allergy Canada, 2024). Yet, in the Australian experience, even when states had mandatory food allergy and anaphylaxis requirements, principals reported that parents were the drivers who initiated local school policies for food allergy exposure prevention and emergency management (Lawlis et al., 2017). However, in Australia, national law now requires that school staff do regular anaphylaxis training as part of the school management policy (Lee, 2022). In Hong Kong, Lee (2022) identified gaps of no national guidelines for food allergy management in schools, nor a national requirement for school anaphylaxis training. In summary, many countries have made great strides with legislative policies to ensure safe environments for young children with food allergies, yet additional work needs to be accomplished.

Emergency Care Plans

In the United States, the American Academy of Pediatrics (AAP) *Management of Food Allergy in Schools: Clinical Report* 2025 and the *Food Allergy Management in Schools (FAMS)* 2024 expert panel recommends implementing sitewide protocols for students with suspected anaphylaxis or allergic reactions as many students may experience a reaction without a known history of food allergy, complementing the previous CDC's 2013 *Voluntary Guidelines for Managing Food Allergies in Schools and Early Care and Education Programs* (CDC, 2013; FAMS, 2024; Sicherer et al., 2025). Individualized allergy and anaphylaxis emergency care plans (sometimes called action plans) for children with known food allergy should include information about the specific allergen(s), signs and symptoms of a reaction, history of anaphylaxis, treatment plan, and emergency contact information (FAMS, 2024; Waserman et al., 2021). In the United States, different forms of individualized plans exist and vary between states and even school districts. A standardized individual emergency care plan that some childcare centers and schools use was developed by Food Allergy Research and Education (FARE, 2025) (Fig. 1). Other emergency care plans are available from the American Academy of Pediatrics and the Asthma and Allergy Foundation of America as well as other organizations (see Resources Page at end of book). International guidelines for emergency care plans are similar (Food Allergy Canada, 2024; National Allergy Council, 2023a, b).

In Australia, the Australian Society of Clinical Immunology and Allergy (ASCIA) developed a universal First Aid Plan for anaphylaxis for patients with and without a known history of food allergy (ASCIA, 2025). Additionally, the ASCIA developed a standard Individualized Emergency Action Care Plan to prepare for patients with a known history of food allergy, allowing for patient-specific dosing and reaction information (Fig. 1).

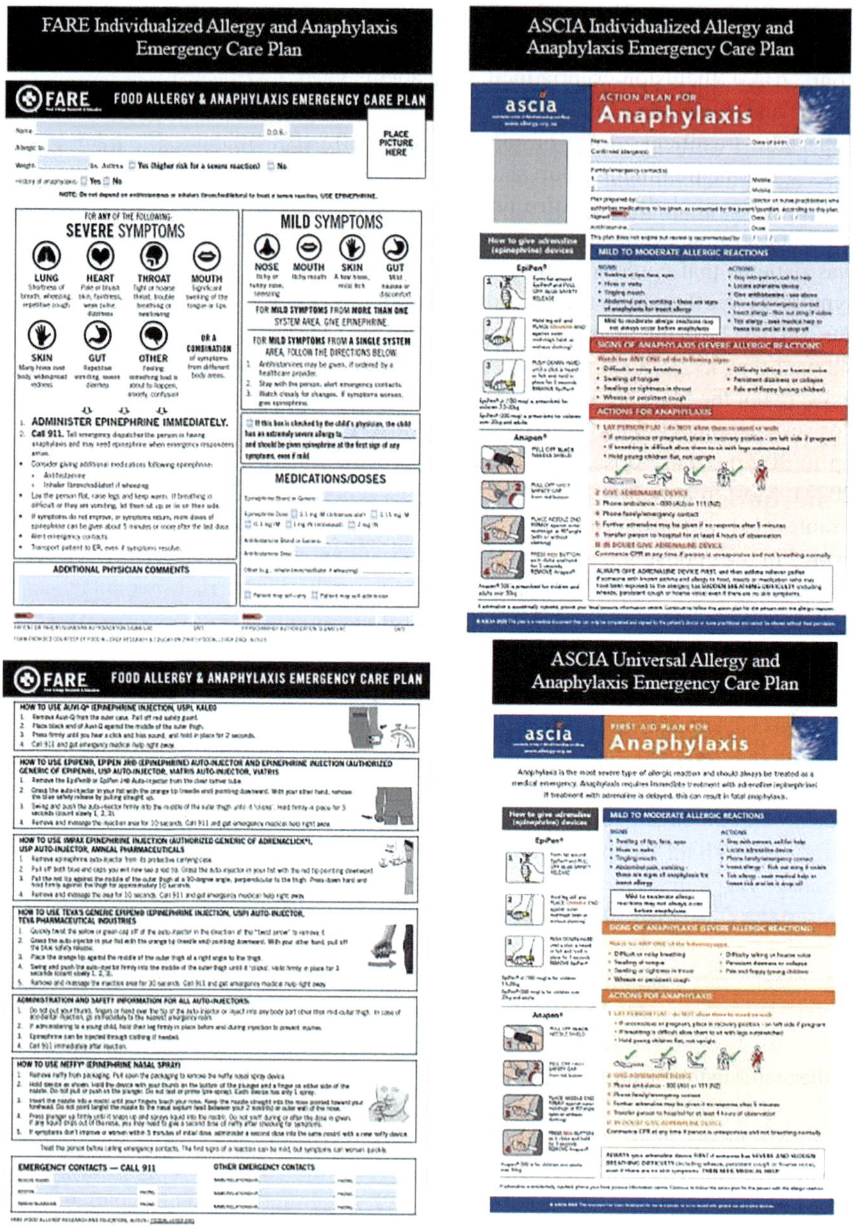

Fig. 1 Sample emergency care plans (FARE, 2025; [ASCIA], 2025). (Used with permission from: FARE and ASCIA)

Studies have shown that personnel often need to rely on and follow emergency care plans for food allergies when the recommendation is to treat the patient with epinephrine, due to a lack of knowledge of administration procedures, timing, or other factors (Foster et al., 2015 n.d.; Avedissian et al., 2018; Devetak et al., 2018). The recommendation to use epinephrine for all symptoms of allergic reaction is often used to mitigate the potential underuse of epinephrine for the treatment of anaphylaxis. Currently, emergency care plans suggest action steps to take for severe and mild allergic reactions with a special box to check if epinephrine should automatically be given to a child with severe allergy even if mild symptoms are noted. Additionally, there is no evidence that the preemptive use of epinephrine when no symptoms are present improves outcomes. With the recent Food and Drug Administration (FDA, 2024) approval of the first epinephrine nasal spray, some allergists believe that schools may be more apt to maintain stock of epinephrine, and school staff may be more comfortable administering it if needed.

More evidence must be published on the effects of implementing allergy emergency care plans or site-wide protocols for managing allergic reactions. At the same time, multiple studies have been conducted on implementing training for childcare and school staff. Studies have shown that well-designed training programs for childcare and school personnel can increase allergy-related attitudes, knowledge, skills, and preparedness. Because of this, it can be reasonable to assume that a well-designed food allergy training program, combined with well-designed individual and universal emergency care plans, promotes prompt treatment administration when needed. Additionally, these may reassure parents and students with food allergy concerns in the childcare center or school (Waserman et al., 2021).

Training programs through the FARE organization and Code Ana are both examples of well-designed programs for schools, parents, nurses, and more. Links to these trainings and more information can be found in the Resources Page at the end of the book.

Access to Epinephrine

Epinephrine is the first-line gold standard of treatment for anaphylaxis. The risk of fatalities, biphasic reactions, and hospitalizations decreases when epinephrine is administered at the first sign of suspected anaphylaxis and within less than 30 min of food-induced anaphylaxis (Golden et al., 2024). Therefore, quick access to epinephrine in daycares and schools is essential to manage an anaphylactic emergency. International recommendations and practice guidelines in Australia and the United States recommend that childcare centers and schools maintain stock of non-patient-specific epinephrine (undesignated or general use adrenaline) where allowed by law and local policies (CDC, 2013; Waserman et al., 2021; Golden et al., 2024; National Allergy Council, 2023a, b). All states enable undesignated epinephrine in schools in the United States, but only 25% of states mandate stocking it (Volerman et al., 2022). Thus, local interest holders, such as nurses, school administrators, community healthcare providers, and parents, may carry the burden of advocating for the development and implementation of regional policies to stock epinephrine in schools (Volerman et al., 2022). In contrast, Hong Kong has no legal regulations requiring undesignated epinephrine in schools (Lee, 2022).

Barriers to implementation can include the financial burden of purchasing and maintaining stock epinephrine and local policies such as prescriber regulations, stringent storage guidelines, and availability of licensed healthcare staff (Santos et al., 2022; Lee, 2022; Kao et al., 2018; Russell et al., 2023). In the United Kingdom, the prescription barrier for undesignated epinephrine was eliminated by amending regulations to allow schools to purchase adrenaline auto-injectors without a prescription (Medicines and Healthcare Products Regulatory Agency, 2017). In addition, the international and several national recommendations suggest that patients at high risk for anaphylaxis should self-carry epinephrine devices when they are mature enough to do so and allowed to do so by site-specific conditions and federal and state laws (CDC, 2013; Waserman et al., 2021; Golden et al., 2024; National Allergy Council, 2023a, b; FAMS, 2024).

A significant proportion of school nurses in the United States work part-time or at two or more elementary schools and may not be present in the school during an emergency (Santos et al., 2022; Willgerodt et al., 2018). According to a nationwide random stratified sample, about 18% of elementary schools in the United States do not have a paid school nurse, 21% have part-time nurses (<30 hours per week), and 62% have full-time nurses (Willgerodt et al., 2018). This means that unlicensed or non-healthcare staff must be trained to recognize an anaphylactic emergency, quickly administer epinephrine, and follow the emergency care plan, including communication to emergency medical services when needed. Furthermore, U.S. schools with full-time nurses are more than twice as likely to have stock epinephrine available than schools with part-time nurses (Kao et al., 2018). With the recent FDA approval of an epinephrine nasal spray for children (Volerman et al., 2022), we expect that the barrier to stocking and using epinephrine may decrease more due to the perception that a nasal spray may be more user-friendly than an injection. The initial FDA approval for nasal epinephrine required children to be both greater than 33 pounds (15 kilograms) and at least 4 years of age. The FDA has since removed the age requirement, which now allows children who meet the weight requirement alone to be eligible for a prescription and the choice for a needle free epinephrine option (Sicherer, 2026).

Registered nurses, physicians, and other healthcare providers provide excellent anaphylaxis and epinephrine device training using freely available and peer-reviewed curricula (CDC, 2013; FAMS, 2024; Russell et al., 2023). Food allergy management educational interventions delivered by healthcare professionals in several countries demonstrated increased knowledge and self-efficacy for food allergy management, including anaphylaxis identification and epinephrine administration (Santos et al., 2022). Emergency response drills with epinephrine devices should be practiced in school (CDC, 2013; National Allergy Council, 2023b; Gereige et al., 2022). With preparation, school nurses are well-poised to be the leaders of such practice sessions by facilitating the simulations and leading debriefing sessions. The training curriculum should be peer-reviewed and evidence-based (see

Resources Page at the end of the book). Education must include an assessment of the learner's understanding and their hands-on skills in using an epinephrine device with follow-up to clarify any misunderstanding and repeat demonstration to assure mastery (Russell et al., 2023; Brach, 2024).

Bullying Prevention

Children who have food allergies are twice as likely to be bullied than non-food allergic children. The presence of food allergy requires a complete lifestyle modification that makes social activities (like lunchtime, recess, field trips, and holiday parties) difficult, causing stress and anxiety for children with food allergies. These social activities are often centered around food, meaning the child must bring allergen-free foods for themselves, not participate, or sit at a separate table.

In the United States, 34% of children with food allergies reported experiencing some form of bullying ranging from physical acts such as waving the allergen in their face, throwing it at them, or intentionally placing it in their food; to non-physical or verbal acts such as teasing, threats, or intimidation; to relational acts such as rumors spread about them or intentionally being excluded from activities. Of the children who report bullying occurred in school, one-fifth of the children report the perpetrator was a teacher and/or school staff member (FAMS, 2024). In a study by Cooke et al. (2022), 12% of parents reported that their child had been bullied because of their food allergies, and 70% reported that their child had not been bullied (Cooke et al., 2022). A study in Australia provided similar results, with 42% of children experiencing some form of bullying and 23% reporting bullying directly related to their food allergy (Fong et al., 2018).

Food allergy bullying can pose severe life-threatening effects on children, which makes the prevention of bullying even more important. Prevention of bullying relies heavily on the school administration. In the United States, there is no anti-bullying legislation at the federal level, but all fifty states have some form of anti-bullying laws, which include requiring districts to implement an anti-bullying policy and defining specific consequences for bullying actions (Prince, 2020). Further, food allergy can be considered a disability with protections provided under Section 504 of the Rehabilitation Act of 1973 (Section 504). Section 504 prohibits harassment based on the individual's disability in federal financial assistance programs (C.F.R. Part 104, 2024).

School nurses are important advocates for students with food allergies to ensure that they are included safely in all school activities. School nurses should review anti-bullying policies with staff, including prevention, risk factors, and any steps to be taken if witnessed (Keller & Stanislo, 2023). Risk factors for bullying include a more severe allergy, being separated or singled out, having to wear allergy identifiers, or receiving special treatment. Additionally, school nurses should assess for signs of bullying in students with food allergies, such as torn clothing; damaged books or backpack; frequent complaints of stomach aches or headaches; unexplained injuries; and behavioral changes such as social isolation, depression, or anger (Bartnikas et al., 2022).

Including students is important to prevent all types of bullying. Common strategies to prevent bullying include recommendations against segregating students with food allergies to a separate area, exposing the student's medical privacy, or attaching a label to the student. Instead, it is recommended that schools, teachers, and other caregivers reduce the risk of exposure in the classroom, find acceptable ways to safely perform food activities to include the student, and participate in food allergy awareness campaigns to improve school culture and education for staff and students (Food Allergy and Anaphylaxis Connection Team, 2024).

Healthcare clinicians can assess bullying in children with food allergies when patients follow up through Patient Reported Outcomes Measures (PROMs). Several PROM tools are available, including Health-Related Quality of Life (HRQL), which many primary care offices utilize in the United States. Several other tools focus directly on food allergy, but only one has been validated for this age group, The Food Allergy Quality of Life—Parent Form (FAQLQ-PF) (DunnGalvin et al., 2008). Early identification and intervention in bullying can lead to an improved quality of life for children with food allergies. Studies further show that the most helpful interventions were parents notifying the school and allowing the school administration to assess the situation and collaboratively work toward a solution for bullying (Bingemann et al., 2020).

Disability Considerations

Children with food allergies have the right to attend daycare or school in a safe and inclusive environment. Nurses can play a role in ensuring these rights are being met. This can be accomplished by educating families and local school authorities about the laws and protections for children with allergies. Nurses can help families advocate for these rights if they are unmet. In the United States and Australia, food allergy is considered a disability, and children are protected under the law. In the United States, Section 504 of the Rehabilitation Act of 1973 is a federal civil rights law that protects students against discrimination due to their disability while at school, including preschools, K-12 schools, colleges, and universities that receive federal financial assistance (Office for Civil Rights, 2024). Having a 504 plan can help ensure reasonable accommodations are in place to receive a free appropriate public education and to keep children safe. Not every student will require a 504 plan; often, a food allergy emergency care plan will suffice. However, even if students do not have a 504 plan in place, they are still protected from discrimination, including harassment. This will require schools to respond to any bullying or harassment a student is experiencing due to their disability (Office for Civil Rights, 2024). If a student with food allergies does not have a 504 plan, it is the responsibility of the school to inform the student and their caregivers of their eligibility to have a meeting with a 504 team (FAMS, 2024). In Australia, students are protected under the Disability Discrimination Act of 1992 as well as the Disability Standards for Education 2005 (the Standards) (Nationally Consistent Collection of Data on School Students with Disability [NCCD], 2024). These laws ensure that students with a disability, including food allergy, are able to access and participate in education the same as their peers (NCCD, 2024). Under these laws, schools will need to provide reasonable adjustments in consultation with parents and caregivers to be sure the student's needs are being met (NCCD, 2024). Nurses, administrators, and other staff members should work with families to help determine what accommodations a child will require while in early childhood settings.

Collaboration with Parents, Caregivers, and School Staff

Collaborating with families, caregivers, school personnel, and community healthcare providers is essential for patient-centered care because student health in the context of chronic conditions is associated with academic performance (Carter-Pokras et al., 2021). School nurses are pivotal in preparing individual health plans for students, such as food allergy emergency care plans, in collaboration with families, community healthcare professionals, and school staff members (CDC, 2013; Gereige et al., 2022). Interpersonal relationships and organizational factors support or hinder this multidisciplinary collaborative work for health promotion and disease management (Gädda et al., 2023; Helleve et al., 2022). School nurse-parent partnerships are characterized by trusting relationships, transparent communication, balanced responsibility, and tailored care in chronic disease management (Uhm & Choi, 2022). School nurses can use these characteristics to collaborate with families to develop individual care plans, implement care, and evaluate it periodically. In addition, using technology and virtual platforms to enhance communication with families and multidisciplinary collaboration, as was begun during the COVID-19 pandemic, will continue to be useful in many communities (Cook et al., 2023). Communicating effectively with families and multidisciplinary staff members involves using health-literate communication strategies, such as the teach-back method and the show-me method (Brach, 2024). The teach-back method of communication uses non-shaming questions to confirm patient or caregiver understanding, putting the responsibility for clear communication on the healthcare professional (Brach, 2024). In the context of food allergy management in schools, the iterative teach-back approach then proceeds with the child, teacher, or caregiver describing how they would tell someone else to implement their emergency care plan. Then, the nurse may detect misunderstandings, rephrase teaching, and re-check for understanding. Clinicians use the teach-back method effectively to improve patient knowledge and retention of information, self-care behaviors, and health-related outcomes (Talevski et al., 2020). Performing patient education using teach-back methods versus conventional methods has been demonstrated to save time (1:39 minutes compared to 3:11 minutes with emergency department discharge instructions) (Agency for Healthcare Quality, 2024; Mahajan et al., 2020). Similarly, the show-me method (Brach, 2024) involves asking the patient or caregiver to demonstrate how to perform a skill, such as how to use an epinephrine device. After observing the demonstration, the nurse can correct any necessary techniques, and the learner can re-demonstrate the skill until competence is achieved.

The Nursing Role

Nurses can significantly impact the well-being of children with food allergies in school and childcare settings by educating staff, children, and families. Nurses have a unique opportunity to build trusting relationships with families and facility staff and to be a resource for creating change and addressing knowledge gaps when they arise. Nurses should act as educators for children, parents/guardians, and facility staff.

Nurses should advocate for institutional policy change to create safe school/childcare environments for their patients. For example, in the United States, all 50 states allow stock epinephrine; however, only 14 states mandate stock epinephrine (Volerman et al., 2022). Nurses can advocate for local and institutional policies requiring undesignated epinephrine. Secondly, there are variations across states on who is responsible for creating policies and procedures for epinephrine in schools, underscoring the need for a national unified approach to managing food allergy in schools (Volerman et al., 2022). Nurses can advocate for the importance of this unification because guidelines, such as the CDC (2013), FAMS (2024), and AAP (Sicherer et al., 2025) comprehensive guidelines, are voluntary and not mandated. Nurses can help advocate for nationally mandated guidelines to ensure their patients remain safe in these settings. In Australia, the National Allergy Council has developed the *Best Practice Guidelines for Anaphylaxis Prevention and Management in Schools,* which aims to create a nationally unified approach to managing allergies (National Allergy Council, 2023b). However, it is important to note each state or territory may have its own existing legislation. This again highlights the need for a national, and perhaps global, unified approach to managing food allergies.

In the United States, the school nurse is pivotal in providing school health services such as acute and emergency care, care coordination, chronic disease management, and family engagement within the CDC Healthy Schools framework (CDC, 2022). The National Association of School Nurses has created a comprehensive, evidence-based guideline and other resources for school nurses to use when caring for students with food allergies (Keller & Stanislo, 2023). This guideline highlights the importance of understanding the basics of an allergic reaction, the importance of creating a safe and supportive environment for those with allergies, and emphasizing that school nurses are essential in implementing preventative measures. Nurses as educators and policy advocates are pivotal in managing food allergies in early childhood settings.

Conclusion

While childcare and school management policies and guidelines vary internationally and even by state, province, or district, the basic principles of food allergy prevention, recognition, and treatment are the same, intended to create a safe and inclusive environment for all children to learn and grow. Nurses play important roles in the collaborative efforts to manage food allergy care among the settings of home, school, childcare, and health care. Nurses advocate for policies and resources at the local and national level, educating non-licensed school and childcare staff and families, maintaining and updating individualized emergency care plans for students, creating and implementing universal emergency response plans, and providing frontline care in response to food allergy reactions. Nurses should remain up to date with the latest best practices for the prevention, recognition, and management of allergic reactions and be aware of their local laws and regulations.

References

Agency for Healthcare Quality. (2024). *Use the Teach-Back Method: Tool #5*. https://www.ahrq.gov/health-literacy/improve/precautions/tool5.html. Accessed 20 Aug 2024.

Asthma and Allergy Foundation of America, Elijah-Alavi Foundation. (2022). *Child Care Policies for Food Allergy: Elijah's Law report for U.S. States and Territories*. https://aafa.org/ElijahsLaw

Australasian Society of Clinical Immunology and Allergy. (2025). *ASCIA Action, First Aid, Management, Transfer, Travel and Treatment Plans*. https://www.allergy.org.au/hp/ascia-plans-action-and-treatment?highlight=WyJwbGFuIl0=. Accessed 12 Aug 2025

Avedissian, T., Honein-AbouHaidar, G., Dumit, N., & Richa, N. (2018). Anaphylaxis management: A survey of school and day care nurses in Lebanon. *BMJ Paediatrics Open*. https://doi.org/10.1136/bmjpo-2018-000260

Bartnikas, L. M., Dupuis, R., Wang, J., & Phipatanakul, W. (2022). Food allergies in inner-city schools: Addressing disparities and improving management. *Annals of Allergy, Asthma & Immunology, 129*, 430–439.

Bingemann, T., Herbert, L. J., Young, M. C., Sicherer, S. H., Petty, C. R., Phipatanakul, W., Bartnikas, L. M. (2020). Deficits and Opportunities in Allergists' Approaches to Food Allergy-Related Bullying. *The Journal of Allergy and Clinical Immunology: In Practice 8*:343–345.e2

Brach, C. (Ed.). (2024). *Health Literacy Universal P.recautions Toolkit* (3rd ed.). Agency for Healthcare Research.

34 C.F.R. Part 104. (2000). Nondiscrimination on the Basis of Handicap in Programs or Activities Receiving Federal Financial Assistance. https://www2.ed.gov/policy/rights/reg/ocr/edlite-34cfr104.html. Accessed 27 Aug 2024

Carter-Pokras, O. D., Bugbee, B. A., Gold, R. S., Lauver, P. E., Aiken, R., & Arria, A. M. (2021). Utilizing student health and academic data: A county-level demonstration project. *Health Promotion Practice, 22*, 193–203.

Centers for Disease Control and Prevention. (2022). *School health services, healthy schools, CDC*. https://www.cdc.gov/healthyschools/schoolhealthservices.html. Accessed 21 Aug 2024.

Centers for Disease Control and Prevention. (2013). *Voluntary guidelines for managing food allergies in schools and early care and education programs*. U.S. Department of Health and Human Services.

Cook, G., Appleton, J. V., Bekaert, S., Harrold, T., Taylor, J., & Sammut, D. (2023). School nursing: New ways of working with children and young people during the Covid-19 pandemic: A scoping review. *Journal of Advanced Nursing, 79*, 471–501.

Cooke, F., Ramos, A., & Herbert, L. (2022). Food allergy-related bullying among children and adolescents. *Journal of Pediatric Psychology, 47*, 318–326.

Devetak, I., Devetak, S. P., & Vesel, T. (2018). Future teachers' attitudes and knowledge regarding the management of the potential students' life-threatening allergic reactions in Slovenian schools. *Slovenian Journal of Public Health, 57*, 124–132.

DunnGalvin, A., De BlokFlokstra, B. M. J., Burks, A. W., Dubois, A. E. J., & Hourihane, J. O. (2008). Food allergy QoL questionnaire for children aged 0–12 years: Content, construct, and cross-cultural validity. *Clinical and Experimental Allergy, 38*, 977–986.

Food and Drug Administration. (2024). *FDA Approves First Nasal Spray for Treatment of Anaphylaxis.* https://www.fda.gov/news-events/press-announcements/fda-approves-first-nasal-spray-treatment-anaphylaxis. Accessed 28 Aug 2024.

Food Allergy and Anaphylaxis Connection Team. (2024). *Bullying: Bullying facts, stats, & resources.* https://www.foodallergyawareness.org/bullying/bullying-facts-stats-and-resources/. Accessed 27 Aug 2024.

Food Allergy Canada. (2024). *National School Policies.* https://foodallergycanada.ca/professional-resources/educators/school-k-to-12/national-school-policies/. Accessed 7 Aug 2024.

Food Allergy Management in Schools Advisory Panel. (2024). Food Allergy Management in Schools (FAMS): Expert recommendations for K–12. https://www.foodallergy.org/resources/food-allergy-management-schools-fams-expert-recommendations-k-12/. Accessed 12 Aug 2025.

Food Allergy Research & Education (2025). *Food Allergy Anaphylaxis Emergency Care Plan.* https://www.foodallergy.org/living-food-allergy/food-allergy-essentials/food-allergy-anaphylaxis-emergency-care-plan. Accessed 12 Aug 2025.

Food Allergy Research and Resource Program University of Nebraska Lincoln. (2024). *Food Allergens: International regulatory chart.* https://farrp.unl.edu/IRChart. Accessed 21 Aug 2024

Fong, A. T., Katelaris, C. H., & Wainstein, B. K. (2018). Bullying in Australian children and adolescents with food allergies. *Pediatric Allergy and Immunology, 29*, 740–746.

Foster, A. A., Campbell, R. L., Lee, S, & Anderson, J. L. (2015). Anaphylaxis Preparedness among Preschool Staff before and after an Educational Intervention. *Journal of Allergy (Cairo)* 2015:23182. https://doi.org/10.1155/2015/231862.

Gädda, F., Hemberg, J., & Nyman-Kurkiala, P. (2023). School health care and multiprofessional collaboration in compulsory school – teaching staff's perceptions. *Cogent Education, 10*, 2241644.

Gereige, R. S., Gross, T., Jastaniah, E., & Council on School Health and Committee on Pediatric Emergency Medicine. (2022). Individual medical emergencies occurring at school. *Pediatrics/American Academy of Pediatrics, 150*, e2022057987.

Golden, D. B. K., Wang, J., Waserman, S., et al. (2024). Anaphylaxis: A 2023 practice parameter update. *Annals of Allergy, Asthma & Immunology, 132*, 124–176.

Gupta, R. S., Warren, C. M., Smith, B. M., Blumenstock, J. A., Jiang, J., Davis, M. M., & Nadeau, K. C. (2018). The public health impact of parent-reported childhood food allergies in the United States. *Pediatrics*. https://doi.org/10.1542/peds.2018-1235.

Hall, H., & Nielsen, E. (2020). *How do children spend their time? Time use and skill development in the PSID.* FEDS Notes. https://doi.org/10.17016/2380-7172.2577.

Helleve, A., Midthassel, U. V., & Federici, R. A. (2022). Finding the balance between collaboration and autonomy among school nurses in interactions with schools. *The Journal of School Nursing, 38*, 184–193.

Kao, L. M., Wang, J., Kagan, O., Russell, A., Mustafa, S. S., Houdek, D., Smith, B., & Gupta, R. (2018). School nurse perspectives on school policies for food allergy and anaphylaxis. *Annals of Allergy, Asthma & Immunology, 120*, 304–309.

Keller A, Stanislo K (2023) *School nursing evidence-based clinical practice guideline: Students with allergies and risk for Anaphylaxis* | NASN Learning Center. In: nasn.org. https://learn.nasn.org/courses/58496. Accessed 20 Aug 2024.

Lawlis, T., Bakonyi, S., & Williams, L. T. (2017). Food allergy in schools: The importance of government involvement. *Nutrition & Dietetics, 74*, 82–87.

Lee, S. C. (2022). Pediatric anaphylaxis management in schools: Current issues and challenges in Asia and Hong Kong. A scoping review. *Pediatric Respirology and Critical Care Medicine, 6*, 54.

Mahajan, M., Hogewoning, J. A., Zewald, J. J. A., Kerkmeer, M., Feitsma, M., & van Rijssel, D. A. (2020). The impact of teach-back on patient recall and understanding of discharge information in the emergency department: The Emergency Teach-Back (EM-TeBa) study. *International Journal of Emergency Medicine, 13*, 49.

Medicines and Healthcare Products Regulatory Agency. (2017). *Explanatory Memorandum to the Human Medicines (Amendment) Regulations 2017 No. 715*. MHRA, Department of Health, United Kingdom. https://www.legislation.gov.uk/uksi/2017/715/pdfs/uksiem_20170715_en.pdf
Muraro, A., Clark, A., Beyer, K., et al. (2010). The management of the allergic child at school: EAACI/GA[2]LEN Task Force on the allergic child at school. *Allergy, 65*, 681–689.
National Allergy Council. (2023a). *Best practice guidelines for anaphylaxis prevention and management in Children's Education and Care*. https://allergyaware.org.au/childrens-education-and-care/best-practice-guidelines-cec. Accessed 7 Aug 2024.
National Allergy Council (2023b) *Best practice guidelines for anaphylaxis prevention and management in Schools*. https://allergyaware.org.au/schools/best-practice-guidelines-schools. Accessed 7 Aug 2024.
Nationally Consistent Collection of Data on School Students with Disability (NCCD). *What is the NCCD? In: Understanding the NCCD*. https://www.nccd.edu.au/wider-support-materials/what-nccd. Accessed 29 Aug 2024
Office for Civil Rights. (2024). *Section 504 Protections for Students with Food Allergies*. U.S. Department of Education. https://www.ed.gov/media/document/ocr-factsheet-food-allergies-2024-33827.pdf
Organisation for Economic Cooperation and Development. (2023). Education at a Glance 2023: OECD Indicators. https://doi.org/10.1787/e13bef63-en
Prince, H. (2020). Anti-bully legislation: Effects for youth in United States schools. *Justice Evaluation Journal, 3*, 245–266.
Russell, A. F., Bingemann, T. A., Cooke, A. T., Ponda, P., Pistiner, M., Jean, T., Nanda, A., Jobrack, J., Hoyt, A. E. W., & Young, M. C. (2023). The need for required stock epinephrine in all schools: A work group report of the AAAAI adverse reactions to Foods Committee. *The Journal of Allergy and Clinical Immunology. In Practice, 11*, 1068–1082.e1.
Santos, M. J. L., Merrill, K. A., Gerdts, J. D., Ben-Shoshan, M., & Protudjer, J. L. P. (2022). Food allergy education and management in schools: A scoping review on current practices and gaps. *Nutrients, 14*, 732.
Sicherer, S. H., O'Leary, S., Pistiner, M., Wang, J., Section on Allergy and Immunology, Council on School Health. (2025). Management of food allergy in schools: clinical report. *Pediatrics, 156*:e2025073168br
Sicherer, S. H. (2026). Prescribing epinephrine for anaphylaxis self-treatment. UpToDate. Retrieved June 9, 2026, from https://www.uptodate.com/contents/prescribing-epinephrine-for-anaphylaxis-self-treatment?source=history#H3898227691.
Talevski, J., Shee, A. W., Rasmussen, B., Kemp, G., & Beauchamp, A. (2020). Teach-back: A systematic review of implementation and impacts. *PLoS One, 15*, e0231350.
Tanno, L. K., & Demoly, P. (2022). Food allergy in the World Health Organization's International Classification of Diseases (ICD)-11. *Pediatric Allergy and Immunology, 33*, e13882.
Uhm, J.-Y., & Choi, M.-Y. (2022). School nurse–parent partnership in school health care for children with type 1 diabetes: A hybrid method concept analysis. *Asian Nursing Research, 16*, 282–291.
Volerman, A., Brindley, C., Amerson, N., Pressley, T., & Woolverton, N. (2022). A national review of State Laws for Stock Epinephrine in Schools. *The Journal of School Health, 92*, 209–222.
Waserman, S., Cruickshank, H., Hildebrand, K. J., et al. (2021). Prevention and management of allergic reactions to food in child care centers and schools: Practice guidelines. *The Journal of Allergy and Clinical Immunology, 147*, 1561–1578.
Willgerodt, M. A., Brock, D. M., & Maughan, E. D. (2018). Public school nursing practice in the United States. *The Journal of School Nursing, 34*, 232–244.

Food Allergy Management in Adolescents and Young Adults

Matthew Doucette, Kathleen Doucette, Carolyn D'Amato, and Mary Heinz

Introduction

Effective management of food allergy (FA) during adolescence and early adulthood is a collaborative endeavor involving the individual, their family, healthcare providers, and educational or workplace institutions (Roberts et al., 2020; Vazquez-Ortiz et al., 2023). Although general management principles span all ages, adolescents and young adults (AYAs) merit additional transitional support because they engage in more risk-taking behaviors and experience the highest incidence of fatal anaphylaxis (Keohane et al., 2022). Studies consistently show suboptimal epinephrine carriage among AYAs, with only 42–72% routinely carrying devices, leaving many unprotected during critical moments (Robinson et al., 2019; Warren et al., 2018).

Key management domains include identifying allergens and recognizing allergen-exposure risks in social, dating, educational, and workplace settings. Qualitative work with AYAs consistently highlights restaurants, bars, and peer gatherings as major sources of accidental exposure (Dyer et al., 2018; Egmose

M. Doucette (✉)
University of Texas Southwestern Medical Center, Dallas, TX, USA
e-mail: Matthew.Doucette@UTSouthwestern.edu

K. Doucette
Fifth Third Bank, Dallas, TX, USA

C. D'Amato
Triton Regional School District, Rowley, MA, USA

M. Heinz
Loyola University Chicago, Chicago, IL, USA
e-mail: mheinz@luc.edu

J. Doucette, J. Howard-Ruben (eds.), *Comprehensive Food Allergy Management for Nurses*, https://doi.org/10.1007/978-3-032-28647-5_8

et al., 2024). Maintaining an up-to-date, individualized written allergy action plan is associated with higher adherence scores on the Food Allergy Management Practices Questionnaire (FAMPQ) and lower reaction rates (Herbert et al., 2016). Nevertheless, prospective registry data show that approximately 50% of food-allergic adults still experience two accidental reactions each year, illustrating how avoidance and autoinjector carriage remain sub-optimal despite education efforts (Versluis et al., 2023).

Educational efforts should therefore empower AYAs to identify exposures, co-create their action plans, and practice self-advocacy in various settings. Studies show that parental empowerment and advocacy in fostering school partnerships are linked with safer behaviors underlining the value of teaching proactive communication (e.g., asking about ingredients or kitchen practices) before AYAs enter college or the workforce (Koo et al., 2023). Nurses' goals include educating, encouraging, and verifying that each individual possesses the practical skills to manage their allergy safely while serving as an active partner at every step. By integrating collaborative planning, risk-focused education, label-reading mastery, self-advocacy coaching, and health-literacy reinforcement, nurses can equip AYAs to navigate the transition to independent FA management with greater safety and confidence.

Allergen Exposure

Allergen exposure is often hidden, and without targeted education, many risks go unnoticed until a reaction occurs. In addition to the well-documented suboptimal epinephrine carriage rates previously highlighted, risk-taking rises in social contexts such as parties or restaurants (Robinson et al., 2019; Sampson et al., 2006; Warren et al., 2018). Simultaneously, a 288-product audit in the European Union (EU) found that 21% of packages changed allergen wording within a single retail cycle and 38% relied on precautionary allergen labeling (PAL), underscoring why AYAs must reread "familiar" labels every time they shop or cook (Blom et al., 2021). Failure to do so is one of the top three contributors to the annual accidental-reaction rate in this age group (Rotella & Oriel, 2022).

Nurses must teach AYAs how to interpret ingredient labels, including less common or ambiguous names for allergens and the implications of precautionary allergen labeling (PAL). The multicenter MIRABEL survey in France, Belgium, and Luxemburg demonstrated that frequent, skilled label reading significantly reduces consumption of PAL-containing products among peanut-allergic teens (Papadopoulos et al., 2018). Similarly, a 2024 web-based survey of U.S. college students with food allergies showed that students who prioritized their dietary restrictions were far more likely to read food labels routinely than their peers, underscoring the protective value of label-reading education (Bosch et al., 2024). An understanding of cross-contact risks, highlighted in a recent qualitative study of 16–18 year-olds in Ireland who described shared kitchens as their most frequent source of allergy risk, should be woven into all label-reading sessions with teens (O'Sullivan et al., 2025).

Moreover, structured training in anaphylaxis recognition and epinephrine device use can begin in childhood; caregivers report that introducing these skills early and reinforcing them in adolescence improves timely epinephrine administration (Keohane et al., 2023). Finally, adequate health literacy is pivotal as AYAs assume full responsibility for their care: Higher facilitator scores on the FAMPQ and targeted interventions that address perceived barriers (severity, unpredictability) predict better adherence to self-care behaviors (Herbert et al., 2016; Jones et al., 2015). Notably, adolescents with FA in Sweden who receive comprehensive education report clinically meaningful improvements in health-related quality of life, particularly in domains related to independence (Protudjer et al., 2016).

A narrative review of the dining industry confirms that inadequate staff training and inconsistent menu labeling keep restaurants the single largest source of severe food-allergic reactions in young adults (Stankovich et al., 2023). Alcohol compounds this danger in two ways: It lowers executive control, further reducing label-checking and epinephrine use, and functions as a cofactor in up to 30% of adult food-anaphylaxis cases, lowering the threshold dose needed to trigger a reaction (Bartra et al., 2023). Alcoholic beverages themselves can harbor hidden allergens such as wheat or barley; furthermore, a well-documented case of anaphylaxis to coriander-flavored beer highlights the need to inquire about craft-drink ingredients just as rigorously as food labels (Brussino et al., 2018). College students may participate in keg parties that involve a large distribution of alcohol. Nut-flavored beer has become a trend. Vriesekoop (2021) noted several allergic reactions related to beer have been reported and range from full-blown anaphylaxis to urticaria (hives) and diffuse erythema (localized reddening of the skin due to inflammation of the blood capillaries).

Educational and workplace settings introduce additional, less obvious exposures. Food proteins aerosolized during laboratory exercises or food-service internships can provoke respiratory or systemic reactions, with inhalation increasingly recognized as an underreported route of sensitization. A narrative review of airborne anaphylaxis highlighted multiple recent case reports of systemic reactions to inhaled food allergens in occupational and school environments, reinforcing the need for preventive strategies (Ridolo et al., 2022). Nurse counseling should therefore include guidance on personal protective equipment, dedicated allergen-free work zones, and clear reporting pathways when reactions occur.

Finally, intimate contact poses a real but often uncomfortable risk to discuss. A clinical update on allergy and sexual behaviors found that kiss-induced reactions still affect roughly one in ten food-allergic individuals when a partner consumes the trigger food shortly before contact (Caminati et al., 2019). Teaching AYAs to discuss the timing of meals and brushing teeth with partners is an essential component of any comprehensive action plan.

By integrating habitual label rereading, scrutiny of personal-care items, surface hygiene, cofactor awareness, workplace precautions, and safe-intimacy conversations, nurses can equip AYAs to recognize and mitigate the subtle exposures that account for the majority of severe reactions during the journey toward independent food allergy self-management.

Unexpected Sources of Specific Allergens

- Egg
  - Egg white or whole egg is widely deployed as a "hidden" ingredient in cookies, pasta, salad dressings and stock cubes, confirming its routine use as a binder or emulsifier in processed and baked goods (Smits et al., 2023).
  - In beverages, ovalbumin remains the clarifier of choice for premium red wines; a oenological study reiterates its effectiveness as a fining agent to tame tannins without compromising quality (Obreque-Slier et al., 2023).
- Tree-nuts
  - Nut oils (e.g., almond, macadamia) appear in >10% of moisturizers and other skincare items marketed for atopic skin (AAAAI, 2020; Ryczaj et al., 2023).
  - Ground nut shells are sometimes used to stuff bean-bag toys, draft stoppers, and certain bird-seed mixes, posing an inhalation or contact risk (Kids with Food Allergies, 2024).
- Milk
  - Casein-derived additives have triggered anaphylaxis from a prescription toothpaste formulated with recaldent/CPP-ACP (Budi & Pebriani, 2020).
  - Trace milk proteins contaminating the lactose excipient in dry-powder inhalers have produced severe reactions in patients allergic to cow's milk (Robles & Motheral, 2014).
- Wheat
  - Glycerol (VG), often derived from wheat starch, is widely used in toothpastes, mouthwashes and lipsticks. In a survey of 66 such items, three toothpastes and one lipstick were found to contain gluten above the 20 mg/kg "gluten-free" threshold, indicating residual wheat protein in products not normally considered food (Wieser et al., 2021).
- Soy
  - Major and minor soybean allergens have been characterized in depth, and even highly refined hydrolysates (e.g., vegetable gums, texturizers) can retain trace peptide fragments above detection thresholds, underscoring the need for clear labeling (Wiederstein et al., 2023).
- Shellfish
  - Shrimp can be found in stuffings such as oyster stuffing and may not be apparent from visual inspection (FAACT, n.d.)
  - Pet foods and some supplements for nutrition or exercise can contain hidden shellfish exposure.
  - Outdoor fertilizer derived from shellfish products can pose a risk.
- Fish
  - Isinglass (fish-bladder gelatin) can leave trace amounts of fish proteins in the finished beer product, posing a potential risk for fish-allergic consumers (Vriesekoop, 2021).
  - Protamine sulfate, derived from fish milt and used to reverse heparin, can rarely trigger anaphylaxis in sensitized individuals, underscoring the need for source verification in fish-allergic patients (Levy et al., 2023).

- Peanut
  - Peanut proteins can be detected in processed foods, such as sauces and baked goods, under labels that do not explicitly declare peanuts, highlighting gaps in current allergen labeling (Tramuta et al., 2022).
  - Undeclared peanut can be found in confectionery, spice blends, and cosmetics labeled "nut-free," pointing to the need for broader surveillance (Luparelli et al., 2023).
- Sesame
  - Some LiP SMACKER© lip gloss products contain sesame seed oil (www.lipsmacker.com).
  - In chocolates, biscuits, and muesli bars, sesame protein was found in 12% of products carrying no "may contain sesame" warning, demonstrating persistent cross-contact issues (Turner et al., 2024).
- Mammalian Meat
  - Alpha-gal Syndrome (AGS) is an IgE-mediated allergy to beef, pork, or lamb and associated products after a tick bite and can occur at any age (Commins, 2020).

Designing and Developing Allergy Action Plans for AYAs

A growing body of literature confirms that a well-written, regularly rehearsed FA action plan does more than organize information; it measurably improves real-world outcomes for AYAs. A newly validated North American pediatric action plan embedded age-specific symptom checklists and stepwise epinephrine dosing; pilot testing showed that caregivers and teens could locate critical instructions 30% faster than with traditional plans, and 94% judged it "easy to follow under stress" (Anagnostou et al., 2025). It is important for nurses managing patients with FA to leverage these structured tools during patient visits to reinforce symptom recognition and self-management in AYAs.

Recognizing symptoms is the critical first step in a successful food allergy response strategy (see Fig. 1). Please see chapter "Understanding the Diagnosis and Management of Food Allergy Part I: IgE-Mediated Food Allergy and Anaphylaxis" for a more comprehensive description of food allergy symptoms. Here is a non-exhaustive list of the symptoms a nurse should educate their AYA patients to look for when they are concerned, they may be having an allergic reaction:

Robust training is the next foundational step. An in-person, nurse-led program delivered to 4818 school and community staff produced durable gains: Knowledge scores and self-reported confidence in recognizing and treating reactions increased by roughly two-thirds while remaining elevated at six-month follow-up (Wahl et al., 2015). Similar benefits appear with high-fidelity simulation; a case-based manikin exercise for healthcare trainees reduced critical-action times, including symptom recognition, epinephrine delivery, and EMS activation by 40–48% (Mawhirt et al., 2018). Even brief, online modules can help: First-aid volunteers who completed a

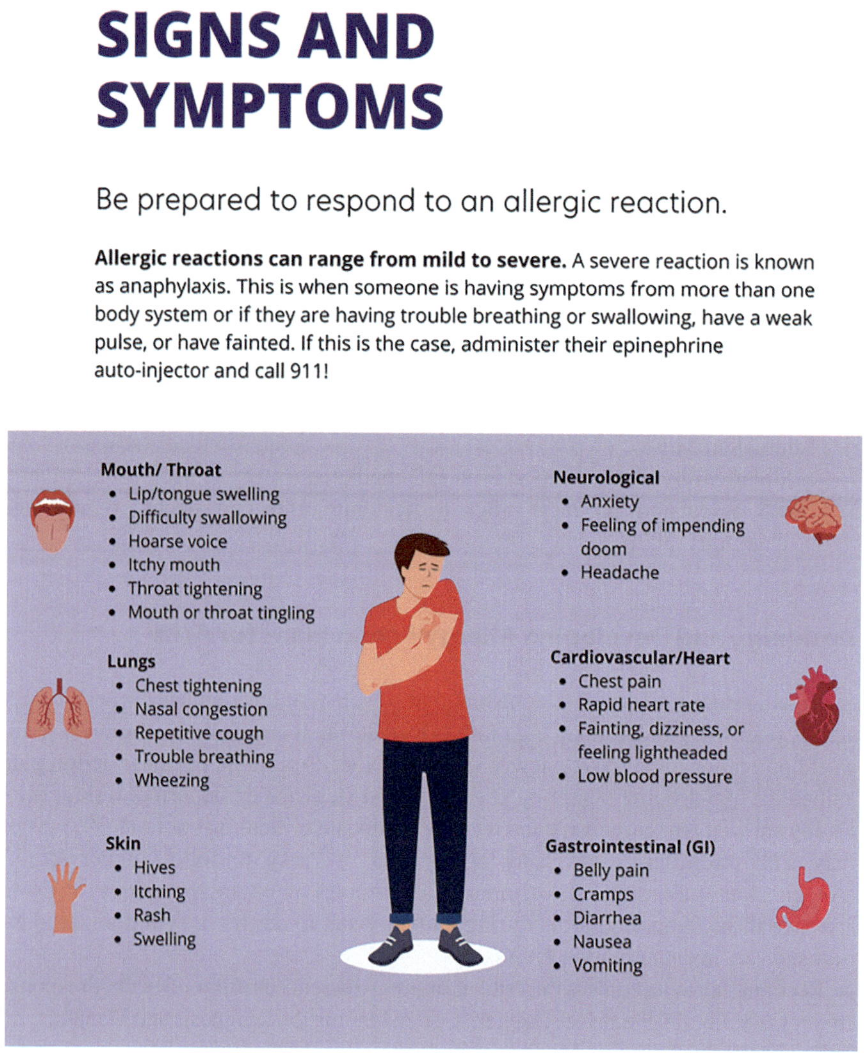

Fig. 1 Signs and symptoms of an allergic reaction. (Reprinted with permission from: Food allergy education guide: Early childhood through college by Center for Food Allergy and Asthma Research. (2024). Retrieved from https://issuu.com/cfaarnu/docs/cfaar_ed_guide_final)

30-minute e-learning course doubled their correct anaphylaxis diagnoses on a post-test and showed parallel gains in autoinjector technique (Meyran et al., 2023). Nurses should feel empowered to lead or recommend these training opportunities for both patients and community members, adapting the delivery format for the resources and learning environment.

Leveraging insights from school-based research can help bridge this preparedness gap. As Downey et al. (2025) illustrate, a nurse educator-led food allergy educational intervention significantly increased knowledge, shifted attitudes, and bolstered support for allergy response policies among non-medical school staff. This demonstrates how strategic, concise training can empower individuals without clinical backgrounds to manage food allergy concerns effectively. Adapting this model to higher education could involve training dining services employees, resident advisors, and student leaders to recognize symptoms, initiate emergency protocols, and use epinephrine devices, thus building a safer and more responsive campus food environment. Colleges can strengthen allergy preparedness by implementing training programs such as AllerTrain Lite and FARECheck (FARE, 2025e; MenuTrinfo, 2025).

Still, training only matters if the medicine is on hand. As mentioned before, only 42–72% of adolescents carried an autoinjector during their most recent food allergy reaction, with "forgetting" cited as the leading barrier (Robinson et al., 2019; Warren et al., 2018). A randomized controlled trial sought to combat this issue: Weekly text-message "nudges" plus small gift-card incentives raised daily on-person carriage from 21% at baseline to 64% after 24 weeks, outperforming usual care by 28 percentage points (Dupuis et al., 2023). Even before prescriptions are filled, gaps appear. Canadian primary-care data show that 27% of first-time autoinjector scripts for young adults are never redeemed (Abrams et al., 2017). Nurses play a crucial role in identifying these barriers early and supporting adherence through follow-up, motivational strategies, and personalized action planning.

Timely epinephrine saves lives beyond the campus as well. A systematic review linked administration within 30 minutes of symptom onset to 70% lower odds of biphasic reactions (Dodd et al., 2021). An observational EMS cohort echoed the message: Patients who received pre-hospital epinephrine were significantly less likely to require escalated care on arrival, whereas those arriving more than 50 minutes after onset had missed opportunities for early dosing in 63% of episodes (Cha et al., 2022; Dribin & Greenhawt, 2024). These data emphasize the urgency nurses must convey to patients and families: Epinephrine should never be delayed nor treated as a last resort.

Device design also matters. In a randomized trial, only 43% of parents could deliver a full dose with their assigned autoinjector six weeks after optimal training; success rates diverged sharply after an untrained device switch, highlighting why AYAs must practice with the exact model they carry (Umasunthar et al., 2015). Subsequent usability work showed that voice-prompt devices (Auvi-Q) were used correctly by 93% of untrained adults versus 51% for a traditional pen, suggesting a role for intuitive technologies in AYA self-care (Kessler et al., 2019).

Collectively, these studies reinforce the allergy action plan's core goals: ensure AYAs can recognize early symptoms, keep epinephrine immediately accessible, empower peers and staff through hands-on training, and plan for rapid EMS or hospital access. By integrating these evidence-based strategies into patient teaching and care coordination, nurses can transform the action plan from a static document into a living tool that supports independence, safety, and confidence for AYAs with FA.

Navigating the Transition to Independent Management of Food Allergies for Students in School-Specific Environments: Guidelines for Nurses

Food allergy affects as many as 11% of college-aged students, and the transition to independent living is accompanied by a strikingly high event rate: Longitudinal campus surveys show that 42–63% of food-allergic undergraduates experience at least one reaction while enrolled (Wu & Wang, 2023). These data frame college selection as a safety intervention; nurses who counsel AYAs and their families should therefore weigh institutional allergy policies alongside traditional academic and social fit.

Eating Safely on Campus: Integrating Dining Hall Vigilance with Proactive Meal Planning

For nurses advising college students with FA, the first step is clarifying where the danger lies. Pooled U.S. mortality reviews show that 46–52% of fatal reactions originate in restaurants or other food-service venues, underscoring the disproportionate risk that mealtimes on campus introduce (Radke, 2017; Stankovich et al., 2023). Within the university setting, surveys of more than 2800 undergraduates reveal that only 12–45% say their dining hall always labels the top allergens, and when reactions do occur in this setting, 56% meet anaphylaxis criteria (Wu & Wang, 2023). These data frame meal planning, in addition to epinephrine carriage, as a core safety intervention.

When families are still evaluating schools, nurses can recommend campuses located near familiar grocery chains or trusted restaurant brands. In a cross-sectional study of 285 Canadian eateries, standardized allergen icons on online menus doubled consumer confidence and reduced self-reported errors compared with independent outlets lacking such disclosure (Nahle et al., 2025). Encouraging prospective students to try the dining program and nearby familiar restaurants during campus visits can give prospective students reassurance that their FA can be accommodated safely.

Food-service education remains patchy: In a CDC multicenter audit, only 44% of managers and 41% of line workers had ever received formal food allergy training, and a mere 7% of kitchens maintained a designated allergen-free station (Radke, 2017). Targeted interventions help: One trial in Turkey showed that a single 32-minute video boosted post-test knowledge scores and safety attitudes among 619 employees in restaurants, schools, and hospitals (Aytulu et al., 2025). Nurses can point dining directors toward accredited curricula such as ServSafe Allergens, AllerTrain U, or FARECheck and recommend recording how often refreshers occur (FARE, 2025e; MenuTrinfo, 2025; Servesafe, 2025).

Experimental work in simulated restaurant kitchens confirms that peanut, egg, and milk proteins are readily transferred from shared spatulas and frying pans to previously uncontaminated foods, underscoring that cross-contact remains a major threat in any shared cooking space (Remington et al., 2020). Laboratory cleaning trials as described in the US Food and Drug Administration Food Code (US Food and Drug Administration, 2023) demonstrate that a wash with detergent, rinse with clean water, sanitizing with chlorine-based products, and then air-drying sequence or multiple quaternary-ammonium wipes eliminate >99% of allergen residue from stainless steel and plastic, whereas a single dry wipe leaves clinically relevant protein behind (Bedford et al., 2020).

Emerging literature on nutritional management of FA emphasizes that dietitian-led counseling not only closes micronutrient gaps but measurably improves quality-of-life indices in adolescents and young adults (Leone et al., 2023). Booking an intake visit before classes start allows the student, dietitian, and nursing team to co-create rotating menus and contingency snacks that align with lecture times and dietary guidelines.

Ignoring precautionary allergen labeling ("may contain peanuts") is ill-advised: A study analyzing food products with ELISA assays found clinically significant peanut protein in nearly one-third of PAL-labeled foods on European shelves (Krejner-Bienias et al., 2023). Nurses should therefore encourage students to compile a living list of trusted brands that publish quantitative testing data and to contact manufacturers when uncertainty arises. As always, each food label should be read each time the food is obtained and ingested.

By guiding families through campus selection, dining-hall auditing, staff training advocacy, early dietitian referral, housing negotiations, dorm-kitchen protocols, label literacy, and fallback on pre-prepared food items that are pantry or freezer staples, nurses can equip food-allergic college students to choose either vetted dining services or self-prepared meals, allowing them to navigate both with confidence grounded in evidence rather than fear.

Creating a Safe "Home Base": Housing Strategies for College Students with Food Allergies

Selecting a living space is as safety-critical as having a well-thought-out meal plan: Teenagers and young adults account for the highest rate of fatal food-induced anaphylaxis, so the environment where they store, cook, and share food must be predictable and controllable (FARE, 2019). Because many undergraduates now report a clinician-diagnosed FA, virtually every residence hall will house at least one affected student each year (Wu & Wang, 2023). Nurses should therefore encourage families to scrutinize campus housing policies as closely as they evaluate academics.

Residence-hall living offers proximity to classes and social life, but the communal model amplifies cross-contact risk: even trace amounts of an allergen transferred by shared utensils or countertops can trigger reactions (Stankovich et al., 2023). Ask whether the school provides "medical singles," priority placement in suites with private or semi-private kitchens, or dorm rooms equipped with microwaves and mini-fridges; many institutions now reserve such spaces for food-allergic students when presented a clinician's letter (FARE, 2019; Wu & Wang, 2023). Nurses should coach students to finalize roommate contracts that designate allergen-free shelves to ensure clean surfaces, sealed bins, labeled cookware, and availability of wipes to clean surfaces when needed (Watson et al., 2015). However, cross-contact does not disappear in private spaces; shared boards, residual steam, and even dish towels can transfer protein. Color-coded utensils, separate drying racks, and detergent-and-water cleaning, not alcohol wipes, form the evidence-based triad of dorm-kitchen hygiene endorsed by collegiate FARE guidelines (Sheehan et al., 2018; FARE, 2025c).

As highlighted previously, effective risk reduction also hinges on training the people who share or supervise that environment. Only 18% of resident advisers (RAs) at one large U.S. university could correctly describe the steps for intramuscular epinephrine before training. Similar to the results in dining halls, a 15-minute AllerTrain RA module raised competency to 92% immediately and 71% at three-month follow-up (Valerie, 2015; Wagner, n.d.). Nurses can encourage housing directors to mandate such brief, evidence-based programs and include dining staff, athletic trainers, and campus security. See Fig. 2 for instructions on how to use the epinephrine auto-injector device and see manufacturer website for epinephrine nasal spray use.

Whatever the setting, colleges have a legal duty to make "reasonable accommodations" under the Americans with Disabilities Act and its 2008 Amendments; the landmark Lesley University settlement confirms that housing and meal-plan fees cannot penalize students who require allergy-related modifications (National Association of College and University Attorneys, 2014). FARE's Access Services Guidance advises campuses to manage requests through a central accessibility office, integrate housing, dining, and health services, and provide clear grievance procedures, all steps shown to reduce reaction rates and improve quality of life (FARE, 2019). The College Resource Center on the Food Allergy and Anaphylaxis Connection Team (FAACT) website provides legal considerations for AYAs and their parents to prepare legal documents for access to medical, financial, and academic records and more via a College Toolkit (FAACT, n.d.). Nurses should direct families to the accommodations office as early as possible and document the accommodations agreed upon.

Qualitative interviews and survey data from U.S. campuses consistently show that juniors and seniors with food allergy seek off-campus apartments to gain greater control of grocery purchasing, pantry organization, and meal preparation, a shift they link to fewer accidental exposures compared with dormitory life (O'Sullivan et al., 2025; Yuan et al., 2024). Yet the same studies emphasize hidden trade-offs: higher rent, utilities, and transportation costs increase financial stress and have been

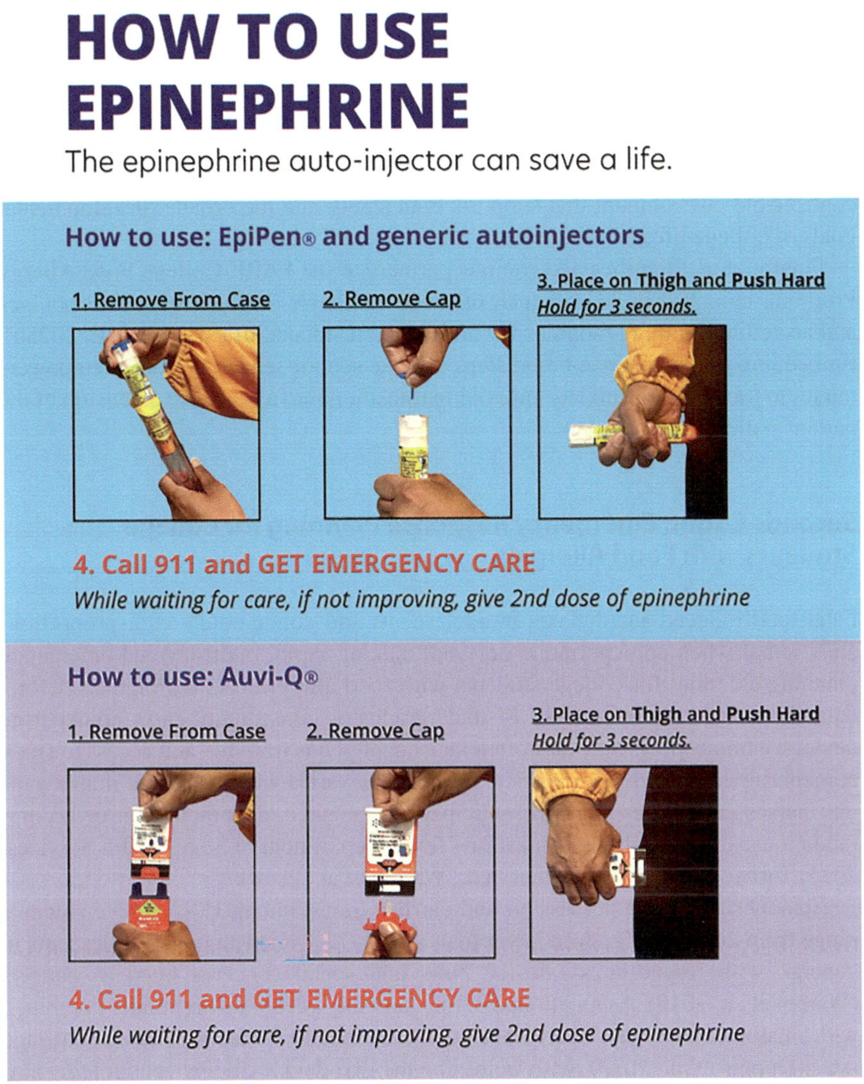

Fig. 2 How to use epinephrine. (Reprinted with permission from: Food allergy education guide: Early childhood through college by Center for Food Allergy and Asthma Research. (2024). Retrieved from https://issuu.com/cfaarnu/docs/cfaar_ed_guide_final)

associated with lapses in strict avoidance and epinephrine-carriage practices (Duncan & Annunziato, 2018; Dyer et al., 2018).

For nurses guiding adolescents and young adults through the transition to campus life, housing decisions deserve the same clinical rigor as medication management. Encourage families to start early with the accessibility services office, secure written accommodation agreements, and verify that roommates, resident advisers, and landlords all understand cross-contact prevention and emergency protocols.

Reinforce the evidence that meticulous cleaning routines, labeled storage, and separate cookware are as critical in a four-person apartment as they are in a communal dorm kitchen. Finally, remind students that autonomy brings new responsibilities: budgeting for allergen-safe food, consistently carrying epinephrine, and holding regular "kitchen huddles" with roommates. When these elements are in place, the living space, whether residence hall or off-campus rental, becomes a predictable, controllable environment that supports both safety and the broader developmental goals of college life.

Finally, direct families and campus partners to the FARE College Food Allergy Program, launched in 2014, which offers a searchable database of school policies and accredited training modules for dining and residence-life staff (FARE, 2025b). Embedding these evidence-based steps into the school-selection process empowers nurses to transform an anxiety-provoking transition into a proactive extension of the patient's allergy care plan.

Seconds Count: Emergency Response Planning for College Students with Food Allergies

Fatal food-induced anaphylaxis in adolescents and young adults is disproportionately lethal when epinephrine is delayed, making rapid, multi-layered emergency planning essential for college students with food allergies. As highlighted before, data show that fewer than half of undergraduates consistently carry epinephrine devices, campus peers and staff often lack anaphylaxis training, and access to stock epinephrine and nearby emergency departments varies widely, all modifiable gaps that nurses can address through anticipatory guidance, documentation of accommodations, and skills-based education (Texas Department of State Health Services, 2025; Turner et al., 2015; Wagner, n.d.; Warren et al., 2018).

Epinephrine device possession and carriage rates among U.S. college students range from 26% to 48%, even lower than the 42–72% cited amongst adolescents in general, with forgetfulness, device bulk, and social concerns cited as barriers (Warren et al., 2018). As mentioned before, a twice-weekly text reminder combined with small incentives can be leveraged to increase daily epinephrine device carriage rates (Dupuis et al., 2023). Also, reinforce the two-device rule by encouraging students to carry two epinephrine devices at all times. Maintaining spare devices that remain in the dorm or apartment in a designated spot to access during an emergency is recommended. Students should log refill dates and enable automatic expiration-date alerts on their phones; in one quality-improvement initiative, pairing device logs with smartphone reminders increased the proportion of participants with at least one valid autoinjector on hand from 38% at baseline to 76% at six-month follow-up in a college-age cohort (Ziyar et al., 2022).

Qualitative work shows that adolescents who disclose their allergy and teach two or more friends to recognize anaphylaxis report higher self-efficacy and faster treatment times during simulated emergencies (Newman et al., 2022; Sampson et al., 2006). Social-support studies also link peer involvement to lower anxiety and better quality-of-life scores on the FAQLQ-Teen form (Greiwe, 2023). Nurses can advise students to hold a five-minute "allergy huddle" with roommates at the start of each term and practice epinephrine use on trainer devices.

At least 15 U.S. states now permit or require colleges to maintain undesignated (stock) epinephrine auto-injectors (EAIs); implementation studies show 100% treatment success with no dosing errors when devices are placed in dining halls and residence-life offices and staff are algorithm-trained (Texas Department of State Health Services, 2025; Jain et al., 2025). Confirm whether the accessibility-services office coordinates epinephrine device placement and ensure written emergency action plans (EAPs) specify stock locations. States adopting mandatory "stock epinephrine" laws saw a 2.5-fold increase in lay-staff administration and a corresponding drop in ambulance transfers for uncontrolled reactions (Russell et al., 2023).

Population-level analyses reveal that anaphylaxis fatality correlates with delayed hospital arrival; mortality falls by 23% when treatment occurs within 30 minutes of symptom onset (Turner et al., 2020). United Kingdom registry data show stable case-fatality rates despite a 615% rise in admissions, emphasizing the life-saving impact of prompt epinephrine and ready access to emergency care (Turner et al., 2015). Map the closest emergency department, confirm 24-hour service, and coach students on calling campus EMS versus direct transport depending on response times.

In the end, a rapid, coordinated response is what turns an allergic emergency from life-threatening to manageable. This readiness rests on many layers: students who keep two current epinephrine devices on hand, friends and campus staff who can recognize anaphylaxis and act, college systems that supply stock epinephrine, knowledge of how to administer devices, and quick access to emergency care (see Fig. 2 for instructions on epinephrine autoinjector use). By helping students weave these layers together, through practical carriage strategies, peer education, and collaboration with housing, dining, and accessibility services, nurses can shift the campus environment from reactive to prepared, freeing young adults with food allergies to focus on learning rather than looming risk.

A nasal epinephrine device was approved in 2024. The device is similar to a Narcan nasal spray device. Instructions for use include holding the device upright with thumb on the bottom of the plunger component and placing fingers on either side of the nasal spray component (ARS Pharmaceuticals Operations, 2025). Spray should be deployed straight into the nostril with head in an upright position and instruct the patient to avoid sniffing the medication. Monitoring for symptom resolution is important and if symptoms persist another nasal spray can be given in the same manner in the same nostril 5 minutes after the initial dose (ARS Pharmaceuticals Operations, 2025).

Safe and Confident Dating for Adolescents and Young Adults with Food Allergies

Romantic relationships introduce new social milestones just as AYAs assume full responsibility for their FA care, making clear, evidence-based guidance essential for nurses. Qualitative interviews show that disclosure worries, fear of appearing "difficult," and anxiety in restaurants are recurrent themes when teens discuss dating with food allergy (Hullmann et al., 2012; O'Sullivan et al., 2025). As highlighted earlier, intimacy poses documented risks, with partner contact triggering reactions in food-allergic individuals when precautions are overlooked (Caminati et al., 2019; Liccardi et al., 2017).

Effective risk reduction begins with early, unapologetic communication. Educational resources for patients consistently emphasize telling new partners about specific allergens and reaction severity before physical contact; doing so not only normalizes safety discussions but also empowers the partner to help avoid accidental exposure (Allergy & Asthma Network, 2025; FARE, 2025d). Nurses should coach AYAs to frame the conversation as routine health information, comparable to carrying an inhaler, rather than a personal shortcoming, a strategy linked to lower dating-related anxiety scores in mixed-methods studies (Hullmann et al., 2012).

Partner preparedness is the next pillar. Simulation and school-based trials show that brief, hands-on epinephrine device instruction markedly improves correct-use rates and confidence among laypersons, benefits that persist for months (Shiraishi et al., 2019). Encourage patients to demonstrate their own device, review anaphylaxis symptoms, and rehearse the emergency action plan together; couples who practice in advance respond faster and are less likely to delay epinephrine during real events (Hullmann et al., 2012; Shiraishi et al., 2019). Carrying two in-date epinephrine devices, one for the patient and one that a companion can access, is recommended.

Intimate contact warrants special precautions because peanuts and other allergens can linger in saliva or semen (Bahna, 2023). Controlled studies found that brushing teeth or chewing gum immediately after ingestion fails to eliminate peanut protein, whereas waiting several hours and consuming an allergen-free meal reduces salivary levels below detection in most cases (Allergy & Asthma Network, 2025; Maloney et al., 2006). Hand hygiene matters too: Laboratory work shows that soap-and-water washing, or commercial wipes, remove Ara h 1, a peanut protein, from skin surfaces, while plain water or alcohol-based sanitizer does not (FARE, 2025b). Nurses should therefore advise couples to combine time intervals with thorough hand- and mouth-cleaning before kissing or engaging in intimate contact. Disposable travel toothbrushes and wipes can facilitate these steps when dining out.

Young adults with latex allergy should feel confident discussing latex-free condoms with partners to prevent reactions and reduce anxiety about safer sex. According to Abma and Martinez (2017), the majority of teenagers reported condom use at their first sexual experience. Latex allergy is strongly associated with cross-reactivity to certain foods ("latex-fruit syndrome"). Gromek et al. (2024) describe the top allergic foods as banana, avocado, kiwi, and papaya, but allergic reactions to associated fruits and vegetables have also been reported.

The U.S. does not require labeling of allergens in cosmetics currently, but the Modernization of the Cosmetics Regulations Act (MoCRA) will increase regulatory guidance for fragrances and cosmetics (U.S. Food & Drug Administration, 2025). Other countries may have various regulations such as labeling fragrances but exposures to allergens in non-food products may provoke symptoms. Nut oils, wheat proteins, and milk derivatives appear in shaving creams, body lotions, and hair products; case-control data link regular use of peanut-containing skin preparations to higher odds of clinical peanut allergy, and patient advocacy groups continue to document reactions from cosmetic lines marketed as "natural" (Adomaite et al., 2020; Lack et al., 2003). Nurses should remind AYAs to inspect ingredient lists, sometimes written in Latin on cosmetics, and, if necessary, suggest hypoallergenic alternatives for both partners. In addition, adolescents and young adults should be mindful of allergens in alcohol products which are not required to contain precautionary or food allergen labeling in the United States.

Restaurant dates pose well-described risks: Cross-contact in commercial kitchens and inconsistent staff knowledge remain leading triggers of adolescent reactions (FARE, 2025a; Blachar et al., 2025). AYAs who feel unsafe can reframe the experience by cooking together at home; this strategy not only strengthens relationship bonds but also affords full control over ingredients. Finally, partner attitudes affect adherence. Psychosocial research indicates that AYAs who perceive their partners as supportive report better quality-of-life scores and fewer near-misses during social eating (O'Sullivan et al., 2025; Blachar et al., 2025). Nurses should validate patients' right to insist on safety boundaries: If a partner belittles precautions or repeatedly forgets agreed-upon measures, this is a red flag rather than an overreaction (Allergy & Asthma Network, 2025). Encouraging AYAs to prioritize their health and modeling language for reinforcing boundaries, renegotiating expectations, or ending unsafe relationships helps strengthen self-advocacy skills that extend beyond dating.

By integrating early disclosure, partner training, evidence-based hygiene protocols, vigilance over personal-care items, and empowerment to set boundaries, nurses can equip adolescents and young adults to experience dating as a source of joy rather than hazard, without compromising on food-allergy safety.

Other Cofactors That Could Increase Risk of Anaphylaxis

Extrinsic factors such as NSAID use, exercise, sleep deprivation, stress, alcohol, infections, and menstruation can all increase the risk of anaphylaxis if a food allergen is ingested. Nurses can advise AYAs proactively about managing these risk factors (Bartra et al., 2023; Chong et al., 2024).

Conclusion

AYAs living with FA must be prepared to navigate the convergence of autonomy, risk-taking, and rapid transitions. This chapter underscores that safe handling of this period depends not only on prescribing an epinephrine device, but also an intentionally layered strategy led by knowledgeable nurses. By combining proactive counseling, skill-based training, and advocacy, nurses can transform high-risk environments, including dining halls, dorm kitchens, laboratories, social settings, and the workplace into safer, more predictable spaces.

Throughout the discussion in this chapter, a few key messages stand out. First, early, structured education in allergen recognition, label literacy, cross-contact prevention, and prompt epinephrine use remains critical to effective self-management. Second, institutional partnerships matter and proactive engagement with accessibility services, dining directors, housing offices, and student affairs personnel creates a framework that supports individual vigilance. Third, coaching AYAs to disclose their allergy confidently, to train peers and partners, and to rehearse emergency plans converts anxiety into actionable preparedness and improves quality-of-life. Finally, technology and policy innovations, including stock epinephrine programs, voice-prompt epinephrine devices, and standardized training modules, offer scalable tools that nurses should encourage within their practice settings.

Overall, these evidence-based interventions position nurses as catalysts of a culture of safety that extends from clinic to campus and beyond. When nurses equip AYAs with practical skills, advocate for inclusive policies, and foster resilient support networks, they enable this population to pursue academic, social, and professional aspirations without disproportionate fear of allergic reactions. The result is a generation of resilient young adults who not only overcome the challenges of food allergy but also lead with unwavering confidence, empowering themselves and inspiring meaningful change in their communities.

References

Abma, J. C., & Martinez, G. M. (2017, June 22). *Sexual activity and contraceptive use among teenagers in the United States, 2011–2015* (National Health Statistics Report No. 104). National Center for Health Statistics. https://www.cdc.gov/nchs/data/nhsr/nhsr104.pdf

Abrams, E. M., Singer, A. G., Lix, L., Katz, A., Yogendran, M., & Simons, F. E. R. (2017). Adherence with epinephrine autoinjector prescriptions in primary care. *Allergy, Asthma & Clinical Immunology, 13*(1), 46. https://doi.org/10.1186/s13223-017-0218-5

Adomaite, I., Vitkuviene, A., Petraitiene, S., & Rudzeviciene, O. (2020). Food allergens in skincare products marketed for children. *Contact Dermatitis, 83*(4), 271–276. https://doi.org/10.1111/cod.13645

Allergy & Asthma Network. (2025). *Dating with food allergies*. Retrieved July 25, 2025, from https://allergyasthmanetwork.org/news/dating-with-food-allergies/

Allergy and Asthma Network. (2025). *Dating with food allergies: What you need to know*. Retrieved July 25, 2025 from https://allergyasthmanetwork.org/news/dating-with-food-allergies/

American Academy of Allergy, Asthma, & Immunology. (2020). *Food allergy: Nuts oils in topical products*. Retrieved July 25, 2025, from https://www.aaaai.org/allergist-resources/ask-the-expert/answers/old-ask-the-experts/nutoil

Anagnostou, A., Abrams, E. M., Anderson, W. C., Carver, M., Eftekhari, S., Golden, D. B. K., Jaffee, H., Lieberman, J. A., Mack, D. P., Mustafa, S. S., Shaker, M. S., Spergel, J. M., Stukus, D. R., Wang, J., & Greenhawt, M. (2025). Development of a validated, updated North American pediatric food allergy anaphylaxis management plan. *Annals of Allergy, Asthma & Immunology, 135*(1), 71–78.e4. https://doi.org/10.1016/j.anai.2025.03.027

ARS Pharmaceuticals Operations. (2025). *Instructions for use neffy (epinephrine nasal spray).* Retrieved August 27, 2025 from https://neffypro.com/resources/#resource-library

Aytulu, T., Gundogdu, B. S., Yayci, E., Ezelsoy, I., Buyuktiryaki, B., Veznikli, M., Isik, S. R., & Sackesen, C. (2025). The evaluation of food allergy knowledge and attitude in different food sectors and the effectiveness of video-based training. *Frontiers in Nutrition, 12.* https://doi.org/10.3389/fnut.2025.1512845

Bahna, S. L. (2023). New insights in hidden food allergies. *Journal of Food Allergy (East Providence, R.I. : Online), 5*(1), 19–24. https://doi.org/10.2500/jfa.2023.5.230003

Bartra, J., Turner, P. J., & Muñoz-Cano, R. M. (2023). Cofactors in food anaphylaxis in adults. *Annals of Allergy, Asthma & Immunology: Official Publication of the American College of Allergy, Asthma, & Immunology, 130*(6), 733–740. https://doi.org/10.1016/j.anai.2023.03.017

Bedford, B., Liggans, G., Williams, L., & Jackson, L. (2020). Allergen removal and transfer with wiping and cleaning methods used in retail and food service establishments. *Journal of Food Protection, 83*(7), 1248–1260. https://doi.org/10.4315/JFP-20-025

Blachar, J., Pickett-Nairne, K., Hicks, A., Moore, W., Venter, C., & Athanasopoulou, P. (2025). Social and dietary impacts of food allergies in adolescents: Insights from a US teen survey. *Pediatric Allergy and Immunology, 36*(6), e70134. https://doi.org/10.1111/pai.70134

Blom, W. M., van Dijk, L. M., Michelsen-Huisman, A., Houben, G. F., Knulst, A. C., Linders, Y. F. M., Verhoeckx, K. C. M., Holleman, B. C., & Lentz, L. R. (2021). Allergen labelling: Current practice and improvement from a communication perspective. *Clinical and Experimental Allergy, 51*(4), 574–584. https://doi.org/10.1111/cea.13830

Bosch, C., Niroula, K., & McKinley, E. (2024). College students with medical dietary restrictions face financial and personal challenges trying to meet nutritional needs. *Psychology, 15*(1), Article 1. https://doi.org/10.4236/psych.2024.151002

Brussino, L., Nicola, S., Giorgis, V., & Rolla, G. (2018). Beer anaphylaxis due to coriander as hidden allergen. *BMJ Case Reports, 2018*, bcr2018225562. https://doi.org/10.1136/bcr-2018-225562

Budi, H. S., & Pebriani, I. (2020). The protein level and molecular weight analysis in different children's toothpaste, which probably induced hypersensitivity. *Contemporary Clinical Dentistry, 11*(3), 245–248. https://doi.org/10.4103/ccd.ccd_394_19

Caminati, M., Giorgis, V., Palterer, B., Racca, F., Salvottini, C., & Rossi, O. (2019). Allergy and sexual Behaviours: An update. *Clinical Reviews in Allergy & Immunology, 56*(3), 269–277. https://doi.org/10.1007/s12016-017-8618-3

Center for Food Allergy & Asthma Research. (2024). *Food allergy education guide: Early childhood through college.* Retrieved from https://issuu.com/cfaarnu/docs/cfaar_ed_guide_final

Cha, L. M.-J., Lee, W. S., Han, M. Y., & Lee, K. S. (2022). The timely Administration of Epinephrine and Related Factors in children with anaphylaxis. *Journal of Clinical Medicine, 11*(19), 5494. https://doi.org/10.3390/jcm11195494

Chong, T., Olivieri, B., & Skypala, I. J. (2024). Food-triggered anaphylaxis in adults. *Current Opinion in Allergy and Clinical Immunology, 24*(5), 341–348. https://doi.org/10.1097/ACI.0000000000001008

Commins, S. P. (2020). Diagnosis & management of alpha-gal syndrome: Lessons from 2,500 patients. *Expert Review of Clinical Immunology, 16*(7), 667–677. Retrieved August 14, 2025. https://doi.org/10.1080/1744666X.2020.1782745.

Dodd, A., Hughes, A., Sargant, N., Whyte, A. F., Soar, J., & Turner, P. J. (2021). Evidence update for the treatment of anaphylaxis. *Resuscitation, 163*, 86–96. https://doi.org/10.1016/j.resuscitation.2021.04.010

Downey, L. A., Heinz, M. C., & Murphey, M. (2025). Nurse-led allergy education for non-medical school staff. *OJIN: The Online Journal of Issues in Nursing, 30*(1) Retrieved August 11, 2025. https://doi.org/10.3912/OJIN.Vol30No01PPT64

Dribin, T. E., & Greenhawt, M. (2024). Epinephrine and anaphylaxis outcomes. *Annals of Allergy, Asthma & Immunology: Official Publication of the American College of Allergy, Asthma, & Immunology, 133*(5), 501–502. https://doi.org/10.1016/j.anai.2024.08.029

Duncan, S. E., & Annunziato, R. A. (2018). Barriers to self-management behaviors in college students with food allergies. *Journal of American College Health: J of ACH, 66*(5), 331–339. https://doi.org/10.1080/07448481.2018.1431898

Dupuis, R., Feuerstein-Simon, R., Brown-Whitehorn, T. F., Spergel, J. M., Volpp, K. G., Marti, X. L., Troxel, A. B., Meisel, Z. F., Mollen, C. J., Kenney, E. L., Block, J., Gortmaker, S. L., & Cannuscio, C. C. (2023). Food allergy management for adolescents using behavioral incentives: A randomized trial. *Pediatrics, 151*(2), e2022058876. https://doi.org/10.1542/peds.2022-058876

Dyer, A. A., O'Keefe, A., Kanaley, M. K., Kao, L. M., & Gupta, R. S. (2018). Leaving the nest: Improving food allergy management on college campuses. *Annals of Allergy, Asthma & Immunology, 121*(1), 82–89.e5. https://doi.org/10.1016/j.anai.2018.04.009

Egmose, B., Huniche, L., Bindslev-Jensen, C., Nielsen, D. S., & Mørtz, C. G. (2024). Exploring young adults' experiences with food allergy during their teenage years: A practice research study. *Scandinavian Journal of Caring Sciences, 38*(4), 844–853. https://doi.org/10.1111/scs.13283

FARE. (2019). *Access service guidance for students with food-related disabilities*. Retrieved August 25, 2025 from chrome-extension://efaidnbmnnnibpcajpcglclefindmkaj/https://www.foodallergy.org/sites/default/files/2020-01/FARE-guidelines-for-access-service-guidance.pdf

FARE. (2025a). *Avoiding cross-contact*. Retrieved July 25, 2025, from https://www.foodallergy.org/resources/avoiding-cross-contact

FARE. (2025b). *Cleaning methods*. Retrieved July 28, 2025 from https://www.foodallergy.org/resources/cleaning-methods

FARE. (2025c). *FARE food allergy college program*. Retrieved July 25, 2025, from https://www.foodallergy.org/our-initiatives/education-programs-training/fare-food-allergy-college-program

FARE. (2025d). *Relationships and dating*. Retrieved July 25, 2025, from https://www.foodallergy.org/resources/relationships-and-dating

FARE. (2025e). *FARECheck*. https://www.foodallergy.org/our-initiatives/education-programs-training/farecheck

Food Allergy & Anaphylaxis Connection Team. (n.d.). *Legal considerations*. Retrieved August 5, 2025, from https://www.foodallergyawareness.org/college-resource-center/legal-considerations/legal-considerations/

Food Allergy & Anaphylaxis Connection Team (FAACT). (n.d.). *Crustacean shellfish*. Retrieved August 26, 2025, from https://www.foodallergyawareness.org/food-allergy-and-anaphylaxis/food-allergens/crustacean-shellfish/?utm_source=chatgpt.com

Greiwe, J. (2023). Quality of life and psychological issues associated with food allergy. *Journal of Food Allergy, 5*(2), 43–48. https://doi.org/10.2500/jfa.2023.5.230011

Gromek, W., Kołdej, N., Świtała, S., Majsiak, E., & Kurowski, M. (2024). Revisiting latex-fruit syndrome after 30 years of research: A comprehensive literature review and description of two cases. *Journal of Clinical Medicine, 13*(14), 4222. https://doi.org/10.3390/jcm13144222. PMID: 39064262; PMCID: PMC11278189.

Herbert, L. J., Lin, A., Matsui, E., Wood, R. A., & Sharma, H. (2016). Development of a tool to measure youths' food allergy management facilitators and barriers. *Journal of Pediatric Psychology, 41*(3), 363–372. https://doi.org/10.1093/jpepsy/jsv099

Hullmann, S. E., Molzon, E. S., Eddington, A. R., & Mullins, L. L. (2012). Dating anxiety in adolescents and young adults with food allergies: A comparison to healthy peers. *Journal of Asthma & Allergy Educators, 3*(4), 172–177. https://doi.org/10.1177/2150129711431888

Jain, A., Haffey, E., Whiteside, K., O'Shea, K., Slack, I., Baker, J., & Schuler, C. (2025). Food allergy and anaphylaxis in a university campus dining program. *Journal of Allergy and Clinical Immunology, 155*(2), AB64. https://doi.org/10.1016/j.jaci.2024.12.202

Jones, C. J., Llewellyn, C. D., Frew, A. J., Du Toit, G., Mukhopadhyay, S., & Smith, H. (2015). Factors associated with good adherence to self-care behaviours amongst adolescents with food allergy. *Pediatric Allergy and Immunology: Official Publication of the European Society of Pediatric Allergy and Immunology, 26*(2), 111–118. https://doi.org/10.1111/pai.12333

Keohane, H., Cronin, C., & Trujillo, J. (2022). Risk taking and self-care behaviours amongst adolescents and young adults with food allergies. *Allergologia et Immunopathologia, 50*(4), 31–49. https://doi.org/10.15586/aei.v50i4.580

Keohane, H., Cronin, C., O'Rourke, E., O'Kelly, C., Ramesh, Y., Flores, L., Velasco, R., & Trujillo, J. (2023). Teaching children with food allergy to recognize anaphylaxis: The caregivers' perspectives. *Pediatric Allergy and Immunology: Official Publication of the European Society of Pediatric Allergy and Immunology, 34*(8), e14006. https://doi.org/10.1111/pai.14006

Kessler, C., Edwards, E., Dissinger, E., Sye, S., Visich, T., & Grant, E. (2019). Usability and preference of epinephrine auto-injectors: Auvi-Q and EpiPen Jr. *Annals of Allergy, Asthma & Immunology, 123*(3), 256–262. https://doi.org/10.1016/j.anai.2019.06.005

Kids with Food Allergies. (2024). *Food allergens may hide in non-food items.* https://kidswithfoodallergies.org/living-with-food-allergies/choosing-safe-foods/unexpected-allergens-in-non-food-items/

Koo, L. W., Baur, C., Horowitz, A. M., & Wang, M. Q. (2023). Parental health literacy, empowerment, and advocacy for Food Allergy safety in schools: A cross-sectional study. *Health Literacy Research and Practice, 7*(3), e165–e175. https://doi.org/10.3928/24748307-20230823-01

Krejner-Bienias, A., Grzela, K., Kulus, M., & Grzela, T. (2023). Peanut contamination in food products: A real danger for allergic people? *Advances in Dermatology and Allergology/Postępy Dermatologii i Alergologii, 40*(5), 625–629. https://doi.org/10.5114/ada.2023.132219

Lack, G., Fox, D., Northstone, K., & Golding, J. (2003). Factors associated with the development of peanut allergy in childhood. *New England Journal of Medicine, 348*(11), 977–985. https://doi.org/10.1056/NEJMoa013536

Leone, L., Mazzocchi, A., Maffeis, L., De Cosmi, V., & Agostoni, C. (2023). Nutritional management of food allergies: Prevention and treatment. *Frontiers in Allergy, 3*, 1083669. https://doi.org/10.3389/falgy.2022.1083669

Levy, J. H., Ghadimi, K., Kizhakkedathu, J. N., & Iba, T. (2023). What's fishy about protamine? Clinical use, adverse reactions, and potential alternatives. *Journal of Thrombosis and Haemostasis, 21*(7), 1714–1723. https://doi.org/10.1016/j.jtha.2023.04.005

Liccardi, G., Caminati, M., Senna, G., Calzetta, L., & Rogliani, P. (2017). Anaphylaxis and intimate behaviour. *Current Opinion in Allergy and Clinical Immunology, 17*(5), 350–355. https://doi.org/10.1097/ACI.0000000000000386

Luparelli, A., Losito, I., De Angelis, E., Pilolli, R., & Monaci, L. (2023). Multi-target detection of nuts and peanuts as hidden allergens in bakery products through bottom-up proteomics and high-resolution mass spectrometry. *Food, 12*(4), Article 4. https://doi.org/10.3390/foods12040726

Maloney, J. M., Chapman, M. D., & Sicherer, S. H. (2006). Peanut allergen exposure through saliva: Assessment and interventions to reduce exposure. *The Journal of Allergy and Clinical Immunology, 118*(3), 719–724. https://doi.org/10.1016/j.jaci.2006.05.017

Mawhirt, S., Fonacier, L., & Aquino, M. (2018). Educational outcomes of an anaphylaxis simulation activity among medical students and residents. *Annals of Allergy, Asthma & Immunology, 121*(5, Supplement), S1. https://doi.org/10.1016/j.anai.2018.09.001

MenuTrinfo. (2025). *AllerTrain Lite*. Retrieved August 14th, 2025, from https://menutrinfo.com/training/allertrain-lite/

Meyran, D., Cassan, P., Nemeth, M., Singletary, E., Raitt, J., Djarv, T., & Carlson, J. N. (2023). The ability of first aid providers to recognize anaphylaxis: A scoping review. *Cureus, 15*(7), e41547. https://doi.org/10.7759/cureus.41547

Nahle, R., Thaivalappil, A., & Young, I. (2025). Food Allergy labeling and disclosure practices on restaurants' online menus in Toronto, Canada. *Journal of Food Protection, 88*(7), 100533. https://doi.org/10.1016/j.jfp.2025.100533

National Association of College and University Attorneys (NACUANOTES). (2014). *Food for thought: Applying the ADA to students with food allergies*. Retrieved August 25, 2025 from chrome-extension://efaidnbmnnnibpcajpcglclefindmkaj/https://www.higheredcompliance.org/wp-content/uploads/2018/10/FoodAllergies.pdf

Newman, K. L., Chater, A., & Knibb, R. C. (2022). Beliefs about food allergies in adolescents aged 11-19 years: A systematic review. *Clinical and Translational Allergy, 12*(4), e12142. https://doi.org/10.1002/clt2.12142

Novembre, E., Gelsomino, M., Liotti, L., Barni, S., Mori, F., Giovannini, M., Mastrorilli, C., Pecoraro, L., Saretta, F., Castagnoli, R., Arasi, S., Caminiti, L., Klain, A., & del Giudice, M. M. (2024). Fatal food anaphylaxis in adults and children. *Italian Journal of Pediatrics, 50*, 40. https://doi.org/10.1186/s13052-024-01608-x

O'Sullivan, M., Curtin, M., Flynn, R., Trujillo, J., & O'Mahony, J. (2025). "When I became older, I started having to manage that more myself"—Experiences of adolescents with food allergies: A qualitative study. *Pediatric Allergy and Immunology, 36*(2), e70048. https://doi.org/10.1111/pai.70048

Obreque-Slier, E., Cortés-Araya, K., Medel-Marabolí, M., & López-Solís, R. (2023). Different effectiveness of protein fining agents when tested for interaction and precipitation with tannic acid, a seed polyphenol extract and seven wines. *OENO one, 57*(2), Article 2. https://doi.org/10.20870/oeno-one.2023.57.2.7264

Papadopoulos, A., Elegbede, C. F., Ait-Dahmane, S., Dubuisson, C., Deschildre, A., & Crépet, A. (2018). Tree nut allergy and anxiety related factors modulate food consumption behaviour in peanut-allergic patients: Results of the MIRABEL survey. *Regulatory Toxicology and Pharmacology: RTP, 99*, 191–199. https://doi.org/10.1016/j.yrtph.2018.09.020

Protudjer, J. L. P., Jansson, S.-A., Middelveld, R., Östblom, E., Dahlén, S.-E., Arnlind, M. H., Bengtsson, U., Kallström-Bengtsson, I., Marklund, B., Rentzos, G., Sundqvist, A.-C., Åkerström, J., & Ahlstedt, S. (2016). Impaired health-related quality of life in adolescents with allergy to staple foods. *Clinical and Translational Allergy, 6*, 37. https://doi.org/10.1186/s13601-016-0128-5

Radke, T. J. (2017). Restaurant food allergy practices—Six selected sites, United States, 2014. *MMWR. Morbidity and Mortality Weekly Report*, 66. https://doi.org/10.15585/mmwr.mm6615a2

Remington, B. C., Blom, W. M., Bassa, B., & Koppelman, S. J. (2020). Risk of shared equipment in restaurants for consumers with peanut allergy: A simulation for preparing Asian foods. *Annals of Allergy, Asthma & Immunology, 125*(5), 543–551.e6. https://doi.org/10.1016/j.anai.2020.07.030

Ridolo, E., Incorvaia, C., & Schroeder, J. W. (2022). Airborne anaphylaxis: Highlighting an invisible enemy. *Current Opinion in Allergy and Clinical Immunology, 22*(5), 283–290. https://doi.org/10.1097/ACI.0000000000000848

Roberts, G., Vazquez-Ortiz, M., Knibb, R., Khaleva, E., Alviani, C., Angier, E., Blumchen, K., Comberiati, P., Duca, B., DunnGalvin, A., Garriga-Baraut, T., Gore, C., Gowland, M. H., Hox, V., Jensen, B., Mortz, C. G., Pfaar, O., Pite, H., Santos, A. F., et al. (2020). EAACI guidelines on the effective transition of adolescents and young adults with allergy and asthma. *Allergy, 75*(11), 2734–2752. https://doi.org/10.1111/all.14459

Robinson, M., Koplin, J. J., Field, M. J., Sasaki, M., Peters, R. L., McWilliam, V., Sawyer, S. M., Patton, G. C., Vuillermin, P. J., Douglass, J., Gurrin, L. C., Tang, M. L. K., Dharmage, S. C., Allen, K. J., & SchoolNuts Investigators. (2019). Patterns of carriage of prescribed adrenaline autoinjectors in 10- to 14-year-old Food-allergic students: A population-based study. *The Journal of Allergy and Clinical Immunology. In Practice, 7*(2), 437–443. https://doi.org/10.1016/j.jaip.2018.06.025

Robles, J., & Motheral, L. (2014). Hypersensitivity reaction after inhalation of a lactose-containing dry powder inhaler. *The Journal of Pediatric Pharmacology and Therapeutics: JPPT, 19*(3), 206–211. https://doi.org/10.5863/1551-6776-19.3.206

Rotella, K., & Oriel, R. C. (2022). Accidental reactions to foods: Frequency, causes, and severity. *Current Treatment Options in Allergy, 9*(3), 157–168. https://doi.org/10.1007/s40521-022-00314-5

Russell, A. F., Bingemann, T. A., Cooke, A. T., Ponda, P., Pistiner, M., Jean, T., Nanda, A., Jobrack, J., Hoyt, A. E. W., & Young, M. C. (2023). The need for required stock epinephrine in all schools: A work group report of the AAAAI adverse reactions to foods committee. *The Journal of Allergy and Clinical Immunology: In Practice, 11*(4), 1068–1082.e1. https://doi.org/10.1016/j.jaip.2022.12.047

Ryczaj, K., Chojnowska-Wójtowicz, M., Dumycz, K., Feleszko, W., & Kulus, M. (2023). Prevalence of major food allergens in skincare products for atopic dermatitis. *Advances in Dermatology and Allergology/Postępy Dermatologii i Alergologii, 40*(6), 762–765. https://doi.org/10.5114/ada.2023.133819

Sampson, M. A., Muñoz-Furlong, A., & Sicherer, S. H. (2006). Risk-taking and coping strategies of adolescents and young adults with food allergy. *The Journal of Allergy and Clinical Immunology, 117*(6), 1440–1445. https://doi.org/10.1016/j.jaci.2006.03.009

ServSafe. (2025). Retrieved on August 25, 2025 from https://www.servsafe.com/?gclsrc=aw.ds&gad_source=1&gad_campaignid=21111869981&gbraid=0AAAAADnsYS-KsZB0_bXS9r5eiJjvB9ibn&gclid=CjwKCAjwtrXFBhBiEiwAEKen12bJjvtur9U7_-qSeEuWF-RchEEs7y5eQV7Ek7tc8EyhfSfF3tvZmxoCtFYQAvD_BwE

Sheehan, W. J., Taylor, S. L., Phipatanakul, W., & Brough, H. A. (2018). Environmental food exposure: What is the risk of clinical reactivity from cross-contact and what is the risk of sensitization. *The Journal of Allergy and Clinical Immunology. In Practice, 6*(6), 1825–1832. https://doi.org/10.1016/j.jaip.2018.08.001

Shiraishi, Y., Ishikawa, Y., Shiraishi, Y., & Matsumura, M. (2019). Effectiveness of epinephrine auto-injector skill training for school nurses. *Journal of General and Family Medicine, 21*(1), 30–31. https://doi.org/10.1002/jgf2.282

Smits, N. G. E., De Dominicis, E., Koops, A. J., Kraan, R., Saner, S., Van Der Fels-Klerx, H. J., & Hoek-van den Hil, E. (2023). Comparison of commercial allergen ELISA kits for egg detection in food matrices. *Heliyon, 9*(10), e19687. https://doi.org/10.1016/j.heliyon.2023.e19687

Stankovich, G. A., Warren, C. M., Gupta, R., Sindher, S. B., Chinthrajah, R. S., & Nadeau, K. C. (2023). Food allergy risks and dining industry—An assessment and a path forward. *Frontiers in Allergy, 4*, 1060932. https://doi.org/10.3389/falgy.2023.1060932

Texas Department of State Health Services. (2025). *Epinephrine auto-injector resources for schools*. Retrieved July 25, 2025, from https://www.dshs.texas.gov/texas-school-health/skilled-procedures-texas-school-health/epinephrine-auto-injector-resources

Tramuta, C., Decastelli, L., Barcucci, E., Ingravalle, F., Fragassi, S., Lupi, S., & Bianchi, D. M. (2022). Detection of peanut traces in food by an official food safety laboratory. *Food, 11*(5), 643. https://doi.org/10.3390/foods11050643

Turner, P. J., Gowland, M. H., Sharma, V., Ierodiakonou, D., Harper, N., Garcez, T., Pumphrey, R., & Boyle, R. J. (2015). Increase in anaphylaxis-related hospitalizations but no increase in fatalities: An analysis of United Kingdom national anaphylaxis data, 1992-2012. *The Journal of Allergy and Clinical Immunology, 135*(4), 956–963.e1. https://doi.org/10.1016/j.jaci.2014.10.021

Turner, P. J., Campbell, D. E., Motosue, M. S., & Campbell, R. L. (2020). Global trends in anaphylaxis epidemiology and clinical implications. *The Journal of Allergy and Clinical Immunology. In Practice, 8*(4), 1169–1176. https://doi.org/10.1016/j.jaip.2019.11.027

Turner, P. J., Bognanni, A., Arasi, S., Ansotegui, I. J., Schnadt, S., Vieille, S. L., Hourihane, J. O., Zuberbier, T., Eigenmann, P., Ebisawa, M., Morais-Almeida, M., Barnett, J., Martin, B., Monaci, L., Roberts, G., Wong, G., Gupta, R., Tsabouri, S., Mills, C., et al. (2024). Time to ACT-UP: Update on precautionary allergen labelling (PAL). *World Allergy Organization Journal, 17*(10), 100972. https://doi.org/10.1016/j.waojou.2024.100972

U.S. Food & Drug Administration (2025, March 26). *Food Allergies*. Retrieved July 28, 2025, from https://www.fda.gov/food/nutrition-food-labeling-and-critical-foods/food-allergies

U.S. Food and Drug Administration. (2023). *Food code: 2022 Recommendations of the United States public health service Food and Drug Administration*. Retrieved August 5, 2025, from https://www.pa.gov/content/dam/copapwp-pagov/en/pda/documents/consumer_protection/foodsafety/retail-food/documents/FDA%20Food%20Code%202022_Full%20Document.pdf

U.S. Food and Drug Administration. (2025). *Modernization of cosmetics regulation act of 2022 (MoCRA)*. Retrieved August 5, 2025, from https://www.fda.gov/cosmetics/cosmetics-laws-regulations/modernization-cosmetics-regulation-act-2022-mocra

Umasunthar, T., Procktor, A., Hodes, M., Smith, J. G., Gore, C., Cox, H. E., Marrs, T., Hanna, H., Phillips, K., Pinto, C., Turner, P. J., Warner, J. O., & Boyle, R. J. (2015). Patients' ability to treat anaphylaxis using adrenaline autoinjectors: A randomized controlled trial. *Allergy, 70*(7), 855–863. https://doi.org/10.1111/all.12628

Valerie. (2015, August 31). AllerTrain RA™- A New Class for Resident Advisers. MenuTrinfo. https://menutrinfo.com/blog/introducing-food-allergen-class-for-resident-advisers-allertrain-ra/

Vazquez-Ortiz, M., Gore, C., Alviani, C., Angier, E., Blumchen, K., Comberiati, P., Duca, B., DunnGalvin, A., Garriga-Baraut, T., Gowland, M. H., Egmose, B., Knibb, R., Khaleva, E., Mortz, C. G., Pfaar, O., Pite, H., Podesta, M., Santos, A. F., Sanchez-Garcia, S., et al. (2023). A practical toolbox for the effective transition of adolescents and young adults with asthma and allergies: An EAACI position paper. *Allergy, 78*(1), 20–46. https://doi.org/10.1111/all.15533

Versluis, A., Le, T.-M., Houben, G. F., Knulst, A. C., & Van Os-Medendorp, H. (2023). Accidental allergic reactions to food in adolescents and adults: An overview of the factors involved and implications for prevention. *Frontiers in Allergy, 4*. https://doi.org/10.3389/falgy.2023.1062049

Vriesekoop, F. (2021). Beer and Allergens. *Beverages, 7*(4), 79. https://doi.org/10.3390/beverages7040079

Wagner, K. (n.d.). *Food allergies on the college campus: Increasing awareness*. Retrieved August 25, 2025 from chrome-extension://efaidnbmnnnibpcajpcglclefindmkaj/https://repository.belmont.edu/cgi/viewcontent.cgi?article=1104&context=dnpscholarlyprojects.

Wahl, A., Stephens, H., Ruffo, M., & Jones, A. L. (2015). The evaluation of a food allergy and epinephrine autoinjector training program for personnel who care for children in schools and community settings. *The Journal of School Nursing: The Official Publication of the National Association of School Nurses, 31*(2), 91–98. https://doi.org/10.1177/1059840514526889

Warren, C. M., Zaslavsky, J. M., Kan, K., Spergel, J. M., & Gupta, R. S. (2018). Epinephrine auto-injector carriage and use practices among US children, adolescents, and adults. *Annals of Allergy, Asthma & Immunology, 121*(4), 479–489.e2. https://doi.org/10.1016/j.anai.2018.06.010

Watson, W. T., Woodrow, A., & Stadnyk, A. W. (2015). Removal of peanut allergen Ara h 1 from common hospital surfaces, toys and books using standard cleaning methods. *Allergy, Asthma, and Clinical Immunology: Official Journal of the Canadian Society of Allergy and Clinical Immunology, 11*(1), 4. https://doi.org/10.1186/s13223-015-0069-x

Wiederstein, M., Baumgartner, S., & Lauter, K. (2023). Soybean (glycine max) allergens – A review on an outstanding plant food with allergenic potential. *ACS Food Science & Technology, 3*(3), 363–378. https://doi.org/10.1021/acsfoodscitech.2c00380

Wieser, H., Segura, V., Ruiz-Carnicer, Á., Sousa, C., & Comino, I. (2021). Food safety and cross-contamination of gluten-free products: A narrative review. *Nutrients, 13*(7), 2244. https://doi.org/10.3390/nu13072244

Wu, A. C., & Wang, A. L. (2023). Preventing anaphylaxis in college students with food allergies. *The Journal of Allergy and Clinical Immunology. In Practice, 11*(4), 1047–1048. https://doi.org/10.1016/j.jaip.2023.02.004

Yuan, I. H., Greenhawt, M., Abrams, E. M., Kim, E. H., Mustafa, S. S., & Iglesia, E. G. A. (2024). Food allergies on a college campus. *Annals of Allergy, Asthma & Immunology, 132*(5), 579–584. https://doi.org/10.1016/j.anai.2024.01.023

Ziyar, A., Kwon, J., Li, A., Naderi, A., & Jean, T. (2022). Improving epinephrine autoinjector usability and carriage frequency among patients at risk of anaphylaxis: A quality improvement initiative. *BMJ Open Quality, 11*(3). https://doi.org/10.1136/bmjoq-2021-001742

Food Allergy Management in the Hospital Setting

Kimberly Zimmanck, Carolynn Sielaff, and Danielle Palmer

General Knowledge About Food Allergies for Hospital Nurses

Most hospital nurses have received little training about food allergies in their educational programs. However, since food allergy prevalence is increasing in children and adults, it is imperative for hospital nurses to have general knowledge about food allergies. There are many situations where patients with food allergies may require hospital care and it is the nurse's role to keep patients safe. Patients are seen in the emergency department (ED) for suspected or actual allergic reactions and anaphylaxis. Patients may be placed in the hospital for observation and/or continued treatment after an allergic reaction. Depending on the patient's clinical status and the hospital's patient placement processes, patients may be placed in acute care or critical care units. In these cases, nurses may need to administer additional medications to manage the allergic reaction. Other patients with known or unknown food allergies who are in the hospital for an unrelated illness, injury, and/or surgery could be at risk of experiencing an allergic reaction or anaphylaxis due to potential allergens present in hospital food or medications. In any situation, knowledge of existing allergies, recognizing signs and symptoms of an allergic reaction, and being prepared to intervene are important for keeping patients safe.

The awareness of anaphylaxis due to any cause has improved over the years; however, many knowledge and practice gaps still exist in hospital settings. The lifetime prevalence of all-cause anaphylaxis in the United States is relatively low at 1.6–5.1% (Golden et al., 2024). While allergic reactions to foods can be life

K. Zimmanck (✉) · D. Palmer
Children's Wisconsin, Milwaukee, WI, USA
e-mail: KZimmanck@childrenswi.org; DPalmer@childrenswi.org

C. Sielaff
Children's Wisconsin with the Medical College of Wisconsin, Milwaukee, WI, USA
e-mail: CSielaff@mcw.edu

J. Doucette, J. Howard-Ruben (eds.), *Comprehensive Food Allergy Management for Nurses*, https://doi.org/10.1007/978-3-032-28647-5_9

threatening, the rate of fatal food allergy related anaphylaxis is rare at any age, although adolescents seem to be at higher risk. However, the role of risk factors is unclear, and it is difficult to predict a severe reaction so all patients are treated equally at risk of fatal anaphylaxis (Golden et al., 2024; Dorris, 2025; Turner et al., 2017). Infants appear to be at decreased risk of fatal anaphylaxis and typically present with cutaneous symptoms (Golden et al., 2024; Dorris, 2025). Overall data on anaphylaxis to food has been reported sporadically with more data available for some countries versus others. However, the literature has identified that failure to administer epinephrine in a timely manner as a contributing factor to fatal anaphylaxis (Dorris, 2025; Turner et al., 2017).

Emergency Department Management

Anaphylaxis is a life-threatening allergic reaction that can present with a broad range of signs and symptoms dependent on multiple variables. According to the World Allergy Organization (WAO), "anaphylaxis is a serious systemic hypersensitivity reaction that is usually rapid in onset and may cause death. Severe anaphylaxis is characterized by potentially life-threatening compromise in airway, breathing and/or the circulation, and may occur without typical skin features or circulatory shock being present" (Cardona et al., 2020). Patients presenting to the ED with suspected allergic reaction or food-induced anaphylaxis must be triaged promptly. Prompt recognition by the triage nurse or provider of urticaria, angioedema, gastrointestinal symptoms, respiratory compromise such as wheezing or cough, and hypotension is essential to activate emergency action. Allergic reactions can quickly progress to anaphylaxis, necessitating timely administration of epinephrine. In some cases, patients may already be experiencing anaphylaxis and/or have already received epinephrine prior to arriving in the ED.

Diagnosis of Acute Anaphylaxis in the ED Setting

Multiple different anaphylaxis diagnosis criteria and grading systems exist (Fig. 1 for one example), meaning there is variability across emergency departments depending on the applicable guidelines. Appropriate diagnosis of anaphylaxis is imperative for appropriate and timely treatment. However, delaying treatment with epinephrine can lead to poor outcomes or death; therefore, rapid treatment of symptoms if anaphylaxis is suspected should take precedence over meeting specific criteria (Golden et al., 2024).

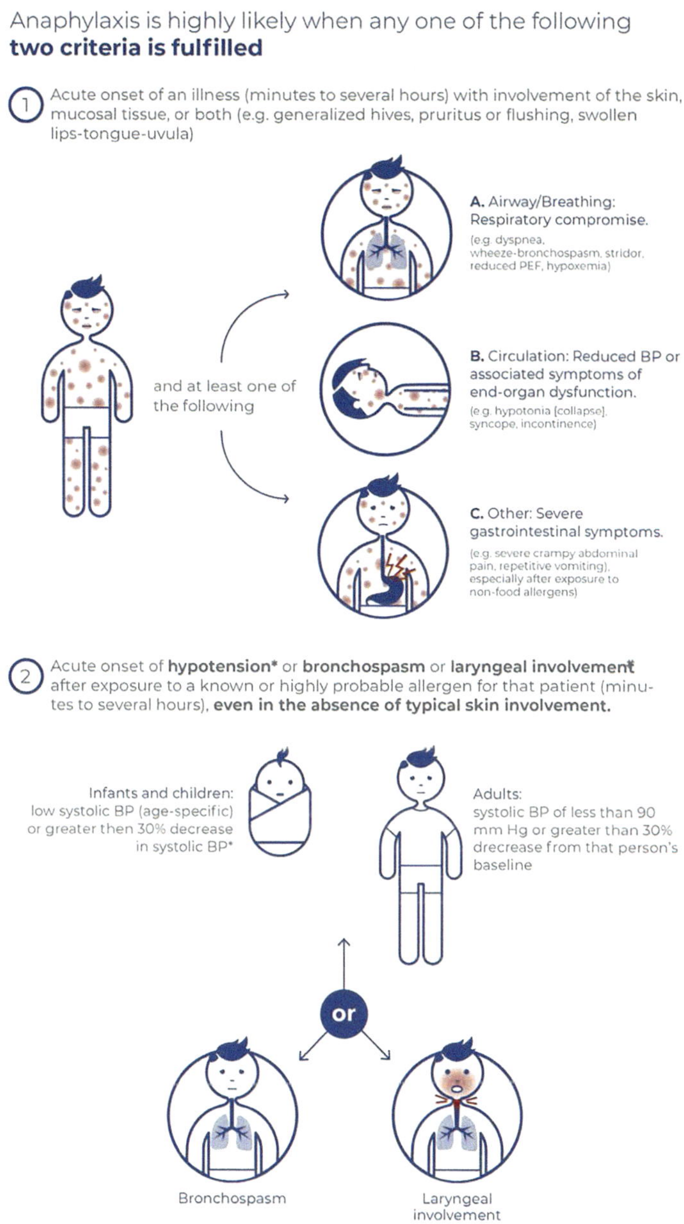

PEF, Peak expiratory flow; BP blood presure.

*Hypotension defined as a decrease in systolic BP greater than 3% from that person's baseline, OR
i. Infants and children under 10 years: systolic BP less than (70mmHg + [2 x age in years])
ii. Adults: systolic BP les than < 90 mmHg

' Laryngeal symptoms include: stridor, vocal changes, odynophagia.

Fig. 1 Diagnostic criteria for the diagnosis of anaphylaxis. (Used with permission from: Cardona et al. (2020). Published under CC BY 4.0 https://creativecommons.org/licenses/by/4.0/)

A thorough clinical history is needed to diagnose anaphylaxis (see Table 1) and should include a review of patient characteristics, a description of the reaction and other factors as outlined below:

Table 1 Clinical history when diagnosing anaphylaxis

Patient characteristics	Reaction description	Concomitant factors	Treatment/response to treatment
Age Gender Medical/atopic history Concurrent medications	Potential triggers Onset of symptoms Duration of symptoms Specific symptoms and pattern	Food Alcohol Viral illness Medications Exercise Menstrual status Stress	Was epinephrine already given? Was an antihistamine given? Was albuterol given? How did the patient respond?

Note: Table created by Kimberly Zimmanck, MS, RN, PCNS-BC, Carolynn Sielaff, MSN, APNP, FNP-C, AE-C, CPN and Danielle Palmer, BSN, RN, CPN. Content adapted from Golden et al. (2024)

Additional Considerations

Depending on the presentation and the patient's history of anaphylaxis, additional labs and testing may be required, especially for patients with recurrent, idiopathic, and/or severe anaphylaxis. For example, a serum tryptase level may be drawn if a mast cell disorder is suspected (Golden et al., 2024).

Infants and toddlers present unique age-specific symptoms that make diagnosis and treatment challenging; there are no age-specific diagnostic criteria. Infants and toddlers cannot communicate their symptoms in the same way that older children and adults can (Fig. 2). Symptoms of anaphylaxis in this age group can easily be attributed to developmentally normal behavior or other clinical conditions. Clinicians must be astute in their assessment and history taking to reduce the risk of missing a diagnosis of anaphylaxis. Of note, if this is the first time an infant or toddler had been exposed to an allergen, anaphylaxis is less likely (Golden et al., 2024; Dorris, 2025). Also see chapter "Food Allergy Management in Early Childhood Settings".

Initial Nursing Interventions

- Assessment and Airway Management
  - *Airway and Breathing Assessment*:
    - Conduct rapid Airway, Breathing, Circulation (ABC) assessment upon patient arrival.
    - Place oxygen for any patient with respiratory distress and/or decreased oxygen saturations.
    - Strongly consider oxygen for all patients with suspected anaphylaxis (Cardona et al., 2020).

AAFA's Recommended Language for Signs and Symptoms of Food Allergy Reactions in Infants and Toddlers

Medical Term	Common Term	What to look for: (Adjusted language for symptoms specific to infants and toddlers)	
Pruritis	• Itchiness	• Tongue thrusting • Tongue pulling • Repetitive lip licking or licking of hands or objects	• Throat itching • Ear pulling, scratching or putting fingers in the ears • Eye rubbing, eye itching
Dyspnea	• Shortness of breath • Difficulty breathing	• Belly breathing • Fast breathing	• Nasal flaring (nostrils open wide) • Chest or neck "tugging"
Stridor	• Noisy breathing • High-pitched sound while breathing (whistling sound)	• Hoarse voice, hoarse cry • Barky/croup-like cough	• Noisy breathing, especially when inhaling
Reduced blood pressure	• Shock	• Wobbly appearance • Lethargic • Floppy or limp • Poor head control • Difficult to wake up • Crankiness	• Withdrawn or clingy • Inconsolable crying • Subdued or less active • Lace-like appearance of the skin • Blue/grey skin around mouth/lips or hands/feet
Hypotonia, Syncope	• Poor muscle tone • Fainting ("passing out")	• Wobbly appearance • Lethargic • Floppy or limp • Poor head control • Difficult to wake up	• Crankiness • Withdrawn or clingy • Inconsolable crying • Less active
Persistent gastrointestinal symptoms	• Gastrointestinal symptoms that are significant	• Abdominal pain • Diarrhea • Hiccups	• Spitting up • Back arching • Vomiting

Asthma and Allergy Foundation of America

KFA Kids with Food Allergies

Fig. 2 Signs and symptoms of food allergy reactions in infants and toddlers. (Used with permission from: Asthma and Allergy Foundation of America (2024). Adapted from Pistiner et al. (2021))

- *Positioning*:
  - Place patient in a supine position with legs elevated to prevent circulatory collapse.
  - If supine position worsens respiratory distress, patient may sit up until able to lay supine.
  - If vomiting, place in semi-supine position on their side.

    - Avoid sudden sitting or standing, which may negatively impact cardiovascular function, potentially leading to cardiovascular collapse and death.
    - If pregnant, patient may sit up or be in semi-supine position on their left side (Cardona et al., 2020).
  - *Additional Airway Support*:
    - Administer bronchodilators for bronchoconstriction.
    - Use inhaled racemic epinephrine for upper airway stridor or obstruction. However, this is considered adjunctive therapy (see Table 2 below) that should not delay or replace the administration of IM epinephrine (Dribin et al., 2025).
    - Prepare for advanced airway management (e.g., intubation) if needed, especially with signs like hoarseness, stridor, or severe distress.
- *Medication Administration—Epinephrine (First-Line Treatment)*
  - Administer 1:1000 epinephrine IM into the anterolateral thigh for suspected/confirmed anaphylaxis.
  - Dosage from vial: 0.01 mg/kg.
    - Max single dose: 0.3 mg for children/teens.
    - Max single dose: 0.5 mg for adults (Golden et al., 2024).
  - Autoinjector doses:
    - AUVI-Q: 0.1 mg (7.5 kg to less than 15 kg), 0.15 mg (15 kg to less than 30 kg) or 0.3 mg (30 kg or greater) (https://dailymed.nlm.nih.gov/dailymed/fda/fdaDrugXsl.cfm?setid=6180fb40-7fca-4602-b3da-ce62b8cd2470&type=display).
    - EPIPEN Jr.: 0.15 mg (15–30 kg) or EPIPEN: 0.3 mg (30 kg or greater) (https://www.epipen.com/hcp/about-epipen-and-generic/dosage-and-administration).
  - Repeat every 5 min if needed for refractory symptoms.
  - Consider IV epinephrine if no response to 2–3 IM epinephrine doses. Note that epinephrine is available in different dosage concentrations, so care in dosage calculation is paramount.
- *Circulation and Fluid Support*
  - Monitoring:
    - Place patient on cardiorespiratory monitoring.
    - Obtain and document vital signs.
  - Obtain intravenous (IV) or intraosseous (IO) access.
  - Fluid Bolus:
    - Administer normal saline bolus(es) for:
      - Orthostasis.
      - Hypotension.
      - Incomplete response to epinephrine.
      - Adults: 1–2 L as quickly as possible.
      - Children: 20 mL/kg boluses, repeated as needed.

Patients experiencing anaphylaxis are at high risk for or are already in distributive shock due to fluid shift from intravascular to extravascular space (ASCIA, 2025; Cardona et al., 2020; Dodd et al., 2021; Golden et al., 2024; Whyte et al., 2022).

The above information is educational and should not be used as a basis for treatment. Nurses should consult evidence-based and up-to-date treatment guidelines to manage anaphylaxis in collaboration with the healthcare team.

Other Supportive Measures

- *Psychosocial Support*: Contact Social Work, Chaplain, Psychology, Child Life, or other appropriate supports for the patient and family.
- *Prepare for Ongoing Management*: See adjunctive therapies section for additional interventions. Prepare for further medication administration and possible admission to acute or critical care.

Adjunctive Therapies

Epinephrine is the first-line treatment of choice for anaphylaxis. Additional adjunctive medications may be given, but the evidence for many of these therapies varies. Adjunctive therapies and indications are included in Table 2 (ASCIA, 2025; Blaiss et al., 2022; Whyte et al., 2022; Cardona et al., 2020; Pourmand et al., 2018). Note that antihistamines are not a first-line treatment, as they do not treat anaphylaxis and its serious complications, including cardiovascular and respiratory symptoms. However, they can be useful for treating cutaneous manifestations like urticaria and pruritis, but after treatment with epinephrine (Blaiss et al., 2022; Shaker et al., 2020).

Criteria for Discharge from the ED

Historically, observation for at least 4–6 hours is recommended for patients with resolved severe anaphylaxis or those who received more than one dose of epinephrine (Pourmand et al., 2018; Walters et al., 2025). Patients should be observed until symptoms have fully resolved, though different organizations may have varying observation guidelines after resolution since biphasic reactions can occur after initial symptoms subside or hours later without further exposure to the allergen (Pourmand et al., 2018; Walters et al., 2025). Those who require additional monitoring or treatment may be admitted to acute care or the ICU.

Newer evidence suggests that patients experiencing mild reactions may be monitored safely outside of the ED, such as in an urgent care setting or even at home. In cases where anaphylaxis has been promptly treated with epinephrine resulting in complete resolution of symptoms, calling emergency services or going to the emergency room may no longer be universal recommendations (Golden et al., 2024).

Table 2 Adjunctive medication for anaphylaxis

Therapy	Indication/considerations
Repeat IM epinephrine	For returning or worsening symptoms after 5 min
Steroids[a] (i.e., glucocorticosteroids—IV hydrocortisone or methylprednisolone)	May prevent protracted symptoms—particularly in patients with asthma; to prevent biphasic reactions, but little to no research evidence
Racemic epinephrine, nebulized	Upper airway obstruction; should not take the place or delay IM epinephrine
Bronchodilators (i.e., albuterol)	For bronchoconstriction
2nd generation antihistamine[b] [e.g., cetirizine (Zyrtec)]	For example, cetirizine/Zyrtec, an H1 receptor antagonist can help improve cutaneous symptoms. Second generation H1-antihistamines are preferred over first generation antihistamines (i.e., diphenhydramine, Benadryl) due to less central nervous system side effects. Ceterizine is also available in an IV formulation for the treatment of acute urticaria for children over 6 months and adults.
H2 receptor antagonist [i.e., famotidine (Pepcid)]	Used in combination with H2 receptor antagonist to block systemic histamine effects
Oxygen	Use 100% high flow oxygen for patients with any respiratory distress or decreased oxygen saturations
IV fluids	Administer 20 mL/kg bolus(es) via large bore IV; insert IO if IV access is unobtainable
Glucagon	For patients on beta blockers (beta blockers may interfere with the effectiveness of epinephrine)
Epinephrine drip	If not responding to IM epinephrine
Other respiratory support (i.e., intubation)	As needed for continued respiratory compromise despite initial treatments (i.e., bronchospasm, airway edema, obstruction)
Other cardiovascular or vasopressor support	As needed for persistent hypotension
Extracorporeal membrane oxygenation (ECMO)	If not responding to traditional resuscitative interventions

Note: Table created by Kimberly Zimmanck, MS, RN, PCNS-BC, Carolynn Sielaff, MSN, APNP, FNP-C, AE-C, CPN and Danielle Palmer, BSN, RN, CPN. Content adapted from ASCIA (Australian Society of Clinical Immunology and Allergy) (2025), Blaiss et al. (2022); Cardona et al. (2020), Pourmand et al. (2018), and Whyte et al. (2022)

[a]There is some evidence that glucocorticosteroids may not be beneficial in the acute management of anaphylaxis and may cause harm, including prolonged reactions, need for inpatient intensive care, and increased length of hospital admission (Cardona et al., 2020; Leiberman et al., 2025)

[b]There is concern that antihistamine administration can delay initial and repeated use of epinephrine, and therefore, antihistamines are not considered first-line treatment (Cardona et al., 2020)

The emerging change in guidelines reflects recent data that shows no significant decrease in the risk of a biphasic reaction when patients immediately use emergency services. Instead, each situation should be assessed on a case-by-case basis. However, it is important to remember that if anaphylaxis is severe, not responding to a single dose of epinephrine, or if symptoms worsen/return, immediate medical attention should be sought. Additionally, some patients are reluctant to use epinephrine because they have been historically required to call 911 or proceed to the ED, which has delayed and/or deterred timely administration of epinephrine. Evidence also suggests that always seeking emergency care is neither cost-effective nor does it improve patient outcomes (Golden et al., 2024).

While the guidelines can vary and treatment options are always evolving, it is important that the patient/family and the provider use shared decision-making to make a plan that is best suited to the individual. When in doubt, patients should be informed to always seek emergency care if they feel it is necessary. If anaphylaxis occurs at school or daycare or a similar setting, epinephrine should be given and emergency services initiated for further evaluation.

Biphasic Reactions

Extended monitoring in the ED is necessary to observe the patient for persistent, refractory, or biphasic anaphylaxis. If symptoms or exam findings of anaphylaxis persist for at least 4 hours, then persistent anaphylaxis is highly likely (Dribin et al., 2020). Refractory anaphylaxis is likely occurring when both (1) anaphylaxis symptoms are present after being appropriately dosed with epinephrine and other symptom-specific treatment (e.g., intravenous fluids for hypotension) and (2) the initial reaction has required three or more doses of epinephrine (appropriately dosed) or requires an epinephrine intravenous infusion (Dribin et al., 2020; Golden et al., 2024). Furthermore, a biphasic reaction is likely occurring when these four criteria are met: (1) new or recurrence of symptoms that are consistent with anaphylaxis, (2) the symptoms from the initial reaction completely resolved prior to the return of symptoms, (3) there has not been re-exposure to the allergen trigger, (4) the return of symptoms occurs within 1–48 h after the time when the initial symptoms fully resolved (Dribin et al., 2020; Golden et al., 2024).

Biphasic reactions are relatively rare. According to one meta-analysis, biphasic reactions were noted on average 6.5% (range 0.4–20%) in 2890 adult patients with anaphylaxis (Golden et al., 2024). Greater severity of initial symptoms, persistence of symptoms, or requiring more than one dose of epinephrine are all associated with a biphasic reaction. Other risk factors include a wide pulse pressure (due to early arteriolar dilation), anaphylaxis from unknown reason or drug reaction in children, or skin signs and symptoms (Golden et al., 2024).

Early administration of epinephrine has been linked to a lower risk of biphasic reactions and overall hospitalization rate, improving clinical outcomes (Golden et al., 2024).

Patients may require close and extended monitoring if they have a history of progressive severe symptoms or history of biphasic reactions. In addition, patients with any comorbid condition that could affect their response to necessary treatment may also require extended observation (Golden et al., 2024).

Criteria for Hospitalization and Hospital Management of Acute Anaphylaxis

In many situations, allergic reactions and anaphylaxis can be managed and observed in the ED without needing hospitalization. However, some reactions do require further observation and/or treatment in a hospital setting. Depending on the patient's clinical status and the hospital's patient placement processes, patients may be managed in acute care or critical care. In general, the following considerations guide placement (Table 3):

While in the hospital, the nurse will continue monitoring the patient's cardiorespiratory status, monitor for a biphasic reaction, and continue to administer any ordered adjunctive therapies as listed above in (Table 2).

Table 3 Follow-up care after allergic reaction diagnosed in the ED

Can be discharged from ED	Needs observation or hospital acute care	Needs critical care
Symptoms have fully resolved	Resolved severe anaphylaxis Received >1 dose of epinephrine Stable airway Stable hemodynamics	Epinephrine drip due to persistent hypotension Continued vasoactive medication infusions Airway/respiratory support (high flow nasal cannula [HFNC], CPAP/BiPAP, intubation)

Note: Table created by Kimberly Zimmanck, MS, RN, PCNS-BC, Carolynn Sielaff, MSN, APNP, FNP-C, AE-C, CPN and Danielle Palmer, BSN, RN, CPN. Content adapted from Medical College of Wisconsin/Children's Hospital and Health System (2024) and Children's Hospital of Philadelphia (2024).

Hospital Management of Acute Anaphylaxis

Hospital management of acute anaphylaxis is similar to management in an ED setting. The biggest difference is that the reaction is triggered while the patient is in the hospital. The first step in managing an acute reaction that occurs in the hospital setting is to remove the potential triggering agent (i.e., food or drug/medication) immediately if an allergic reaction or anaphylaxis is suspected. The hospital nurse should then notify a medical provider immediately to assess the patient and to determine if anaphylaxis is suspected. If this is the case, the nurse will prepare to give IM epinephrine immediately. Nurses must also be aware of internal hospital processes for activating rapid response and code teams for patients requiring urgent or emergent airway and/or physiologic support. The nurse should document details related to the reaction such as suspected trigger, initial symptoms and symptom progression, medications given, and the patient's response to interventions.

See the biphasic reactions section for patients that are being observed in the hospital, following a reaction at home, or in the community.

Psychosocial Support in the Hospital

Patients who have experienced anaphylaxis may need additional psychosocial support. Nurses who recognize this need should advocate for Psychology, Social Work, Chaplain, and/or Child Life to be involved in the patient's and family's plan of care while in the hospital and after discharge (See chapter "Social Emotional Impact of Food Allergy").

Hospital Discharge Criteria

Refer to Criteria for Discharge from the ED earlier in this chapter.

Nursing Education for Patients/Families

Nurses play an important role in the education of patients and families about food allergies, especially when it is a new diagnosis. For all patients and families, it is important to assess their knowledge level. Inpatient nurses should plan to teach the topics in the list below at a health literacy and knowledge level to keep the patient safe at home until their follow-up allergy appointment. Patients should have outpatient primary care and allergy follow-up appointments where they will learn these and other concepts in more depth.

- Food avoidance and reading food labels.
- Emergency action plan (i.e., FARE plan see chapter "Food Allergy Management in Early Childhood Settings").
- Recognizing anaphylaxis.
- Administering epinephrine.
- Accessing emergency care (911 or ED).

It is recommended that nurses educate patients and families on the importance of always carrying two epinephrine devices. While the inpatient nurse might not have access to the commercial epinephrine devices, it will still be important for them to be familiar with the products available for home use, as they may need to teach their patient and family/caregiver how to properly use them.

Refer to previous chapters in the book for additional details on patient and family education and how to administer a specific type of epinephrine autoinjector or nasal epinephrine device.

Perioperative Anaphylaxis

Perioperative anaphylaxis has a greater risk of death than anaphylaxis in other settings, with a rate of 15.3 per 100,000 (Golden et al., 2024). Evaluation of perioperative anaphylaxis is complicated and difficult due to many medications being administered in a short period of time. Evidence suggests that antibiotics and paralytics, or neuromuscular blocking agents, are the more common triggers of anaphylaxis perioperatively. For patients who have experienced perioperative anaphylaxis in the past, repeat anesthesia is possible with shared patient/provider decision-making (Golden et al., 2024).

Radiology and Contrast Considerations

Intravenous iodinated contrast media (ICM) is widely used in radiology settings with reports of 0.2–0.7% of patients experiencing hypersensitivity reactions (Wang et al., 2025). Reactions can occur immediately after ICM use or can be delayed. Until recently, there was no consensus on how to proactively manage or premedicate patients at risk of experiencing adverse reactions to ICM (Wang et al., 2025). The current recommendation is to avoid premedication with corticosteroids for patients with a history of mild acute hypersensitivity reactions. If possible, use an alternate contrast agent if the previous inciting agent is known. For patients with a history of severe, immediate reaction to ICM, the first recommendation is to consider alternative radiologic studies that do not require ICM. If ICM must be used, premedication and switching the contrast agent is recommended if possible. For patients with an isolated history of shellfish or iodine allergy, no premedication is necessary because these patients have not been found to have an increased risk of adverse reactions versus patients without this type of allergy (Wang et al., 2025).

Food Allergens in Medications and Medication Allergies

While some patients may be allergic to medications, such as antibiotics, other patients are at risk of an allergic reaction due to a food product as an inactive ingredient in a medication. Severe allergic reactions to inactive medication ingredients are rare, but individuals with food allergies should talk with their clinician and pharmacist to ascertain the risks. In addition to pharmacists checking ingredients, nurses need to be aware that food allergens may also be in medications that are prescribed for hospitalized patients. Information about medication ingredients is not always readily available and should be requested by the patient and/or caregiver when food allergies are present. Any medication administered should be evaluated by the pharmacist for the presence of relevant allergens. If a patient is experiencing an allergic reaction or anaphylaxis from an unknown substance, medications should always be considered as a cause.

A study at the Massachusetts Institute of Technology and Brigham and Women's Hospital showed that around 93% of all medications, prescription and over the counter (OTC), contain potential allergens such as corn, peanut oil, or lactose (Trafton, 2019). For example, a commonly prescribed oral steroid, prednisone, contains lactose, which is derived from milk. Lactose is the most common inactive ingredient, with 44.82% of medications containing this ingredient, which could contain milk protein through cross-contact. Other common additives include corn starch, gelatin, dyes, sugars, and oils (peanut, soybean, sesame) (Reker et al., 2019).

Table 4 Medications that may contain food allergens

Medication	Potential food allergen
Propofol	Egg and soybean oil
Vaccines	Egg and milk[a]
Inhalers	Lactose
Some insulins	Fish
Glucosamine	Shellfish
Multivitamins/ supplements	Fish oil
Progesterone	Compounded in sesame oil/peanut oil
Lip Smackers[b]	Sesame

Note. Table created by Kimberly Zimmanck, MS, RN, PCNS-BC, Carolynn Sielaff, MSN, APNP, FNP-C, AE-C, CPN and Danielle Palmer, BSN, RN, CPN. Content adapted from Kelso (2014) and Reker et al. (2019)

[a]The influenza vaccine, which contains trace amount of egg protein, has been deemed safe in recent years for those with an egg allergy who are >6 months of age (Blanton et al., 2024). No serious reactions (including death, anaphylaxis or hospitalization) were reported, and less severe reactions were reported in <1.5% of cases studied (Blanton et al., 2024)

[b]"Lip Smackers" has been used to flavor masks for pediatric anesthesia in some facilities

Some common medications that contain food allergens are listed in Table 4. Note that this is not an all-encompassing list, and it is important to check the most recent label for current ingredients as they can change over time (Kelso, 2014; Reker et al., 2019).

Food Safety During Hospitalization

With food allergies on the rise, inpatient nurses will likely care for patients who have one or more food allergens. Food allergies can impact the care of a patient while in the hospital and nurses will need to advocate for safe food options. On admission, nurses will verify allergies with the patient and/or family to ensure that the electronic medical record has their most current allergens listed, which may include foods and/or drugs (medications). Many hospitals require patients to wear bracelets or bands denoting their allergy status. In addition, to maintain patient safety, it is essential that inpatient nurses have the knowledge to respond quickly in the event of an accidental food allergen exposure (Bromiley et al., 2025).

Hand hygiene is always important in hospital and health care settings. For patients with food allergies, nurses should clean hands with soap and water prior to and after handling any food products. Friction with hand washing and rinsing with water removes food proteins. Hand sanitizers do not eliminate food allergens from hands or surfaces.

Nurses must be aware of how patients can access allergy-safe food while in the hospital, following their institution's policies, procedures, and workflows and working in collaboration with clinical dieticians and food services staff. The kitchen that prepares hospital meals must also take precautions to prevent cross-contact. Training of food service staff is recommended using a formal training program, such as

MenuTrinfo, AllerTrain, or AllerTrainU, as stated in previous chapters. Hospitals have different methods for identifying allergy-safe food, such as food allergy menus or apps. If the nurse is obtaining food from unit or hospital stock, the label should be reviewed to ensure the food item is safe. If possible, the nurse can also have the patient/family review the food label as well.

One hospital in Turkey developed a protocol where meals for patients with food allergies are prepared in a designated area, and kitchen staff received additional education (Harari et al., 2021). In Australia, one hospital-based food service integrated a food allergy resource kit to help manage patients with food allergies safely. This resource kit had several precautions including making sure food allergies are documented upon admission, using computerized food systems, a designated food preparation area and separate delivery pathway for meals, a special "food allergy" diet order instead of a "regular diet," strict cleaning processes to prevent allergen cross-contact, and processes for double checking to ensure safe meals are delivered (Harari et al., 2021). Dieticians are an excellent resource if available, and some institutions' policies may include the dietician for help with meal planning for any patient with a food allergy (State of Queensland, 2018).

Discharge Education

Prior to discharge from the ED or hospital, there are some important education elements the nurse should cover with the patient and/or family. If the allergen that triggered the allergic reaction is known, the nurse can share avoidance strategies specific to that allergen. Using return demonstration, nurses can train patients and families on how to use the prescribed epinephrine autoinjector or nasal spray devices. Nurses should provide an emergency action plan, such as the Food Allergy & Anaphylaxis Emergency Care Plan (FARE, 2025) or other plan as discussed in previous chapters, with a description of steps to take in case of an allergic or anaphylactic reaction prior to consultation with their primary care or allergy specialist. Nurses can recommend the patient follow-up within 5 days to a week with their primary care provider for further instructions and education on their suspected allergen. Allergists can provide additional options for testing and management.

Conclusion

Nurses in the hospital setting including the ED and inpatient/ICU units are essential to identifying food-induced anaphylaxis and ensuring prompt treatment, as well as safe recovery and follow-up. Current evidence and guideline updates emphasize rapid recognition, immediate IM epinephrine, careful monitoring for relapse or biphasic reactions, appropriate escalation to IV support and ICU care when needed, and coordinated discharge planning. Nurses can provide education on prescribed epinephrine devices, emergency action plans, and allergy referral. Institutional emergency anaphylaxis protocols and nurse training are strategies to narrow the gap between guideline recommendations and bedside nursing care of those with anaphylaxis.

References

ASCIA (Australian Society of Clinical Immunology and Allergy). (2025). *Acute management of anaphylaxis: Guidelines*. https://www.allergy.org.au/hp/papers/acute-management-of-anaphylaxis-guidelines

Asthma and Allergy Foundations of America. (2024). *AAFA's recommended language for signs and symptoms of food allergy reactions in infants and toddlers*. Retrieved from https://aafa.org/asthma-allergy-research/our-research/food-allergy-anaphylaxis-in-infants/

Blaiss, M. S., Bernstein, J. A., Kessler, A., Pines, J. M., Camargo, C. A., Jr., Fulgham, P., Haumschild, R., Rupp, K., Tyler, T., & Moellman, J. (2022). The role of cetirizine in the changing landscape of IV antihistamines: A narrative review. *Advances in Therapy, 39*(1), 178–192. https://doi.org/10.1007/s12325-021-01999-x. Epub 2021 Dec 4.

Blanton, L., Hummell, D., Moro, P., Broder, K., Taliano, J., & Grohskopf, L. (2024). Safety of influenza vaccines in persons with egg allergy—A systematic review. *Journal of Allergy and Clinical Immunology, 153*(2), AB60.

Bromiley, L., Roberts, S., Affleck, K., Clarke, A., Tomecek, L., & Angus, R. L. (2025). Patient expectations and understanding of hospital food service provision when declaring a food allergy. *Journal of Human Nutrition and Dietetics: The Official Journal of the British Dietetic Association, 38*(1), e13382. https://doi.org/10.1111/jhn.13382

Cardona, V., Ansotegui, I. J., Ebisawa, M., El-Gamal, Y., Rivas, M. F., Fineman, S., Geller, M., Gonazalez-Estrada, A., Greenberger, P. A., Borges, M. S., Senna, G., Sheikh, A., Tanno, L. K., Thong, B. Y., Turner, P. J., & Worm, M. (2020). World allergy organization anaphylaxis guideline 2020. *World Allergy Organization Journal, 113*(10). https://doi.org/10.1016/j.waojou.2020.100472. Elsevier.

Children's Hospital of Philadelphia. (2024). *Anaphylaxis clinical pathway – Emergency department (clinical pathway resource)*. Children's Hospital of Philadelphia. https://www.chop.edu/clinical-pathway/anaphylaxis-emergent-care-clinical-pathway

Dodd, A., Hughes, A., Sargant, N., Whyte, A. F., Soar, J., & Turner, P. J. (2021). Evidence update for the treatment of anaphylaxis. *Resuscitation, 163*, 86–96. https://doi.org/10.1016/j.resuscitation.2021.04.010

Dorris, S. (2025). Fatal and near fatal anaphylaxis to food in children and young adults. *Immunology and Allergy Clinics of North America, 45*(3), 445–455. https://doi.org/10.1016/j.iac.2025.05.001

Dribin, T. E., Sampson, H. A., Camargo, C. A., Jr., Brousseau, D. C., Spergel, J. M., Neuman, M. I., Shaker, M., Campbell, R. L., Michelson, K. A., Rudders, S. A., Assa'ad, A. H., Risma, K. A., Castells, M., Schneider, L. C., Wang, J., Lee, J., Mistry, R. D., Vyles, D., Vaughn, L. M., Schumacher, D. J., et al. (2020). Persistent, refractory, and biphasic anaphylaxis: A multidisciplinary Delphi study. *The Journal of Allergy and Clinical Immunology, 146*(5), 1089–1096. https://doi.org/10.1016/j.jaci.2020.08.015

Dribin, T. E., Muraro, A., Camargo, C. A., Jr., Turner, P. J., Wang, J., Roberts, G., Anagnostou, A., Halken, S., Liebermann, J., Worm, M., Zuberbier, T., & Sampson, H. A., & GA(2)LEN Anaphylaxis Study Team (2025). Anaphylaxis definition, overview, and clinical support tool: 2024 consensus report-a GA^{2}LEN project. The *Journal of Allergy and Clinical Immunology, 156*(2), 406–417.e6 https://doi.org/10.1016/j.jaci.2025.01.021. Epub 2025 Jan 27. PMID: 39880313; PMCID: PMC12301991.

Food Allergy Research & Education (FARE). (2025). *Food allergy & anaphylaxis emergency care plan*. FoodAllergy.org

Golden, D. B. K., Wang, J., Waserman, S., Akin, C., Campbell, R. L., Ellis, A. K., Greenhawt, M., et al. (2024). Anaphylaxis: A 2023 practice parameter update. *Annals of Allergy, Asthma & Immunology, 132*(2), 124–176. https://doi.org/10.1016/j.anai.2023.09.015

Harari, R., Toren, O., Tal, Y., & Ben-Porat, T. (2021). Food allergy safety: A descriptive report of changing policy in a single large medical center. *Israel Journal of Health Policy Research, 10*, 32. https://doi.org/10.1186/s13584-021-00466-w

Kelso, J. M. (2014). Potential food allergens in medications. *The Journal of Allergy and Clinical Immunology, 133*(6), 1509–1518. https://doi.org/10.1016/j.jaci.2014.03.011. PMID: 24878443.

Leiberman, J., Abrams, E., Katari, P., & Ben-Shoshan, M. (2025). Updates in food anaphylaxis management. *Journal of Allergy and Clinical Immunology in Practice, 13*(4), 723–729. https://doi.org/10.1016/j.jaip.2024.12.044

Pistiner, M., et al. (2021). Caregiver-reported presentation of severe food-induced allergic reactions in infants and toddlers. *The Journal of Allergy and Clinical Immunology. In Practice, 9*(1), 311–320.e2.

Pourmand, A., Robinson, C., Syed, W., & Mazer-Amirshahi, M. (2018). Biphasic anaphylaxis: A review of the literature and implications for emergency management. *The American Journal of Emergency Medicine, 36*(8), 1480–1485. https://doi.org/10.1016/j.ajem.2018.05.009

Reker, D., Blum, S. M., Steiger, C., Anger, K. E., Sommer, J. M., Fanikos, J., & Traverso, G. (2019). "Inactive" ingredients in oral medications. *Science Translational Medicine, 11*(483), eaau6753. https://doi.org/10.1126/scitranslmed.aau6753

Shaker, M. S., Wallace, D. V., Golden, D. B. K., Oppenheimer, J., Bernstein, J. A., Campbell, R. L., Dinakar, C., Ellis, A., Greenhawt, M., Khan, D. A., Lang, D. M., Lang, E. S., Lieberman, J. A., Portnoy, J., Rank, M. A., Stukus, D. R., Wang, J., Collaborators, Riblet, N., Bobrownicki, A. M. P., Bontrager, T., Dusin, J., Foley, J., Frederick, B., Fregene, E., Hellerstedt, S., Hassan, F., Hess, K., Horner, C., Huntington, K., Kasireddy, P., Keeler, D., Kim, B., Lieberman, P., Lindhorst, E., McEnany, F., Milbank, J., Murphy, H., Pando, O., Patel, A. K., Ratliff, N., Rhodes, R., Robertson, K., Scott, H., Snell, A., Sullivan, R., Trivedi, V., Wickham, A., Chief Editors, Shaker, M. S., Wallace, D. V., Workgroup Contributors, Shaker, M. S., Wallace, D. V., Bernstein, J. A., Campbell, R. L., Dinakar, C., Ellis, A., Golden, D. B. K., Greenhawt, M., Lieberman, J. A., Rank, M. A., Stukus, D. R., Wang, J., Joint Task Force on Practice Parameters Reviewers, Shaker, M. S., Wallace, D. V., Golden, D. B. K., Bernstein, J. A., Dinakar, C., Ellis, A., Greenhawt, M., Horner, C., Khan, D. A., Lieberman, J. A., Oppenheimer, J., Rank, M. A., Shaker, M. S., Stukus, D. R., & Wang, J. (2020). Anaphylaxis-a 2020 practice parameter update, systematic review, and grading of recommendations, assessment, development and evaluation (GRADE) analysis. *The Journal of Allergy and Clinical Immunology, 145*(4), 1082–1123. https://doi.org/10.1016/j.jaci.2020.01.017. Epub 2020 Jan 28. PMID: 32001253.

State of Queensland. (2018). *Food allergen management in foodservice: A best practice*. https://docslib.org/doc/15903/food-allergen-management-in-foodservice-a-best-practice-guideline. https://nationalallergycouncil.org.au/images/doc/Food_Allergen_Best_Practice_Guideline.pdf.

The Medical College of Wisconsin/Children's Hospital and Health System. (2024). *Anaphylaxis acute presentation (acute care)*. The Medical College of Wisconsin/Children's Hospital and Health System.

Trafton, A. (2019). *"Inactive" ingredients may not be, study finds*. https://news.mit.edu/2019/inactive-ingredients-reactions-study-0313#:~:text=They%20found%20that%20for%20most,people%20with%20irritable%20bowel%20syndrome

Turner, P. J., Jerschow, E., Umasunthar, T., Lin, R., Campbell, D. E., & Boyle, R. J. (2017). Fatal anaphylaxis: Mortality rate and risk factors. *The Journal of Allergy and Clinical Immunology. In Practice, 5*(5), 1169–1178. https://doi.org/10.1016/j.jaip.2017.06.031

Walters, B., Short, H. B., Ravida, N., Fabe, M., Boehmer, S., & Reyes, L. (2025). Evaluating practice patterns of observation periods status post epinephrine administration for anaphylaxis. *The Journal of Emergency Medicine, 77*, 69–76. https://doi.org/10.1016/j.jemermed.2025.07.001

Wang, C., Ramsey, A., Lang, D., Copaescu, A. M., Krishman, P., Kurwilla, M., Mervak, B., Newhouse, J., Sumkin, A., & Saff, R. (2025). Management and prevention of hypersensitivity reactions to radiocontrast media: A consensus statement from the American College of Radiology and the American Academy of Allergy, Asthma, and Immunology. *Radiology, 315*(2). https://doi.org/10.1148/radiol.240100

Whyte, A. F., Soar, J., Dodd, A., Hughes, A., Sargant, N., & Turner, P. J. (2022). Emergency treatment of anaphylaxis: Concise clinical guidance. *Clinical Medicine (London, England), 22*(4), 332–339. https://doi.org/10.7861/clinmed.2022-0073

Social Emotional Impact of Food Allergy

Lindsay Green, Alison Bauer, Josie Howard-Ruben, and Julianne Doucette

Introduction

Living with a food allergy or raising children who have a food allergy can pose a significant psychological burden and present challenges that may also impact mental health across the lifespan. The need to avoid certain foods, the challenge of preparing special meals safely, the fear of accidental exposure, the restrictions on a whole host of daily activities, fear about using epinephrine devices, and burdensome medical procedures such as lab draws, skin prick tests, and oral food challenges, as well as newer therapies with risks and side effects, all contribute to this burden. In families where a child has a severe food allergy or has experienced anaphylaxis, the health-related quality of life is often worse than in families without food allergies (Flokstra-de Blok et al., 2010; Protudjer et al., 2021). Studies have highlighted the significant impact of food allergies on the quality of life for families and children (Abrams et al., 2020), noting that the need to constantly avoid foods that could trigger an allergic reaction can be socially limiting, financially burdensome, and emotionally challenging. Building family strengths and capabilities to

L. Green (✉)
University of Northern Colorado, Greeley, CO, USA
e-mail: Lindsay.green@unco.edu

A. Bauer
Carlow University, Pittsburgh, PA, USA
e-mail: akbauer@carlow.edu

J. Howard-Ruben
Rush University College of Nursing, Chicago, IL, USA
e-mail: josie_howard-ruben@rush.edu

J. Doucette
College of Nursing, Rush University, Chicago, IL, USA
e-mail: Julianne_Doucette@rush.edu

J. Doucette, J. Howard-Ruben (eds.), *Comprehensive Food Allergy Management for Nurses*, https://doi.org/10.1007/978-3-032-28647-5_10

face these challenges can help to ameliorate these issues. Just like other chronic health conditions, food allergies can be managed, and lifestyle limitations can be minimized with education, support, and resources, including mental health and psychosocial support. Nurses can help patients and families learn new skills and behaviors to develop a healthy perspective on managing their food allergies.

Approximately 40% of children with food allergy have experienced at least one food-related allergic reaction (Greiwe, 2023; Abrams et al., 2020), which may also contribute to anxiety and fear. Managing a food allergy requires continuous vigilance by both the individual with the allergy and the caregivers of affected children (Schelly et al., 2023). While some anxiety is expected and can be protective by encouraging avoidance of allergens, excessive anxiety can become maladaptive and lead to unhealthy coping strategies (Schelly et al., 2023). Often, the wait time for a definitive food allergy diagnosis can be particularly stressful, especially if it takes a prolonged time to see the specialist or the patient lacks access to an allergist (Feng & Kim, 2019). Social isolation, negative self-perceptions, and the risk of bullying contribute to the development of social anxiety, depression, and low self-esteem in children with food allergies (Quach & John, 2018). Furthermore, the severity of food restrictions correlates with a greater impact on the family's quality of life (Moen et al., 2019). However, helpful strategies for coping with the anxiety and fear associated with food allergies can be learned by parents, children, and adults.

Social media misinformation is rampant and can create both unwarranted concerns and also greater awareness of rare but severe outcomes, exacerbating anxiety and leading to unnecessary behaviors that negatively impact families (Dahlsgaard et al., 2020). However, social media can also be a source of connection and support for families dealing with food allergies, with many online groups offering resources, encouragement, information, and normalization of aspects of food allergy management.

Caregiver Experience

A recent survey revealed a noteworthy psychosocial burden across a variety of demographic and clinical variables in a sample of caregivers for children with food allergies using the six-item Food Allergy Independent Measure (FAIM) (Engel et al., 2025). The FAIM assesses for expectation of adverse outcomes, as well as dietary and social restrictions and is deemed to be helpful as a screening instrument to identify those who would benefit from mental health referrals.

The burden of living with a food allergy is often heavier for caregivers of children than for adults managing their own condition (Santos et al., 2023). Parents of children with food allergies often experience heightened anxiety, stress, and depression, leading to a lower quality of life (Schelly et al., 2023). Parent or caregiver mental health is affected by the number and severity of a child's food allergies and the time since diagnosis (Abrams et al., 2020). Anxiety is typically highest immediately following a child's diagnosis, but tends to improve over time as strategies for managing food allergies are developed (Quach & John, 2018). Parents of children with multiple food allergies may feel overwhelmed and have an intense fear of leaving their child with another caregiver (Abrams et al., 2020). Overall, caregivers may experience constant anxiety over the possibility of their child having a life-threatening reaction, even though fatal anaphylaxis, while devastating, is rare (Turner et al., 2017). Since food is an essential part of daily living, the constant concern over potential allergic reactions creates ongoing emotional distress, contributing to these challenges (Greiwe, 2023).

Mental health concerns related to food allergies, including panic, fear, and anxiety, are widespread and affect caregivers regardless of whether their child has one or multiple food allergies (Casale et al., 2024). A qualitative study involving 40 parents found that every parent experienced anxiety when managing their child's food allergy (Chooniedass et al., 2020). These parents reported a range of emotions, including grief, frustration, guilt, isolation, and anxiety. The persistent vigilance required to prevent accidental allergen exposure contributes to increased stress and diminished coping among parents (Chooniedass et al., 2020). Mothers often experience higher levels of anxiety and stress compared to other family members since caring for a child living with a food allergy often involves making significant lifestyle adjustments such as avoiding certain environments, modifying the home, and managing the daily stress of activities like grocery shopping and dining out (Feng & Kim, 2019; Schelly et al., 2023).

A model proposed by Westwell-Roper et al. (2022) outlines the context of parental anxiety related to a child's food allergies, based on a systematic review of 98

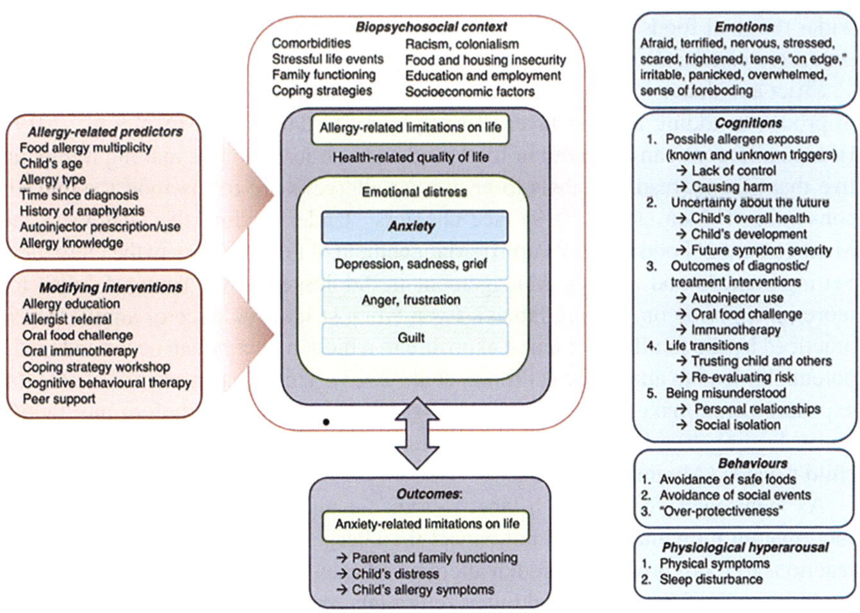

Fig. 1 Simplified schematic summary of features of parental FA-specific anxiety. (Used with permission from: Westwell-Roper et al. (2022))

qualitative or quantitative studies exploring distress or anxiety in parents of children with food allergies. Figure 1 captures the elements of parental distress and FA-specific anxiety.

Parenting Children with Food Allergies

Caregivers may perceive their child's life as constantly threatened, leading to a family life characterized by fear (Moen et al., 2019). Research indicates that anxiety peaks during developmental transitions, particularly between the ages of 6 and 11, when children gain more independence but may not yet have the skills to fully protect themselves (Kanter et al., 2022). In some cases, family activities are often restricted, with some parents opting to homeschool their children to mitigate the risks of food exposure in the school setting (Marsac & Wurth, 2021).

For some parents, managing a child's food allergy can lead to additional lifestyle limitations, such as avoiding dining out or traveling, which can have a ripple effect on the entire family's quality of life (Quach & John, 2018). Parents must navigate the complexities of keeping their children safe while maintaining social relationships, such as attending birthday and holiday parties, playdates, and sleepovers (Quach & John, 2018). Another challenge that caregivers face is the lack of understanding from others regarding the seriousness of food allergies. For instance, some people may not fully grasp that a food allergy requires avoiding not only the allergenic food itself but also any products that may contain traces of it. For example, a milk allergy does not just mean avoiding drinking milk; it also involves avoiding a wider range of foods where milk is an ingredient such as baked goods, sauces, and processed snacks (Dulger et al., n.d.).

Strict avoidance of allergens is complicated by the presence of hidden allergens in products, adding another layer of complexity to daily life (Moen et al., 2019). Hidden allergens can be found in food products in trace amounts making it imperative that parents read all labels to ensure no allergens are in the food the child is consuming (Moen et al., 2019) (see chapters "Understanding the Diagnosis and Management of Food Allergy Part III: Management of Food Allergy in the Outpatient Setting" and "Food Allergy Management in Adolescents and Young Adults" for more information on reading labels). Even when strict avoidance of an allergen is practiced by the family, accidental exposure to a hidden allergy can occur and could potentially lead to anaphylaxis (Tomei et al., 2023). This constant fear of accidental exposure often makes food allergy management a top priority before any family event, leading to a lifestyle centered around accommodating and adapting to the child's needs (Abrams et al., 2020).

As mentioned, reading each label to look for an allergen is necessary even in food that an individual would not expect the allergen to be present. Many allergic reactions to foods are due to hidden allergens (Tomei et al., 2023). Hidden allergens could be in the form of food additives, colorants, preservatives, thickening agents, flavorings, and cow's milk proteins, to name a few (Tomei et al., 2023). However, the vigilance required, reading all ingredient labels, watching for unlisted ingredients, and preventing cross-contact, can add to the stress and anxiety parents feel (Quach & John, 2018). Cross-contact is another risk factor for individuals with food allergies and occurs when an allergen is transmitted to safe food (Tomei et al., 2023). This can occur when someone uses a cutting board or utensils that previously had an allergen on it and was not sufficiently cleaned. Mothers, who often are primarily responsible for meal planning and preparation, reported that sharing parental responsibilities helped reduce the burden, leading to an improved quality of life for the entire family (Moen et al., 2019). Single mothers may experience an increased burden of managing a child's food allergy without a partner, which can significantly impact their quality of life.

Understanding the challenges parents face when raising a child with food allergies is essential for healthcare providers. By sharing knowledge, promoting self-efficacy, and collaborating with a multidisciplinary team, providers can help families feel more secure and supported (Moen et al., 2019). Healthcare providers can provide advice to families on how to deal with food safety issues and limit allergen cross-contact of foods (Tomei et al., 2023). Nurses can recommend use of resources developed by the Centers for Disease Control and Prevention (CDC), the Food Allergy Research and Education (FARE) organization, and Anaphylaxis UK to offer suggestions for managing food allergies (Tomei et al., 2023), as well as other organizations with a focus on food allergy (see the Resources Page at the end of the book). For parents of newly diagnosed children, comprehensive education that reduces anxiety and stress and increases the sense of control can be beneficial. Support groups and learning adaptive coping strategies can also help (Polloni & Muraro, 2020).

The stress and anxiety associated with managing a child's food allergy are pervasive, with significant mental health implications for caregivers. A study revealed that while 70% of parents of children with food allergies would have found mental health support beneficial, only 24% sought such support (Abrams et al., 2020). This gap shows the need to integrate mental health resources into food allergy management (Abrams et al., 2020).

Impact of Food Allergy on Children

Many children safely and successfully manage the burden of food allergies with little disruption of their lives, as they have learned the skills needed to cope with managing food allergies and are resilient in their approach to daily living. However, there are many factors to consider related to the impact of food allergies on daily living as children grow. For younger children, food allergies can hinder participation in sports, birthday parties, camps, and playdates due to transferring responsibility to adults who may not be familiar with handling food allergies and the risk of accidental exposures (See chapter "Food Allergy Management in Early Childhood Settings") (Feng & Kim, 2019). Parents may need to reduce work hours, quit jobs, or relocate due to food allergy concerns (Feng & Kim, 2019).

Children with food allergies have higher levels of anxiety than their peers without allergies and are at a higher risk of developing social anxiety disorder (Kanter et al., 2022). Healthcare workers should screen for heightened anxiety levels in school-age children by assessing the duration and extent of avoidance behaviors, especially when there is a low likelihood of accidental allergen exposure, as excessive avoidance may compromise daily functioning and encourage unhealthy preoccupation with worst-case scenarios (Dahlsgaard et al., 2020). School-age children are particularly vulnerable to increased anxiety, depression, post-traumatic stress, and impaired quality of life and are more than twice as likely to report bullying compared to their peers without food allergies (Marsac & Wurth, 2021). Additionally, children with food allergies may experience social isolation, such as sitting at separate lunch tables at school, or exclusion from food-related activities, which can further increase their fear of humiliation, social rejection, and social anxiety (Kanter et al., 2022).

Since children with food allergies often experience bullying, this experience can significantly impact their mental health, leading to feelings of sadness, anxiety, low self-esteem, embarrassment, and loneliness (Quach & John, 2018). As these children grow into adolescents, they are four times more likely to develop mental health conditions, such as attention deficit hyperactivity disorder (ADHD), depression, and anxiety (Quach & John, 2018). Studies have shown an association of allergic conditions, including food allergy, with ADHD in children. The exact mechanism linking these conditions is not well understood, but healthcare providers should be aware of the risk for ADHD in children with allergic conditions (Xu et al., 2022).

Many children are fearful of the initial evaluation for food allergy, often entailing blood draws, itchy skin tests, and sometimes stressful oral food challenges. Furthermore, newer treatments and epinephrine auto-injectors are injectable medications with needles, which understandably can cause fear in children. Epinephrine auto-injectors come with a training device which nurses can use to practice proper technique, with some using an orange to simulate intramuscular injection. Shemesh et al. described initial reduced anxiety in a group of adolescents who participated in self-injection sessions using trainer devices monitored by clinicians to practice self-injection (Shemesh et al., 2017). On follow-up, the reduction in anxiety was not significant, suggesting repeated practice could be most efficacious. One strategy to reduce anxiety is a proximity challenge, or exposure to an allergen in a controlled setting (across the room or by touching), to instill coping behaviors in the patient by providing confidence in their ability to face adversity and overcome the fear (Dahlsgaard & Lewis, 2025). This type of intervention has proven successful in reducing anxiety in patients and is a viable option for those with food allergy-induced anxiety.

During their teenage years, adolescents assume greater responsibility for managing their food allergies but still rely on caregivers for help (Schelly et al., 2023). Caregivers continue to provide reminders to their adolescents to carry medications and give guidance on checking food labels to ensure safety (Schelly et al., 2023). Often, adolescents are not as concerned with their food allergy as their parents, as they have a lower perception of the risk of anaphylaxis (Moen et al., 2019). One study shows that 24% of teenagers and adults with food allergies have experienced harassment related to their food allergy, and most incidents have occurred at school (Greiwe, 2023). In adolescents, these experiences impact quality of life and can lead to mental or behavioral health disorders, including anxiety, behavioral problems, depression, ADHD, and isolation (Greiwe, 2023). Participants in an online program for adolescents identified multiple psychosocial needs categorized as "connecting with peers, sharing experiences, navigating social situations, coping with emotional challenges, increasing knowledge, and gaining confidence" (Engel et al., 2022). These broad areas of concern expressed by teens underscore the need for healthcare workers to address not only the medical needs of these patients (e.g., reviewing epinephrine device use), but also to explore their psychosocial needs and provide referrals, education, and resources to help address them.

College students with food allergies face unique challenges, including constant attention to avoidance of allergens, which can lead to "disclosure fatigue," where they become tired of discussing their allergies and consequently, avoid doing so, leading to risky behaviors (Schelly et al., 2023). Nurses and healthcare providers must recognize that these social pressures can create barriers to safe eating practices, even in those who previously adhered to them (Schelly et al., 2023). Developing a plan to navigate the college environment is crucial and may include working with accommodation services, establishing backup plans when safe food options are unavailable, communicating with dining services, working with housing services, addressing disclosure fatigue, and preparing for situations where social pressures can be overwhelming (Schelly et al., 2023; see chapter "Food Allergy Management in Adolescents and Young Adults").

Psychosocial Impact on Adults with Food Allergy

Adults with food allergies face their own set of challenges, including anxiety about food safety, high food costs, difficulty maintaining a healthy diet, and stress in social settings (Polloni & Muraro, 2020). The avoidance of food is a large stressor for adults with food allergy (Santos et al., 2023). For adults who have experienced anaphylaxis, anxiety is heightened, and the condition is perceived as more severe (Polloni & Muraro, 2020). Many adults with a food allergy are comfortable with avoiding foods and administering an epinephrine device since they have been living this lifestyle for many years (Santos et al., 2023); however, a significant number of people globally report adult-onset allergies and may require more intense education and support to help them learn food allergy management strategies (Bingemann et al., 2024). Adults with food allergies who feel proficient at managing their own health outcomes report higher anxiety levels, likely due to their need to constantly monitor their environment for potential threats (Polloni & Muraro, 2020).

Factors such as younger age, lower education and income level, history of allergic reactions, use of an epinephrine device, multiple food allergies, and frequent emergency department visits were associated with a lower quality of life in the adult population (Shemesh, 2023). Additionally, those with an allergy to dairy, soy, wheat, and sesame or multiple food allergies suffered from a decreased quality of life (Bingemann et al., 2024). A European study identified adults of female gender with a dairy or fish allergy at higher risk of decreased quality of life (Bingemann et al., 2024). Furthermore, in a U.S. based study, the same authors found that adults whose food allergy persisted from childhood into adulthood reported poorer quality of life compared with those who developed food allergies later in life (Bingemann et al., 2024). Any person or caregiver of persons with a food allergy is at risk of the psychosocial impacts; therefore, nurses need to be alert to signs and symptoms of increased psychosocial distress and decreased quality of life.

Psychological Burden of Food Allergy and the Role of the Nurse

The psychological and emotional burden of this chronic disease affects all facets of life and may change based on stage of life, social situation, and unique individual circumstances. The social and emotional aspects of this disease can create a heightened response to many situations surrounding food, including socializing, relationships, and all components of life and daily living. While patients and caregivers alike can benefit from mental health resources, access to this group of providers may be limited. The American Academy of Allergy, Asthma & Immunology (AAAAI) Committee on Integrative Medicine issued a report focusing on the mental health needs of patients and families coping with food allergies and developed a plan for addressing this gap in care (Herbert et al., 2025).

In a study conducted by Food Allergy Research and Education (FARE) with information derived from their patient registry, approximately 62% of patients experienced mental health concerns related to food allergies (Casale et al., 2024). Similarly, the Global Access to Psychological Services for Food Allergy (GAPS) study reviewed the implications of food allergies and psychological distress from a global perspective, incorporating responses from 20 other countries, finding that two-thirds of all adults with food allergies and almost three-quarters of all caregivers reported psychological distress (Knibb et al., 2024). This same study found that only 19.4% of adults expressed that they were screened or assessed for food allergy-related psychological concerns during a food allergy appointment. Additionally, only 13.9% of caregivers and 15.8% of the children reported being screened or assessed for food allergy-related psychological concerns during their appointment (Knibb et al., 2024). Another study showed that less than one in 10 individuals with food allergies were screened for mental health concerns during any food allergy appointment (Casale et al., 2024). While there is a growing recognition of the psychological impact of food allergies on both individuals and caregivers, routine mental health screenings are not a part of standard practice in allergy care (Casale et al., 2024).

With the number of patients and caregivers indicating an adverse emotional response to coping with food allergies, there is a need for nursing care that includes advocacy, education, psychological support, and guidance for the food allergic patient and their caregivers.

Identification of Mental Health Concerns by Screening

Screening for potential mental health concerns is the first step clinicians can take to identify those in need of additional support and resources. In fact, universal screening of patients and caregivers managing food allergies could help identify those most in need of additional services to improve health-related quality of life.

Several general screening tools can be applied to this population to screen for anxiety and depression. In children, the Screen for Child Anxiety Related Disorders (SCARED) and the Generalized Anxiety Disorder 7-item scale (GAD-7) identify anxiety symptoms. The Patient Health Questionnaire (PHQ-9) is a common tool for depression screening available in an adult version for those 18 years and older, an adolescent version for those 12 years and older, an adapted version for children, and a parent report version (Spitzer et al., n.d). The Preschool Feelings Checklist is used with a younger population down to age three to identify depression (Verdi et al., 2025).

In addition, there are food allergy-specific tools measuring anxiety, such as the Scales of Food Allergy Anxiety, Child-Rated (SOFAA-C), a 21-item questionnaire assessing food allergy-related anxiety over the past week, for those 8–18 years of age (Greiwe, 2023; Verdi et al., 2025). The tool is also available in a parent version. Other food allergy-specific tools include the Parental Food Allergy-Associated Anxiety and Coping Tool (IMPAACT), the Food Allergy Anxiety Scale (FAAS), and the Worry About Food Allergy Measure (WAFA) (Verdi et al., 2025). Nurses can advocate for mental health screening to identify those patients or caregivers in need of additional resources.

Additionally, the Food Allergy Quality of Life Questionnaire (FAQLQ) form is a food allergy-specific questionnaire often utilized in clinical research on food allergy-related quality of life and can be administered to the patient or parent with forms available for the child, teenager, adult, and parents of those 0–17 years old (Greiwe, 2023). The purpose of the FAQLQ questionnaire is to assess the burdens of food allergies from all perspectives (child/family/parent/caregiver), and how this affects the quality of life. Another tool useful in research is the Food Allergy Self-Efficacy Scale for Parents (FASE-P), used in the UK and US to understand food allergy self-efficacy of caregivers (Bingemann et al., 2024).

Additional screenings may also be appropriate for patients with food allergies. For example, screening for post-traumatic stress disorder (PTSD) in individuals who have experienced or witnessed anaphylaxis is important. PTSD develops after someone has experienced a scary, shocking, or dangerous event, and they feel frightened or stressed even when they are not being harmed (Food Allergy and Anaphylaxis Connection Team, n.d.-a, n.d.-b). A systematic review identified eating disorders, including bulimia nervosa, anorexia, and avoidant restrictive food intake disorders, among individuals with food allergies, although the exact prevalence is unclear (Ciciulla et al., 2023). Clinicians should screen for these conditions, recognize signs and symptoms, and provide appropriate referrals when needed (Ciciulla et al., 2023).

Once patients or caregivers are identified as having anxiety and/or depression or other mental health concerns, shared decision-making regarding options for coping and treatment can be initiated. Nurses can provide practical suggestions for coping, conduct motivational interviewing, suggest counseling, and initiate referrals to psychologists, psychiatric mental health nurse practioners or psychiatrists for cognitive behavioral therapy, medication, or other options, depending on the psychosocial or mental health concern.

Providing Coping Mechanisms and Resilience

Coping with a food allergy diagnosis varies significantly among families, influenced by factors such as the parents' age, the child's gender and developmental stage, socio-economic status, the number and history of food allergies, and the time since diagnosis (Bingemann et al., 2024; Bozen et al., 2020; Quach & John, 2018). A small study of allergists noted the relationship between parental anxiety and how children cope with their allergies and emphasized the importance of good communication and reliable information about food allergies (Bozen et al., 2020). Parents play a key role in helping children develop healthy coping behaviors by helping their children navigate these challenges (Rubeiz & Ernst, 2021). Bingemann et al. (2024) reported on practical interventions aimed at ameliorating the psychosocial impact of food allergies and suggested broad strategies including acknowledgement of the burden (of food allergies), evidence-based education, anxiety management, access to support and advocacy groups, mental health referrals, and peer mentorship. Some successful programs mentioned by the authors to improve coping include the Food Allergy Parent Mentoring Program, which explored whether mothers with a knowledgeable food allergy mentor had reduced psychosocial symptoms (Bingemann et al., 2024; Ramos et al., 2021). In the US, the Food Allergy and Anaphylaxis Connection Team (FAACT) sponsors camps, retreats, and educational programs that provide support, peer connection, and food allergy education for individuals with food allergies and their families (https://www.foodallergyawareness.org/events-and-programs/).

Resiliency in managing food allergies is influenced by various factors, including the individual's age and social support. In early childhood, the burden primarily falls on caregivers and parents, who can enhance self-efficacy by practicing communication about anaphylactic symptoms, being assertive about allergen avoidance, and practicing with epinephrine devices (Rubeiz & Ernst, 2021). Individual resiliency, especially in the setting of a chronic and possibly life-long disease, may change throughout one's life. Having the ability to recognize difficulties, as well as the openness to grow both physically and mentally while managing stress and emotions, aids in defining and establishing resiliency. Resiliency and self-esteem provide confidence, control, and autonomy in a patient with food allergies, all of which are crucial to navigate the psychosocial aspects of this disease. There are many ways to help build resiliency in those with food allergies through communication, advocacy, and support. Rubeiz and Ernst suggest education, problem-solving activities, exercises to improve self-efficacy, social support, and finding meaning in their food allergy experience (2021), which are all behaviors nurses can facilitate.

Concepts to Reduce Anxiety and Improve Coping Through Mindset

The Food Allergy Counselor (https://www.foodallergycounselor.com/), Tamara Hubbard, MA, LCPC, is a licensed therapist and a mother of children with food allergies who recently wrote a book titled *May Contain Anxiety: Managing the Overwhelm of Parenting Children with Food Allergies.* Hubbard (2025) which outlines a helpful approach for assisting parents to manage food allergy-related anxiety and other issues. Based on evidence-based Acceptance and Commitment Therapy principles, and steeped in a growth mindset, the strategies suggested for patients emphasize being "psychologically flexible" (p. 196) and in a state of "relaxed readiness" (p. 196) as they care for their child with food allergies. According to Hubbard, psychological flexibility implies the ability to confront the challenges associated with food allergies in the moment and to adapt to those challenges constructively, based on a realistic perspective of risks. Relaxed readiness highlights the need for vigilance, while weighing risks, allowing people coping with food allergies, including parents, "to live fully while staying prepared to act (when needed) rather than constantly living in fear or, on the contrary, navigating life without any precautions" (p. 15). Using the principles espoused here, Hubbard offers a blueprint for creating a mindful allergy parenting plan. While the strategy is aimed at parents of children with food allergies, the tools would be useful to adults with food allergies as well.

The Role of Brief Cognitive Behavioral Therapy in the Office Setting

Verdi et al. (2025) described a method of brief cognitive behavioral therapy (bCBT) that can be implemented in the office setting to address negative thoughts about food allergies (2025). This type of CBT aims to shape thinking by examining feelings and intrusive thoughts and reframe for improved health and coping (Verdi et al., 2025). Brief CBT is a technique that can be deployed in the clinic setting to encourage a healthy and constructive way of coping with food allergies. Verdi et al. (2025) described the use of "curious questions" with patients or families to encourage discussion of any false thinking with a food allergy expert who can help them reframe thinking based on facts and alleviate some fear. The authors suggest the clinician should evaluate the current stage of readiness before providing advice to the patient or caregiver, so the suggestions are targeted and more likely to result in positive change.

Dahlsgaard et al. (2023) found that anxiety symptoms improved after implementing a “Food Allergy Bravery” (FAB) intervention, which introduced allergens, via smelling or physically touching, to children aged 8–12 years with significant anxiety due to food allergy. This type of confidence-building with close exposure or proximity to the allergen could be conducted in the office setting.

Social Support for Patients and Families with Food Allergy

There are many different opportunities for patients and families to join social support groups, both in person and more commonly, through a variety of social media platforms. These communities are each unique and can share strategies for coping from a parental/guardian and/or child perspective and provide ways to navigate life with food allergies. When working with patients and families, it is imperative to emphasize the importance of selecting support groups that will promote a positive collegial environment to engage and learn from each other. The Food Allergy Research and Education (FARE) organization provides a tool on their website for searching support groups in the US, Australia, Canada, and Mexico (https://www.foodallergy.org/living-food-allergies/join-community/find-support-group).

Physicians such as Dr. Zach Rubin @rubin_allergy provide YouTube videos and information via Instagram and other social media sites, and Dr. David Stukus provides podcasts for clinicians and shares content on Instagram @AllergyKidsDoc for patients and families. Other social media groups that may be helpful include No Nut Traveler on Facebook and Instagram, Friends Helping Friends Food Allergies Support Facebook Group, Food Allergy Treatment Talk Facebook Group and other sites, such as Allergic Living. It is also important to highlight that support groups are versatile; it might take time to find and connect with one that fits the patient and/or their support system’s needs. The benefit of communal understanding and rapport from others living through the same diagnosis helps fuel interconnectedness and the feeling of being accepted, thereby improving psycho-emotional well-being (Greiwe, 2023). Additional information about these sites is on the Resources Page.

Referral to Counseling and Mental Health Professionals

Finding support from others who share similar circumstances is important to help foster a sense of community; however, there are times when a more individualized approach to psychosocial well-being is warranted and essential to navigate one’s needs. As food allergies continue to increase, there has been more attention from healthcare professionals focusing on the needs of those with food allergies, including counseling and mental health services. Our healthcare infrastructure has an ongoing shortage of psychiatric and mental health providers in general and specifically for those affected by food allergies. In the GAPS study (2024), the biggest barrier to seeking mental health treatment for food allergy-related concerns was cost/lack of insurance, lack of referral options from their primary care clinician, and, lastly, practitioner availability (Knibb et al., 2024). The GAPS study was designed to be a multi-level study, with the next objective of creating an online intervention for psychological support for both adults and caregivers navigating life with food allergies.

Behavioral health resources directly focused on the food allergy community include the FAACT Behavioral Health Resource Center, including information for parents, caregivers, and patients related to self-care recommendations, coping skills, resilience, anxiety, depression, post-traumatic stress disorder information, and more (https://www.foodallergyawareness.org/behavioral-health/). One unique offering is Camp TAG (The Allergy Gang), a sleepover camp held annually for children aged 4–13 designed to be a safe setting for children with food allergies and other allergic disorders (e.g., FPIES, celiac diseases) and non-allergic siblings (https://www.foodallergyawareness.org/camp-tag/camp-tag-the-allergy-gang/). The organization holds a yearly FAACT Allergy Summit to link patients, caregivers, allergy advocates, medical professionals, and pharmaceutical companies for educational sessions including sessions on managing stress and anxiety (FAACT, n.d.-a, n.d.-b). For general information, visit www.foodallergyawareness.org.

As noted above, Hubbard offers a comprehensive website dedicated to providing resources for those managing anxiety and stress related to food allergies as she was the founder of the *Academy of Food Allergy Counseling* and features a page on the website for locating therapists knowledgeable about food allergy all over the US and some in other countries.

Other Organizations with a Focus on Food Allergy Quality of Life Through Education

Other organizations provide support for patients and families coping with food allergies in general, but do not focus on providing counseling or behavioral health information. FARE, a non-profit organization has a goal of improving the quality of life for those affected personally or by means of caregiving for individuals with food allergies through advocacy, research, and education (Food Allergy Research and Education [FARE], 2024). FARE supports those newly diagnosed with food allergies through direct education, support groups, and training. The organization fosters camaraderie among those with food allergy and their caregivers through their annual educational sessions at FARE Food Allergy Summit. Overall, the organization aims to help patients and caregivers to further understand the food allergy diagnosis, modifications to lifestyle with established guides, emergency care plans, tools for recognizing signs and symptoms of reactions, and preparation of living with food allergies. These are some of a vast array of educational features on their website to support patients coping with food allergy and healthcare providers supporting patients (FARE, 2024). To learn more and find all the services supplied by FARE, please visit, https://www.foodallergy.org.

The Allergy and Asthma Network shares information about food allergies in addition to other common co-diagnoses, including environmental and seasonal allergies, asthma, anaphylaxis, eczema, and atopic dermatitis (Asthma and Allergy Network, 2024). They provide Food Allergy Stages: Effective Age-Based Food Allergy Guidance aimed at providing clinicians, patients, and their families with management and coping strategies. There are many areas of support that this network provides for this target population, including current news, webinars, events, policy and advocacy at state and federal levels, information on insurance coverage and health equity, research, and professional development with digital content (Asthma and Allergy Network, 2024). To learn more, visit www.allergyasthmanetwork.org.

FAACT also provides general information in addition to their behavioral health resources for those living with food allergy, including education on managing food allergies from elementary school through college. The website includes information on accommodations, legal documents such as 504 plans, and a civil rights advocacy center. For information, visit www.foodallergyawareness.org.

Nurses can consult these organizations for current social-emotional guidance as the resources may change over time.

Nursing Interventions to Improve Food Allergy Care from a Social Emotional Perspective

Another way to prepare patients and caregivers for communication and social situations is to practice scenarios simulating common food allergy situations. The scenarios can help build confidence by anticipating situations and thinking through how they would respond to situations while in a controlled environment with a clinician available to answer questions.

Scenario Options:

1. If you accidentally ingest an allergen, what steps would you take next? Who would you notify? Feel free to write out your plan once you have one suitable to your needs.
2. If someone is making you feel uncomfortable regarding your food allergies, what do you think you would say? How do you think you would respond?
3. If you want to try a new food, beauty product, or soap, what do you need to do first? Should someone be around the first time that you try something new? If so, who?
4. What if you are unsure of an ingredient on a label, how would you figure out what it is?

5. If you need to explain how to use an epinephrine device to a friend, what are the steps you would tell them? Do you have a trainer device and do you practice using it? How many devices do you carry?
6. Do you have an emergency medication kit? If so, what are the contents? What medications do you take and in which order? How frequently do you check to make sure you are appropriately stocked, and that medication expiration dates are current?
7. When you go out to a restaurant, are there any special considerations? How do you prepare for your visit?

Nursing engagement is pivotal in the process of helping patients and families build resilience. Having a strong personal knowledge base about food allergies and the associated physiology allows nurses to translate the science behind food allergies into language the patient and family can understand. Understanding treatment options specific to the practice setting helps facilitate patient and family teaching. Access to patient education materials, demonstration devices, such as manufacturer-specific epinephrine trainers, or a scale for oral immunotherapy dosing, and applicator bottles for sublingual immunotherapy, are all useful tools to help increase patient and caregiver knowledge and reduce anxiety. Return demonstration helps to evaluate the effectiveness of patient and family teaching, helps to alleviate overall concerns, and identifies those that need additional education or support.

Conclusion

The multifaceted challenges posed by food allergies extend well beyond the immediate health risks associated with allergen exposure. This chapter highlights the significant social and emotional impacts experienced by individuals with food allergies, their families, and caregivers. The anxiety and fear that accompany food allergies often manifest in heightened stress, social isolation, and mental health struggles. For children, these issues can translate into increased social anxiety, bullying, and a diminished quality of life. Adults managing their own allergies face similar emotional burdens, including the stress of constant vigilance and the economic strain of managing food safety.

As the prevalence of food allergies continues to increase, it is essential for healthcare professionals, especially nurses and nurse practitioners, to recognize and address the comprehensive needs of this population. This includes not only managing the physical aspects of food allergies but also providing support for the emotional and social challenges that accompany them. By fostering a supportive environment, screening for psychosocial conditions, enhancing access to mental health resources, and promoting effective coping strategies, we can improve the quality of life for individuals living with food allergies and their families. Continued research and advocacy are critical in addressing the complex interplay between food allergies and mental health, ensuring that affected individuals receive the holistic care and support they need.

References

Abrams, E., Simons, E., Roos, L., Hurst, K., & Protudjer, J. (2020). Qualitative analysis of perceived impacts on childhood food allergy on caregiver mental health and lifestyle. *Annals of Allergy, Asthma & Immunology, 124*(6), 594–599. https://doi.org/10.1016/j.anai.2020.02.016

Asthma and Allergy Network. (2024). Retrieved from Asthma and Allergy Network: www.allergyasthmanetwork.org

Bingemann, T. A., LeBovidge, J., Bartnikas, L., Protudjer, J. L. P., & Herbert, L. J. (2024). Psychosocial impact of food allergy on children and adults and practical interventions. *Current Allergy and Asthma Reports, 24*(3), 107–119. https://doi.org/10.1007/s11882-023-01121-x

Bozen, A., Kanaley, M., Negris, O., Gupta, R., & Lombard, L. (2020). Pediatric allergists' perspectives on the psychosocial challenges of food allergy and factors that support coping. *Annals of Allergy, Asthma & Immunology, 124*(5), 515–516. https://doi.org/10.1016/j.anai.2020.02.003

Casale, T. B., Warren, C., Gupta, S., Schuldt, R., Wang, R., Iqbal, A., Seetasith, A., & Gupta, R. (2024). The mental health burden of food allergies: Insights from patients and their caregivers from the Food Allergy Research & Education (FARE) Patient Registry. *World Allergy Organization Journal, 17*(4), 100891. https://doi.org/10.1016/j.waojou.2024.100891

Chooniedass, R., Soller, L., Hsu, E., To, S., Cameron, S., & Chan, E. (2020). Parents of children with food allergy: A qualitative study describing needs and identifying solutions. *American College of Allergy, Asthma & Immunology, 125*(6), 674–679. https://doi.org/10.1016/j.anai.2020.05.014

Ciciulla, D., Soriano, V., McWilliam, V., Koplin, J., & Peters, R. (2023). Systematic review of the incidence and/or prevalence of eating disorders in individuals with food allergies. *The Journal of Allergy and Clinical Immunology: In Practice, 11*(7), 2196–2207. https://doi.org/10.1016/j.jaip.2023.04.010

Dahlsgaard, K. K., & Lewis, M. O. (2025). Want to help your patients with food allergy anxiety? Do proximity challenges. *Annals of Allergy, Asthma & Immunology, 134*(5), 525–532. https://doi.org/10.1016/j.anai.2025.02.020

Dahlsgaard, K. K., Lewis, M. O., & Spergel, J. M. (2020). New issue of food allergy: Phobia of anaphylaxis in pediatric patients. *Journal of Clinical Immunology, 146*(4), 780–782. https://doi.org/10.1016/j.jaci.2020.07.010

Dahlsgaard, K. K., Lewis, M. O., & Spergel, J. M. (2023). Cognitive-behavioral intervention for anxiety associated with food allergy in a clinical sample of children: Feasibility, acceptability, and proof-of-concept in children. *Annals of Allergy, Asthma & Immunology, 130*(1), 100. https://doi.org/10.1016/j.anai.2022.09.021

Dulger, Z., Sheridan, E., Cohen, L., Le, H., & Walker, C. (n.d.). *Food allergy research and education. Stressing the importance of food allergies.* https://www.foodallergy.org/resources/stressing-importance-food-allergies

Engel, M. L., Rich, S. K., Warren, C. M., & Gupta, R. S. (2022). Psychosocial needs of adolescents with food allergies registering for a national online social program. *Annals of Allergy, Asthma & Immunology: Official Publication of the American College of Allergy, Asthma, & Immunology, 129*(1), 122–124. https://doi.org/10.1016/j.anai.2022.04.010

Engel, M. L., Warren, C. M., Herbert, L. J., Pappalardo, A. A., Ramos, A., & Gupta, R. S. (2025). The psychosocial burden of pediatric food allergy in the United States: A population-based survey. *The Journal of Allergy and Clinical Immunology. In Practice, 13*(3), 630–638.e4. https://doi.org/10.1016/j.jaip.2024.12.007

Feng, C., & Kim, J. (2019). Beyond avoidance: The psychosocial impact of food allergies. *Clinical Reviews in Allergy & Immunology, 57*, 74–82. https://doi.org/10.1007/s12016-018-8708-x

Flokstra-de Blok, B. M., Dubois, A. E., Vlieg-Boerstra, B. J., Oude Elberink, J. N., Raat, H., DunnGalvin, A., Hourihane, J. O., & Duiverman, E. J. (2010). Health-related quality of life of food allergic patients: comparison with the general population and other diseases. *Allergy, 65*(2), 238–244. https://doi.org/10.1111/j.1398-9995.2009.02121.x

Food Allergy & Anaphylaxis Connection Team. (n.d.-a). *Allergy summit*. https://www.foodallergyawareness.org/faact-allergy-summit/faact-allergy-summit/
Food Allergy & Anaphylaxis Connection Team. (n.d.-b). *Post-traumatic stress disorder (PTSD)*. https://www.foodallergyawareness.org/anxiety-and-food-allergies/post-traumatic-stress-disorder-ptsd/#:~:text=For%20individuals%20with%20food%20allergy,stress%20scenario%2C%20PTSD%20can%20develop
Food Allergy Research and Education. (2024). Retrieved from Food Allergy Research and Education: www.foodallergy.org
Greiwe, J. (2023). Quality of life and psychological issues associated with food allergy. *Journal of Food Allergy, 5*(2), 43–48. https://doi.org/10.2500/jfa.2023.5.230011
Herbert, L. J., Cushman, G., Hahn, A., Hubbard, T., Kubala, S. A., LeBovidge, J., Proctor, K., Protudjer, J. L. P., Ramos, A., Rosenberg, L. B., Rotter, N., & Voorhees, S. (2025). Integration of mental health care into food allergy practices: A work group report of the AAAAI Integrative Medicine Committee. *The Journal of Allergy and Clinical Immunology. In Practice, 13*(12), 3227–3236. https://doi.org/10.1016/j.jaip.2025.08.034
Hubbard, T. (2025). *May contain anxiety: Managing the overwhelm of parenting children with food allergies*. Johns Hopkins University Press.
Kanter, A. B., Yasik, A. E., Zaccario, M. L., & Saviano, J. C. (2022). Self-reported anxiety ratings in children with and without food allergies and teacher knowledge of food allergies. *Journal of School Health, 92*(6), 541–549. https://doi.org/10.1111/josh.13181
Knibb, R., Herbert, L., Jones, C., Protudjer, J., Screti, C., Roleston, C., & Marchisotto, M. (2024). Global availability and uptake of psychological services for adults, caregivers and children with food allergy. *Allergy, 79*, 2787–2797. https://doi.org/10.1111/all.16204
Marsac, M., & Wurth, M. (2021). Opportunities to support emotional health in school-age children with food allergy. *Annals of Allergy, Asthma & Immunology, 126*(6), *722–741*. https://doi.org/10.1016/j.anai.2021.02.017
Moen, Ø. M., Opheim, E., & Trollvik. (2019). Parents experiences raising a child with food allergy: A qualitative review. *Journal of Pediatric Nursing, 46*, 52–63. https://doi.org/10.1016/j.pedn.2019.02.036
OpenAI. (2025). Retrieved from ChatGPT [Large language model]: https://chatgpt.com
Polloni, L., & Muraro, A. (2020). Anxiety and food allergy: A review of the last two decades. *Clinical & Experimental Allergy, 50*(4), 420–441. https://doi.org/10.1111/cea.13548
Protudjer, J. L. P., Golding, M., Salisbury, M. R., Abrams, E. M., & Roos, L. E. (2021). High anxiety and health-related quality of life in families with children with food allergy during coronavirus disease 2019. *Annals of Allergy, Asthma & Immunology: Official Publication of the American College of Allergy, Asthma, & Immunology, 126*(1), 83 88.e1. https://doi.org/10.1016/j.anai.2020.09.010
Quach, L., & John, R. (2018). Psychosocial impact of growing up with food allergies. *The Journal for Nurse Practitioners, 14*(6), 477–483. https://doi.org/10.1016/j.nurpra.2018.03.017
Ramos, A., Cooke, F., Miller, E., & Herbert, L. (2021). The food allergy parent mentoring program: a pilot intervention. *Journal of Pediatric Psychology, 46*(7), 856–865. https://doi.org/10.1093/jpepsy/jsab019
Rubeiz, C., & Ernst, M. (2021). Psychosocial aspects of food allergy. *Immunology and Allergy Clinics of North America, 41*(2), 177–188. https://doi.org/10.1016/j.iac.2021.01.006
Santos, A. F., Worm, M., Kurita, S., Wong, T., Contato, D., Pirillo, E., Esteban, A. E., Tassinari, P., Perna, F., & Chinthrajah, R. S. (2023). Living with food allergies: The experiences of adult patients and caregivers. *Frontiers in Allergy, 4*, 1272851. https://doi.org/10.3389/falgy.2023.1272851
Schelly, D., Ohl, A., & Meramo, H. (2023). College students with food allergy: From hypervigilance to disclosure fatigue. *Journal of Pediatric Nursing, 70*, 32–39. https://doi.org/10.1016/j.pedn.2022.11.027
Shemesh, E. (2023). *Food allergy: Impact on health-related quality of life*. https://www.uptodate.com/contents/food-allergy-impact-on-health-related-quality-of-life

Shemesh, E., D'Urso, C., Knight, C., Rubes, M., Picerno, K. M., Posillico, A. M., Atal, Z., Annunziato, R. A., & Sicherer, S. H. (2017). Food-allergic adolescents at risk for anaphylaxis: A randomized controlled study of supervised injection to improve comfort with epinephrine self-injection. *The Journal of Allergy and Clinical Immunology in Practice, 5*(2), 391–397.e4. https://doi.org/10.1016/j.jaip.2016.12.016

Spitzer, R. L., Williams, J. B., & Kroenke, K. (n.d.). *Patient Health Questionnaire-9 (PHQ-9).* Retrieved from American Psychological Association: www.apa.org/depression-guideline/patienthealth-questionnaire.pdf

Tomei, L., Muraro, A., Giovannini, M., Barni, S., Liccioli, G., Paladini, E., Sarti, L., Pessina, B., Skypala, I., Novembre, E., & Mori, F. (2023). Hidden and rare food allergens in pediatric age. *Nutrients, 15*(6), 1386. https://doi.org/10.3390/nu15061386

Turner, P. J., Jerschow, E., Umasunthar, T., Lin, R., Campbell, D. E., & Boyle, R. J. (2017). Fatal Anaphylaxis: Mortality Rate and Risk Factors. The journal of allergy and clinical immunology. *In practice, 5*(5), 1169–1178. https://doi.org/10.1016/j.jaip.2017.06.031

Verdi, M., Candido, D., Madan, J., Bernstein, J. A., Bukstein, D., Anagnostou, A., Greenhawt, M., Mustafa, S. S., Wang, J., Nowak-Wegrzyn, A., Abrams, E. M., Oppenheimer, J., Conway, A. E., White, A. A., Doherty, T. A., Morse, R. P., & Shaker, M. (2025). Addressing anxiety and depression in the allergy clinic through motivational interviewing, brief cognitive behavioral therapy, and curious questions. *The Journal of Allergy and Clinical Immunology in Practice, 13*(8), 1960–1969.e2. https://doi.org/10.1016/j.jaip.2025.05.020

Westwell-Roper, C., To S, Andjelic, G., et al. (2022). Food-allergy-specific anxiety and distress in parents of children with food allergy: A systematic review. *Pediatric Allergy and Immunology, 33*, e13695. https://doi.org/10.1111/pai.13695

Xu, G., Liu, B., Yang, W., Snetselaar, L. G., Chen, M., Bao, W., & Strathearn, L. (2022). Association of food allergy, respiratory allergy, and skin allergy with attention deficit/hyperactivity disorder among children. *Nutrients, 14*(3), 474. https://doi.org/10.3390/nu14030474

Role of Technology in the Management of Food Allergy

Olga Kagan

Introduction

Technology has become an integral part of healthcare delivery and is continually evolving to meet the needs of patients, clinicians, and other interest holders within the healthcare ecosystem, including in the allergy specialty. While allergy nursing is not yet a recognized specialty within the profession of nursing, the number of nurses with an interest in allergy is steadily growing as evidenced by the increasing number of nurses employed in allergy practices to oversee novel treatments (Greiwe et al., 2020; Infante, 2024), the expansion of research conducted and disseminated by nurses domestically and internationally, and the rising involvement of nurses in advocacy and education in the allergy sphere (Kagan et al., 2023; Hathaway & James, 2023; Zimmanck et al., 2024). Nurses often lead the development of digital educational tools and programs (Broome et al., 2022; Kagan, 2024). They are also tasked with roles and responsibilities that include employment of patient and clinician-facing technologies, such as electronic health records (EHR), remote patient monitoring software, telenursing, patient portals, as well as tools that facilitate communication, professional development, resource allocation, and administrative tasks. Finally, nurses remain stewards of the profession and are embracing technology as an innovative component of healthcare including leveraging artificial intelligence to improve healthcare. However, they are also aware of the potential risks and concerns about upholding ethical standards while using technology in practice.

O. Kagan (✉)
City University of New York School of Professional Studies, New York, NY, USA

Barbara H. Hagan School of Nursing and Health Sciences, Molloy University, Rockville Centre, NY, USA

Food Allergy Nursing Association, Great Neck, NY, USA

J. Doucette, J. Howard-Ruben (eds.), *Comprehensive Food Allergy Management for Nurses*, https://doi.org/10.1007/978-3-032-28647-5_11

Technology Overview

Existing and emerging technologies are everyday tools including software and hardware that help nurses provide more equitable, cost-effective, seamless, and easily accessible care to ensure better quality of life and outcomes for patients and families. A term that is commonly used is eHealth (i.e., electronic health) which encompasses a variety of internet and computerized tools, such as telehealth, wearables, and mHealth (mobile health) (See Table 1).

Technology-enabled care (TEC), a collective term often used for telecare, telehealth, telemedicine, mHealth, digital, and eHealth services, has the potential to solve many challenges facing the healthcare sector. A review of 21 studies on patient experiences with TEC highlights issues with technology features that could lead to both: (1) frustration due to technical difficulties and (2) user empowerment because of increasing awareness about their health condition, as well as feeling more safe and self-efficient (Leonardsen et al., 2020). In a consumer-driven healthcare system, patients are encouraged to serve as key interest holders and must be involved in developing TEC solutions that can lead to better health outcomes and improved patient satisfaction. Nurses also play a crucial role in the advancement of technology in healthcare.

Table 1 Glossary of eHealth tools and technologies

App: Abbreviation for application software. Computer program designed to perform a specific activity. They can run on computers, portable devices (mobile app), or web servers (web app)
Artificial intelligence (AI): Simulation of processes associated with human intelligence by computers. It includes natural language processing, speech recognition, or machine vision
Big data: Recording and analysis of datasets that are too large, multidimensional, diverse, and complex to be adequately processed by traditional software solutions
eHealth: Abbreviation for electronic health. It includes a diverse group of tools that use computers and the internet to improve the efficacy and efficiency of the healthcare industry
Health informatics: Integration of healthcare and computer science. It comprises electronic health records, computerized physician order entry, clinical decision support systems, and software solutions for administrative tasks
mHealth: Abbreviation for mobile health. Integration of mobile devices (e.g., smartphones) in the practice of healthcare
Natural language processing (NLP): NLP is the ability of a computer program to understand human language as it is spoken
Social media: Interactive web-based applications where users can share text posts, comments, and multimedia files. They can be used to develop personal or professional social networks
Telemedicine: Delivery of health-related services performed via electronic information and telecommunication technologies. They can be real-time interactive services or store-and-forward, which means acquiring data that is subsequently transmitted to a specialist for assessment
Wearable: Hands-free electronic device that can be worn as an accessory, clothing, or as a part of the body (e.g., smart watches, bracelets, and epidermal electronics resembling tattoos)

Nurses use healthcare technology (HT) in many ways to care for patients. In an allergy population, nurses utilize technology to enhance patient education, monitor patients, and conduct research. They educate and monitor patients using mobile health (mHealth) applications (Matricardi et al., 2020) (see Fig. 1). For example, nurses can track symptoms and adherence to medications (Alvarez-Perea et al., 2021) with mobile apps that have patient self-reported data, allowing for timely interventions (Tripodi et al., 2020). These interventions or routine follow-ups can be administered via telenursing using HIPAA-compliant video conferencing platforms or other secure bidirectional portals (AAAAI, 2025), especially in remote areas where access to clinicians is limited (Henry, 2022). Nurses can recommend and help patients use wearable devices that monitor environmental allergens like pollen and air quality. These devices provide real-time data, enabling nurses to advise patients on preventive measures.

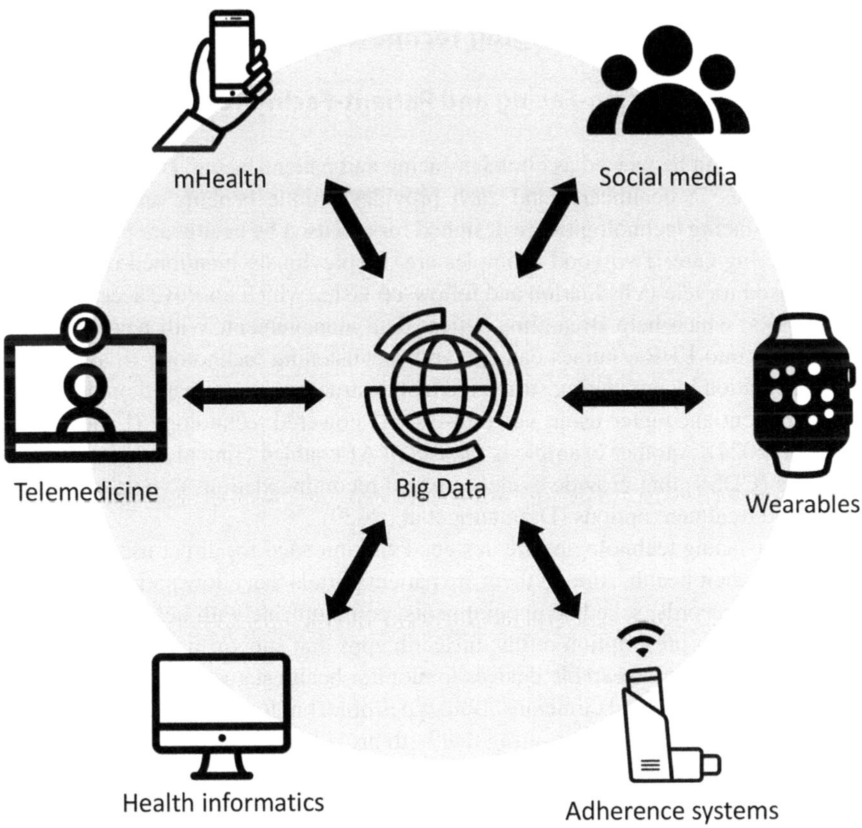

Fig. 1 eHealth. eHealth includes a variety of technologies that can be applied to the healthcare industry. The information generated by these tools can be used as a source of big data which, in turn, may improve the system. (Used with permission from: Alvarez-Perea et al. (2021), John Wiley & Sons Ltd on behalf of European Academy of Allergy and Clinical Immunology. Published under CC BY 4.0 https://creativecommons.org/licenses/by/4.0/)

Furthermore, with the proliferation of artificial intelligence (AI), nurses can enhance practice through scholarship by utilizing AI-powered tools to analyze patient data and identify patterns in allergy triggers (Khan et al., 2024), supporting evidence-based care with a more personalized approach and improving patient outcomes (Infante, 2024; Bousquet et al., 2021). Nurses involved with clinical trials or those working with novel treatments aimed at delivering precision care are responsible for collecting samples for advanced diagnostic tests, such as molecular diagnostics, which provide detailed information about specific allergens and help tailor immunotherapy treatments (Cleveland Clinic, 2019). As technology continues to evolve, nurses will be responsible for staying current on the most up-to-date technologies and seeking professional development opportunities. Emerging technologies will drive the redesign of nursing work and new models of care that employ AI-driven technology as an integral part of the care team.

Use of Existing and Emerging Technologies in Allergy

Overview of Clinician-Facing and Patient-Facing Technologies

Technology can be viewed as clinician-facing and patient-facing. Both serve different purposes in healthcare, and each provides unique benefits and challenges. Clinician-facing technologies are designed for and used by healthcare professionals in delivering care. Two good examples are the previously mentioned digital platforms used for tele-consultation and follow-up visits, which improve access to care, and EHRs, which help streamline patient data management. With newer features integrated into EHRs, nurses can use ambient listening technology to assist with documentation by populating structured and unstructured notes based on the verbal nurse-patient encounter using voice-to-text AI-powered technology (Landi, 2024; Capoot, 2024). Another example is the use of AI-enabled clinical decision support systems (CDSS) that provide evidence-based recommendations to help with diagnosis and treatment options (Dramburg et al., 2020).

Patient-facing technologies are designed and intended for direct use by patients to manage their health. Among them are patient portals that allow patients to access their health records, schedule appointments, communicate with healthcare providers, and request prescription refills; mHealth apps that support patients with tracking their health; and wearable devices to monitor health status, providing real-time data to both patients and clinicians. Both types of technology are crucial for a holistic approach to healthcare, ensuring that both providers and patients have the tools they need to achieve better health outcomes. However, the main differences between the clinician-facing tech and patient-facing tech are that the former focuses on improving clinical workflows and decision-making and can enhance diagnostic accuracy and treatment efficiency, while the latter aims to empower patients in managing their health and helps improve patient engagement and adherence to treatment plans (Bonderud, 2021).

Examples of Patient-Facing Technologies

Evidence-Based and Expert Tools

The COVID-19 pandemic propelled the development and adoption of digital healthcare technologies and has benefited patients, clinicians, and scientists in allergy directly and indirectly. There are several examples of patient-facing tools that can improve patient and caregiver experiences during allergy visits; reinforce allergy education via interactive learning tools; and assist patients in management of allergies at home and beyond. In one feasibility study, the use of virtual reality (VR) during the pediatric oral food challenge (OFC) produced positive feedback in helping alleviate anxiety (Collins et al., 2022). A nurse-led interactive anaphylaxis learning guide, also referred to as a web-based audio-visual anaphylaxis recognition-and-response tool, was developed by an interdisciplinary team at the American Academy of Allergy Asthma and Immunology (AAAAI). The tool is used to reinforce knowledge among patients and caregivers in prompt recognition and effective response to common presentations of anaphylaxis in pre-hospital/pre-emergency medical services community-based scenarios in children and adults (AAAAI Guide, 2024; Kagan, 2024). Patient engagement in self-management and shared decision-making is enabled by employing self-reported mHealth apps for asthma (e.g., ASTHMAXcel, 2025) or digital diaries (Hsia et al., 2021) to track and communicate symptoms, triggers, and/or medication use either short-term or longitudinally, which enables a more precise collection of information prior to meeting with healthcare providers (Tripodi et al., 2020; Alvarez-Perea et al., 2021; Bédard et al., 2019). Mobile apps have the capability to address patient/caregiver evidence-based education, encourage behavior change, facilitate targeted notifications, and gather patient reported outcomes in a timely and more efficient manner (Broome et al., 2022).

Patient Portals

Additionally, patient portals, initially driven by financial incentives in Medicare and Medicaid programs as part of Meaningful Use (Beal et al., 2021), promote informed patient participation and decision-making through improved online access. Meaningful Use was an initiative by the US Office of the National Coordinator for Health Information Technology (ONC) and the Centers for Medicare & Medicaid Services (CMS) that set specific objectives for eligible providers and hospitals to demonstrate the effective and secure use of electronic health records (EHRs) to improve healthcare quality, safety, and efficiency, and to reduce health disparities, engage patients, and improve care coordination, in order to qualify for EHR incentive payments (HealthIT, 2025). EHR-linked web and mobile versions of patient portals serve as powerful tools that provide patients and caregivers with real-time access to health information and enhanced communication with clinicians. Most importantly, a recent study found that portal use was positively received by individuals with lower socioeconomic status and education levels, helping address certain social determinants of health (SDOH) (El Yaman et al., 2023); however, disparities related to race, age, sex, and digital literacy remain (Yoon et al., 2024). Patients can also subscribe to text messaging alerts or email prescription refill or expiration date reminders offered by most pharmacies, third-party apps, and the makers of epinephrine devices (EpiPen®, 2024; Epipen.ca, 2025; AUVI-Q, 2024).

Social Media and Online Communities

Outside of the expert provided tools, patients and caregivers engage with health content via web-based moderated support groups, such as online health communities, social media groups, digital patient-focused content, digital media publications like *Allergic Living*, and with resources and forums offered by patient advocacy organizations like Food Allergy Research and Education (FARE, 2024). The nurse's role in allergy is to ensure that patient-facing digital tools provided to patients and caregivers are evidence-based, equitable, and accessible to all, including to underrepresented and underserved communities, such as people with disabilities and language barriers. It is also important that nurses conduct SDOH screening during the initial and follow-up clinic visits to personalize referrals, education, and resources to ensure proper and effective use of patient-facing tools beyond the clinic setting.

Examples of Clinician-Facing Technology

Electronic Health Records (EHR)

In the US, electronic health records (EHRs) offer secure access to patient records and facilitate the exchange of information in real-time (HealthIT.gov, 2025a, b, c, d, e). Current EHR regulations, such as the 21st Century Cures Act and updates to the Office of the National Coordinator for Health Information Technology Health IT Certification Program (ONC), aim to enhance interoperability, transparency, and access to electronic health information. These regulations promote responsible AI use, equity, and secure, efficient data exchange, supporting improved care delivery across hospitals and outpatient medical offices (health data, technology, and interoperability).

As of 2021, 78% of office-based physicians and nearly 98% of hospitals have adopted certified EHR systems (National Trends), which include those in allergy and immunology practices. Several factors drive the adoption of EHRs in healthcare including:

1. *Federal Incentives*: Programs like the HITECH Act of 2009 (Health IT legislation), which offer financial incentives for EHR implementation.
2. *Improved Patient Care*: Enhanced medication management, better care coordination, and instant access to data.

3. *Public Health Reporting*: Streamlined data collection, surveillance, and reporting capabilities.
4. *Streamlined Workflows*: Automation of administrative tasks, reduction of paperwork, and decreased documentation burden.

Leveraging the EHR can also improve clinical care by contributing to accurate allergy documentation and improved patient safety. For example, one organization adopted a multidisciplinary approach to identify and standardize free-text allergen entries in the EHR as a part of health system-wide patient safety initiative to improve documentation and to ensure consistent clinical decision support, including allergy alerts (Li et al., 2022). In this study, more than two-thirds of free-text entries were entered by medical assistants and registered nurses necessitating a multidisciplinary collaboration between prescribing and non-prescribing professionals to improve allergy documentation. The standardized entries improved documentation through consistent use of terminology and avoidance of misspellings and abbreviations. Structured allergen entries can be easily communicated to other departments such as pharmacy and nutrition services. This collaboration can assist in bridging the knowledge gaps in standardized allergy data entry, differentiate coded and free-text entries, and identify educational opportunities (Li et al., 2022).

When clinicians are presented with documentation challenges, it is imperative to include nurses as part of the team in establishing systematic, unbiased, consistent, and safe guidelines for documenting allergies. The EHR also offers administrative and care coordination benefits for allergy nurses such as staffing, scheduling, recordkeeping, notetaking, and follow-up reminders. Data that nurses generate within EHRs can be analyzed and used to provide a more accurate insight into health trends, patient satisfaction, gaps in practice, research, and education, among other use cases.

Artificial Intelligence and Chatbots

Integration of AI within EHRs has the potential to enhance real-time, data-driven decision-making capabilities, assisting clinicians in diagnosing and managing allergic diseases such as eosinophilic esophagitis (EoE) (Pandya et al., 2024). Advancements in machine learning algorithms offer more personalized diagnoses and treatments based on individual patient data. For example, if an AI model is trained on data from EHRs, clinical trials, systematic reviews, and aggregated data repositories, it can predict the probability of a particular diagnosis and recommend best practice treatments (Pandya et al., 2024).

As AI evolves, so do the AI language models and products emerging in the healthcare arena. For instance, AI-powered chatbots are software tools created to mimic human conversation by using natural language (Clark & Bailey, 2024). A more specific example is the generative pretrained transformer (GPT) tool from OpenAI (open artificial intelligence) (OpenAI et al., 2024) in partnership with Microsoft that offers powerful generative AI-powered chatbots like GPT-5 (generative pretrained transformer 5.0 model version) (GPT-5, 2025). Many are already familiar with more common versions of chatbots, such as Siri or Alexa, as well as Microsoft Copilot (Microsoft Copilot, 2025), and Google Gemini (Gemini, 2025) AI assistants. These tools leverage advanced machine learning algorithms that can generate natural language responses to inquiries that are more detailed and nuanced either via web browsers or on handheld devices.

Allergy nurses may interface with chatbot technology as its effectiveness becomes more established in clinical practice. Access to information, such as symptom assessment, health education, medication reminders, or appointment scheduling, is available 24/7 and even allow access to information when healthcare providers are not available (Clark & Bailey, 2024). Nurses must stay abreast of the AI-driven technology in their practice and employ available resources such as *5 Rights of AI in Healthcare* (see Fig. 2) to ensure its ethical and proper use (HIMSS, 2024; Ross et al., 2024). *5 Rights of AI in Healthcare*, modeled after the often quoted "5 Rights of Medication Administration," is based on the recommendations from the World Health Organization (WHO, 2024) for the ethical and safe use of AI in health. It also aligns with the White House Blueprint for an AI Bill of Rights issued in 2022 (OSTP, 2025) and aims to provide clinicians with a clear and practical framework for applying and managing AI in healthcare settings, including telehealth, remote patient monitoring, and other models of care that increasingly leverage AI technology.

Telehealth

Clinicians and patients now have new ways to communicate, including telehealth, which could be cost-effective in improving allergy management and enhancing quality of life of those affected. Telehealth is defined as "the use of electronic information and telecommunication technologies to support long-distance clinical healthcare, patient and professional health-related education, health administration, and public health" (HRSA, 2021). This includes video and phone consultations and electronic prescription renewals. Through telehealth, healthcare professionals (HCPs) can maintain close contact with their patients to address individual needs and optimize disease and treatment management (Dramburg et al., 2022). Studies suggest that patients who use telehealth reported fewer hospital admissions and emergency department visits resulting in improvement in quality of life, a reduction in healthcare utilization, and better management of chronic diseases (Mun et al., 2024; Zhang & Saltman, 2022; Mammen et al., 2021). Telehealth makes it easier for patients to access allergy specialists without the need for in-person visits. This is particularly beneficial for managing chronic conditions like allergies (Matricardi et al., 2020). Telehealth may also be leveraged to access mental health resources for psychological support for patients and families managing food allergies.

As the use of telecommunication technology continues to demonstrate many benefits (Ayuso Margañon et al., 2023) in providing healthcare from a distance, offering cost savings, improving access to healthcare services that would often not

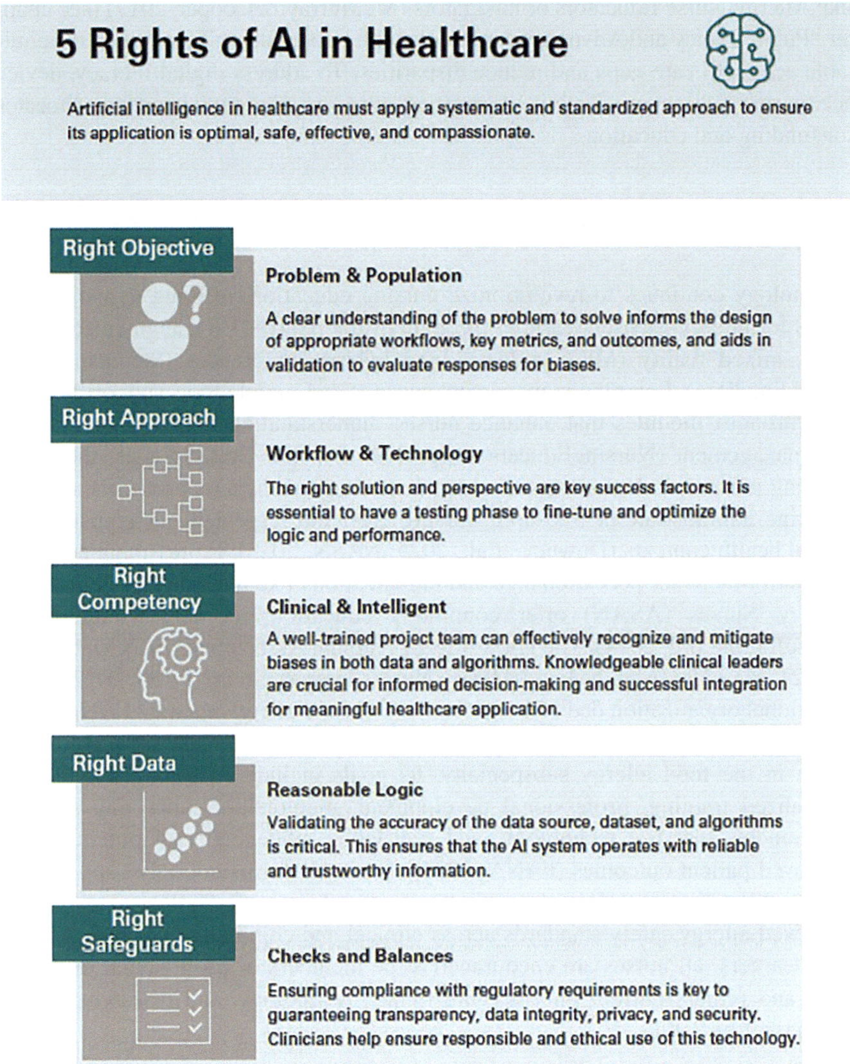

Fig. 2 5 Rights of AI in Healthcare. (Reproduced with permission from: Ross et al. (2024), Wolters Kluwer Health https://journals.lww.com/nursingmanagement/fulltext/2024/07000/implications_of_artificial_intelligence_for_nurse.4.aspx)

be available in remote or rural communities (AHRQ, 2023), or in 25% of US schools where nurses are not employed (Willgerodt et al., 2018), it becomes imperative to consider alternative models of care. For example, future models of care could include blended care, which is the combination of in-person healthcare visits with remote or online sessions (Dramburg et al., 2022), school-based telehealth services (National Association of School Nurses, 2022, 2023), and more specialized roles like Allergy Nurse Educators or navigators (McMurray & Cooper, 2017) (see chapter "Public Policy and Advocacy for People with Food Allergy"), to bridge the equitable access to care gaps and reduce disparities. To address digital literacy, device access, and internet connectivity disparities, nurses need to remain active advocates for funding and education.

Allergy Nursing Education

Technology continues to revolutionize nursing education, offering dynamic platforms for allergy-focused learning through virtual reality (VR), augmented reality (AR), mixed reality (MR), podcasts, and hybrid conferences (Stegman, 2025; Coughlin, 2024). Learning management systems and mobile tools support flexible, asynchronous modules that enhance nurses' understanding of allergy prevention and management (NursingEducation.org, 2024). In the United States, there is a growing push to embed allergy content, including anaphylaxis protocols and epinephrine administration, into core nursing curricula, especially in pediatric and school health contexts (Downey et al., 2025; NASN, 2023). Professional networking platforms foster peer exchange and organizations like the American Society of Allergy Nurses (ASAN) offer continuing education via annual conferences (NurseJournal.org, 2024). The Food Allergy Nursing Association (FANA), founded in 2024 originally from the Food Allergy Nurses Interest Group (FANI, 2022), is the first global organization dedicated exclusively to food allergy nursing. FANA's mission is to advance nursing education, research, leadership, innovation, and collaboration in the food allergy subspecialty. Its goals include equipping nurses with specialized training, professional development, mentorship, supporting scalable care models that use technology, and translating evidence-based practices into improved patient outcomes (FANA, 2024). These platforms not only support continuing education but also empower nurses to advocate for policy changes and improved allergy safety standards across clinical and community settings. As lifelong learners, all nurses are encouraged to be members of professional organizations and remain current on emerging trends, technology, and research in their respective specialties.

Allergy Nursing Research

Artificial intelligence (AI) tools are transforming nursing research rapidly, offering substantial advantages that enhance productivity and provide advanced analytical capabilities. A key benefit lies in AI's robust support for data analysis, especially with large and complex datasets like electronic health records (EHR) (Boussina et al., 2024). AI algorithms can identify subtle patterns, predict patient outcomes, and uncover correlations that might be missed by traditional methods, leading to more precise nursing interventions (Alowais et al., 2023). This capability facilitates a shift from deterministic to probabilistic care, which can inform preventive actions and improve outcomes. Furthermore, AI tools considerably accelerate and enhance the literature review process by analyzing and synthesizing vast amounts of research literature in minutes, saving nurse researchers' considerable time (Kagan & Keny, in press). Natural language processing (NLP), a type of AI, enables AI to analyze patient records, identify trends, and extract key information from numerous articles, synthesizing and organizing it based on researchers' queries (Becker, 2025). While AI's role in suggesting methodologies or sample sizes is still evolving, generative AI tools can indirectly assist in study design by facilitating idea generation, refining research questions, and structuring research synthesis (Becker, 2025; Brown & Sabbaghan, 2025; Fisher, 2025).

However, the integration of AI in nursing research also introduces considerable challenges and critical considerations. Ethical dilemmas, trustworthiness, bias, and fairness are top concerns, requiring allergy nurse researchers to ensure transparency in data use, that actively mitigate potential biases in AI-generated content and maintain essential human oversight (Kagan & Keny, in press). AI "hallucinations," instances where AI systems produce fabricated or inaccurate information (Chelli et al., 2024), necessitate rigorous human verification and validation of AI outputs to prevent the introduction of unreliable information into academic work. Concerns also arise regarding plagiarism and the originality of submitted work, as researchers bear full responsibility for ensuring their work is original and properly attributed, despite AI's ability to generate novel content (Chelli et al., 2024). Finally, transparency is vital, with many academic journals and publishers establishing clear guidelines that require explicit disclosure of AI tool use in research and manuscript preparation specifying the tool, version, purpose, and validation steps (SciPub+, 2025; Taylor and Francis, 2023; CSH, 2025), though minor uses like grammar checks may be exempt (Cheng et al., 2025). AI tools cannot be credited as authors, as authorship entails human accountability. Responsible implementation and human oversight remain crucial for maximizing AI's potential while addressing these challenges. While each journal has its own guidelines, Cheng and colleagues offer a checklist as a guide for authors to use as shown in Fig. 3 and it is clear that discussion on acceptable ethical use will continue.

Nurses who serve as peer reviewers and journal editors are witnessing a gradual integration of AI into editorial workflows. For instance, the Journal of the American Medical Informatics Association's proposed Manubot AI Editor which uses large language models to suggest scholarly revisions with human oversight (Pividori & Greene, 2023). Publishers like MDPI are also developing AI tools to support editorial quality, while exploring safe applications for peer review under strict confidentiality constraints (McKenna, 2024), despite current tools not yet fully perfected in their accuracy and robustness (Descamps et al., 2024). In 2025, widely accepted AI tools in nursing include enterprise-integrated assistants like Microsoft Copilot and Google Gemini, as well as AI-enhanced platforms such as Grammarly, Covidence, and Turnitin. As competition grows and user adoption increases, these tools are expected to become more reliable and robust, with leading platforms setting industry standards.

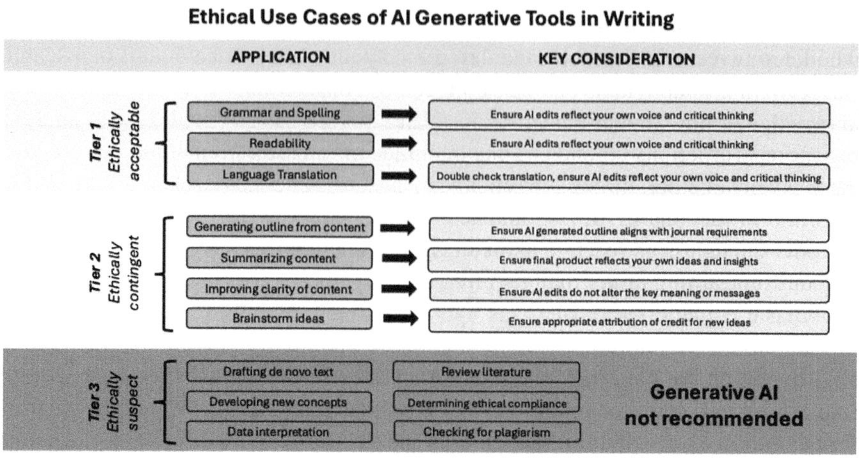

Fig. 3 Ethical use cases of AI generative tools in writing. (Used with permission from: Cheng et al. (2025). Published under CC BY 4.0 https://creativecommons.org/licenses/by/4.0/)

Conclusion

The integration of technology into food allergy management continues to shift how and where care is delivered, offering a host of benefits for both clinicians and patients. In this chapter, we explored digital health technologies, including EHRs, telehealth, mHealth apps, and AI. These are not just supplementary tools but are essential components of a modern, efficient, and patient-centered healthcare system. These technologies empower nurses to deliver more precise, timely, and personalized care, from using AI to analyze patient data for personalized treatment plans to leveraging telehealth for remote follow-ups in underserved communities. The future of allergy nursing will be defined by the proactive adoption of these innovations. Nurses must embrace a role as active participants in the healthcare innovation ecosystem, contributing to the development and implementation of new technologies. This includes advocating for user-centered, evidence-based tools that are validated and accessible to all patients, regardless of their socioeconomic status or digital literacy. By championing ethical AI use, promoting digital health equity, and continuously seeking professional development, nurses can ensure technology serves as an influential force for improving patient outcomes, bridging care gaps, and enhancing the overall quality of life for individuals with food allergies. The ongoing evolution of technology provides a unique opportunity for the nursing profession to lead the charge in creating safer, more effective, and more equitable allergy care for everyone.

Conflict of Interest No conflict of interest to disclose.

References

AAAAI. (2024). *Anaphylaxis interactive learning guide*. https://www.aaaai.org/tools-for-the-public/anaphylaxis. Accessed 20 Sept 2024.

AAAAI. (2025). *mHealth and allergy/immunology*. Retrieved from https://www.aaaai.org/allergist-resources/digital-medicine-ehr/mhealth. Accessed 3 Aug 2025.

AHRQ. (2023). *Telehealth's potential to benefit rural healthcare delivery*. Agency for Healthcare Research and Quality. https://www.ahrq.gov/data/infographics/rural-telehealth-2.html. Accessed 24 Jul 2025.

Allergic Living. (2025). https://www.allergicliving.com/. Accessed 3 Aug 2025.

Alowais, S. A., Alghamdi, S. S., Alsuhebany, N., Alqahtani, T., Alshaya, A. I., Almohareb, S. N., Aldairem, A., Alrashed, M., Bin Saleh, K., Badreldin, H. A., Al Yami, M. S., Al Harbi, S., & Albekairy, A. M. (2023). Revolutionizing healthcare: The role of artificial intelligence in clinical practice. *BMC Medical Education, 23*(1), 689. https://doi.org/10.1186/s12909-023-04698-z

Alvarez-Perea, A., Dimov, V., Popescu, F., & Zubeldia, J. M. (2021). The applications of eHealth technologies in the management of asthma and allergic diseases. *Clinical and Translational Allergy, 11*, e12061. https://doi.org/10.1002/clt2.12061

ASTHMAXcel. (2025). *ASTHMAXcel an algorithmic software tool to help manage asthma*. https://www.asthmaxcel.net/. Accessed 3 Aug 2025.

AUVI-Q. (2024). https://www.auvi-q.com/pdf/AUVI-Q_Direct_Delivery_Info_Card.pdf#:~:text=Get%20a%20reminder%2030%20days%20before%20the%20expiration,days%20before%20the%20expiration%20date%20of%20your%20AUVI-Q. Accessed 23 Sept 2024.

Ayuso Margañon, R., Llistosella, M., Ayuso Margañon, S., Rojano Navarro, M., Bou Gràcia, N., & Sillero, A. (2023). Nursing practice and telehealth in school health services: A scoping review. *Healthcare (Basel), 11*, 3124.

Beal, L. L., Kolman, J. M., Jones, S. L., Khleif, A., & Menser, T. (2021). Quantifying patient portal use: Systematic review of utilization metrics. *Journal of Medical Internet Research, 23*, e23493.

Becker, B. (2025). *Research guides: Artificial Intelligence (AI) in education: Home* [Internet]. https://guides.library.uab.edu/ai/home. Accessed 3 Aug 2025.

Bédard, A., Basagaña, X., Anto, J. M., et al. (2019). Mobile technology offers novel insights into the control and treatment of allergic rhinitis: The MASK study. *The Journal of Allergy and Clinical Immunology, 144*, 135–143.e6.

Bonderud, D. (2021). *Telehealth's benefits for patient-centered care—and where it's going*. Technology Solutions That Drive Healthcare. https://healthtechmagazine.net/article/2021/05/telehealths-benefits-patient-centered-care-and-where-its-going-perfcon. Accessed 3 Aug 2025.

Bousquet, J., Jutel, M., Pfaar, O., et al. (2021). The role of mobile health technologies in stratifying patients for AIT and its cessation: The ARIA-EAACI perspective. *The Journal of Allergy and Clinical Immunology. In Practice, 9*, 1805–1812.

Boussina, A., Krishnamoorthy, R., Quintero, K., Joshi, S., Wardi, G., Pour, H., et al. (2024). Large language models for more efficient reporting of hospital quality measures. *NEJM AI, 1*(11). https://doi.org/10.1056/AIcs2400420

Broome, S. B., Williams, K. W., & Hendrix, K. H. (2022). App providing psychosocial and educational supports benefits caregivers of children with newly diagnosed food allergies. *Journal of Food Allergy, 4*(3), 163–171. https://doi.org/10.2500/jfa.2022.4.220035

Brown, B., & Sabbaghan, S. (2025). Applying interview-research methods using generative AI technology: An action research study with graduate students in mock research teams. *The Canadian Journal of Action Research, 25*(1), 53–70. https://molloy.idm.oclc.org/login?url=https://www.proquest.com/scholarly-journals/applying-interview-research-methods-using/docview/3181717565/se-2. Accessed 3 Aug 2025.

Capoot, A. (2024). *Doctors are turning medical generative AI into a booming business*. CNBC. https://www.cnbc.com/2024/03/16/himss-2024-ambient-clinical-documentation-steals-the-show.html. Accessed 3 Aug 2025.

Chelli, M., Hadan, H., Wang, D. M., Mogavi, R. H., Tu, J., Zhang-Kennedy, L., et al. (2024). *The great AI witch hunt: Reviewers perception and (mis)conception of generative AI in research writing*. Available from: https://browse-export.arxiv.org/pdf/2407.12015v1

Cheng, A., Calhoun, A., & Reedy, G. (2025). Artificial intelligence-assisted academic writing: Recommendations for ethical use. *Advances in Simulation, 10*(1), 22. https://doi.org/10.1186/s41077-025-00350-6. Accessed 3 Aug 2025.

Clark, M., & Bailey, S. (2024). *Chatbots in health care: Connecting patients to information: Emerging health technologies*. Canadian Agency for Drugs and Technologies in Health.

Cleveland Clinic. (2019). *Molecular allergology: The case for a new model of care in allergy management.* https://consultqd.clevelandclinic.org/molecular-allergology-the-case-for-a-new-model-of-care-in-allergy-management. Accessed 3 Aug 2025.

Collins, W., Adlou, B., Rodriguez, A., et al. (2022). Feasibility of virtual reality technology to improve experience during pediatric oral food challenge. *Journal of Allergy and Clinical Immunology, 149*, AB108.

Coughlin, V. (2024). *Exploring the use of podcasts for clinical nursing education*. American Nurses Association. https://www.nursingworld.org/content-hub/resources/workplace/INNO_exploring-the-use-of-podcasts-for-clinical-nursing-education/.

CSH. (2025). *LibGuides: AI tools for research: AI use policy for journals* [Internet]. https://cshl.libguides.com/aitools/aijournalpolicies. Accessed 3 Aug 2025.

Descamps, J., Lavoué, V., Trojani, C., Azar, M., Deckert, M., Raynier, J. L., et al. (2024). Hallucination rates and reference accuracy of ChatGPT and bard for systematic reviews: Comparative analysis. *Journal of Medical Internet Research, 26*(1), e53164. https://www.jmir.org/2024/1/e53164/. Accessed 3 Aug 2025.

Downey, L. A., Heinz, M. C., & Murphey, M. (2025). Nurse-led allergy education for non-medical school staff. *The Online Journal of Issues in Nursing, 30*(1). https://ojin.nursingworld.org/table-of-contents/volume-30-2025/number-1-january-2025/articles-on-previously-published-topics/nurse-led-allergy-education-for-non-medical-school-staff/

Dramburg, S., Marchante Fernández, M., Potapova, E., & Matricardi, P. M. (2020). The potential of clinical decision support systems for prevention, diagnosis, and monitoring of allergic diseases. *Frontiers in Immunology, 11*, 2116.

Dramburg, S., Matricardi, P. M., Pfaar, O., & Klimek, L. (2022). Digital health for allergen immunotherapy. *Allergol Select, 6*, 293–298.

El Yaman, N., Zeitoun, J., Diab, R., Mdaihly, M., Diab, R., Kobeissi, L., Abou Ljoud, S., Antoun, J., & Bardus, M. (2023). Utilization of patient portals: a cross-sectional study investigating associations with mobile app quality. *BMC Medical Informatics and Decision Making, 23*, 177.

Epipen.ca. (2025). *Epipen expiry reminder.* https://www.epipen.ca/epipen-expiry-reminder. Accessed 3 Aug 2025.

EpiPen®. (2024). *EpiPen® expiry date alerts.* https://cloud.email.viatrisconnect.com/EpiPen-Expiry-Alert-Registration. Accessed 23 Sept 2024.

FARE. (2024). *Find a support group—Food allergy support in your area.* https://www.foodallergy.org/living-food-allergies/join-community/find-support-group. Accessed 20 Sept 2024.

Fisher, K. (2025). *Research guides: A guide for graduate nursing: Using AI tools to enhance research* [Internet]. https://researchguides.csuohio.edu/MSN/AIChelli. Accessed 3 Aug 2025.

Food Allergy Nurses Interest Group I (FANI). (2022). *Why we need certified allergy nurse educators.* Allergic Living. https://www.allergicliving.com/2022/04/04/why-we-need-certified-allergy-nurse-educators/. Accessed 3 Aug 2025.

Food Allergy Nursing Association. (2024). *About FANA: Mission, goals, and values.* https://www.foodallergynursing.org/general-9

Gemini. (2025). *Gemini—Chat to supercharge your ideas.* https://gemini.google.com. Accessed 3 Aug 2025.

GPT-5. (2025). https://openai.com/index/gpt-4/. Accessed 8 Aug 2025.

Greiwe, J., Oppenheimer, J., Bird, J. A., Fleischer, D. M., Pongracic, J. A., & Greenhawt, M. (2020). AAAAI work group report: Trends in oral food challenge practices among allergists in the United States. *The Journal of Allergy and Clinical Immunology: In Practice, 8*, 3348–3355.

Hathaway, K., & James, J. (2023). *FARE summit session: Shared decision in food allergy.*

Health Resources Services Administration (HRSA). (2021). *What is telehealth?* https://www.hrsa.gov/rural-health/telehealth/what-is-telehealth

HealthIT. (2025). *What is meaningful use? HealthIT.gov.* https://www.healthit.gov/faq/what-meaningful-use. Accessed 21 July 2025.

HealthIT.gov. (2025a). *What are electronic health records (EHRs)?* https://www.healthit.gov/topic/health-it-and-health-information-exchange-basics/what-are-electronic-health-records-ehrs. Accessed 21 June 2025.

HealthIT.gov. (2025b). *ONC's cures act final rule.* https://www.healthit.gov/topic/oncs-cures-act-final-rule. Accessed 3 Aug 2025.

HealthIT.gov. (2025c). *Health data, technology, and interoperability: Certification program updates, algorithm transparency, and information sharing (HTI-1) final rule.* https://www.healthit.gov/topic/laws-regulation-and-policy/health-data-technology-and-interoperability-certification-program. Accessed 3 Aug 2025.

HealthIT.gov. (2025d). *National trends in hospital and physician adoption of electronic health records.* https://www.healthit.gov/data/quickstats/national-trends-hospital-and-physician-adoption-electronic-health-records. Accessed 3 Aug 2025.

HealthIT.gov. (2025e). *Health IT legislation.* https://www.healthit.gov/topic/laws-regulation-and-policy/health-it-legislation. Accessed 3 Aug 2025.

Henry, T. A. (2022). *6 Tips to succeed with telehealth in allergy and immunology care.* American Medical Association. https://www.ama-assn.org/practice-management/digital/6-tips-succeed-telehealth-allergy-and-immunology-care. Accessed 3 Aug 2025.

HIMSS. (2024). *Five rights of AI in healthcare.* https://www.himss.org/resources/five-rights-ai-healthcare. Accessed 3 Aug 2025.

Hsia, B., Mowrey, W., Keskin, T., Wu, S., Aita, R., Kwak, L., Ferastraoarou, D., Rosenstreich, D., & Jariwala, S. P. (2021). Developing and pilot testing ASTHMAXcel, a mobile app for adults with asthma. *The Journal of Asthma, 58*, 834–847.

Infante, D. (2024). The future of food allergy management: New technologies and treatments. *News-Medical.* https://www.news-medical.net/health/The-Future-of-Food-Allergy-Management-New-Technologies-and-Treatments.aspx. Accessed 17 Sept 2024.

Kagan, O. (2024). *Anaphylaxis education for all—AAAAI Podcast: conversations from the world of allergy.* https://www.buzzsprout.com/2049216/episodes/15702414

Kagan, O., & Keny, C. (in press). Transforming research & quality improvement with AI. In Wang, J., Love, R., Hightow-Weidman, L. (Eds). The nurse's guide to humanizing AI: Nursing's essential handbook to human-centered AI. Wolters Kluwer. ISBN: 9781975280369.

Kagan, O., Kelly, S., Venter, C., Hubbard, T., Hoyt, A., & Fleischer, D. (2023). *FARE summit session: Team work makes the dream work: How to build a perfect food allergy care team!*

Khan, M., Banerjee, S., Muskawad, S., Maity, R., Chowdhury, S. R., Ejaz, R., Kuuzie, E., & Satnarine, T. (2024). The impact of artificial intelligence on allergy diagnosis and treatment. *Current Allergy and Asthma Reports, 24*, 361–372.

Landi, H. (2024). *HIMSS24: How epic is building out AI, ambient tech in EHRs.* https://www.fiercehealthcare.com/ai-and-machine-learning/himss24-how-epic-building-out-ai-ambient-technology-clinicians. Accessed 3 Aug 2025.

Leonardsen, A.-C. L., Hardeland, C., Helgesen, A. K., & Grøndahl, V. A. (2020). Patient experiences with technology enabled care across healthcare settings—A systematic review. *BMC Health Services Research, 20*, 779.

Li, L., Foer, D., Hallisey, R. K., et al. (2022). Improving allergy documentation: A retrospective electronic health record system–wide patient safety initiative. *Journal of Patient Safety, 18*, e108–e114.

Mammen, J. R., et al. (2021). Development and preliminary results of an Electronic Medical Record (EMR)-integrated smartphone telemedicine program to deliver asthma care remotely. *Journal of Telemedicine and Telecare, 27*(4), 217–230. https://doi.org/10.1177/1357633X19870025

Matricardi, P. M., Dramburg, S., Alvarez-Perea, A., et al. (2020). The role of mobile health technologies in allergy care: An EAACI position paper. *Allergy, 75*, 259–272.

McKenna, J. (2024). *Artificial Intelligence in Scientific Publishing*. MDPI Blog [Internet]. https://blog.mdpi.com/2024/04/03/ai-in-scientific-publishing/. Accessed 3 Aug 2025.

McMurray, A., & Cooper, H. (2017). The nurse navigator: An evolving model of care. *Collegian, 24*, 205–212.

Microsoft Copilot. (2025). *Start your Copilot journey*. https://www.microsoft.com/en-us/microsoft-copilot/meet-copilot?ef_id=_k_07294eb0aa311e94b752284a7099a715_k_&OCID=AIDcmm9xzw3cn3_SEM__k_07294eb0aa311e94b752284a7099a715_k_&msclkid=07294eb0aa311e94b752284a7099a715. Accessed 3 Aug 2025.

Mun, M., Park, Y., Hwang, J., & Woo, K. (2024). Types and effects of telenursing in home health care: A systematic review and meta-analysis. *Telemedicine Journal and E-Health, 30*, 2431–2444.

National Association of School Nurses. (2022). *Telehealth, the role of school nursing*. https://www.nasn.org/nasn-resources/professional-practice-documents/position-statements/ps-telehealth. Accessed 3 Aug 2025.

National Association of School Nurses. (2023). *School nursing evidence-based clinical practice guideline: Students with allergies and risk for anaphylaxis*. https://www.maine.gov/doe/sites/maine.gov.doe/files/inline-files/School%20Health%20Services%20-%20NASN%20%20Allergies%20%20Anaphylaxis%20Toolkit%20-%2008.2023.pdf

NurseJournal.org. (2024). *Professional networking in nursing*. https://nursejournal.org/resources/networking-in-nursing/

NursingEducation.org. (2024). *What is the role of technology in nursing education?* https://nursingeducation.org/insights/role-of-technology/

OpenAI, Achiam, J., & Adler, S., et al. (2024). *GPT-4 technical report*. https://doi.org/10.48550/arXiv.2303.08774

OSTP. (2025). Blueprint for an AI bill of rights. *The White House*. https://www.whitehouse.gov/wp-content/uploads/2022/10/Blueprint-for-an-AI-Bill-of-Rights.pdf. Accessed 3 Aug 2025.

Pandya, A., Waller, M., & Portnoy, J. M. (2024). How can artificial intelligence help with management of allergic conditions? *The Journal of Allergy and Clinical Immunology: In Practice, 12*, 1017–1018.

Pividori, M., & Greene, C. S. (2023). A publishing infrastructure for AI-assisted academic authoring. *bioRxiv*. https://doi.org/10.1101/2023.01.21.525030. Accessed 3 Aug 2025.

Ross, A., Freeman, R., McGrow, K., & Kagan, O. (2024). Implications of artificial intelligence for nurse managers. *Nursing Management, 55*, 14–23.

SciPub+. (2025). *Elsevier vs. Springer Nature: Comparing AI Policies for Academic Authors* [Internet]. [cited 2025 Jul 23]. Available from: https://scipubplus.com/hub/blog/elsevier-vs-springer-nature-comparing-ai-policies-for-academic-authors/

Stegman, J. (2025). How immersive technology is reshaping nursing education amid critical shortages. *Healthcare IT Today*. https://www.healthcareittoday.com/2025/04/30/how-immersive-technology-is-reshaping-nursing-education-amid-critical-shortages/

Taylor and Francis. (2023). *Disclosing artificial intelligence use in scientific research and publication: When should disclosure be mandatory, optional, or unnecessary?* https://www.tandfonline.com/doi/full/10.1080/08989621.2023.2201977. Accessed 3 Aug 2025.

Tripodi, S., Giannone, A., Sfika, I., et al. (2020). Digital technologies for an improved management of respiratory allergic diseases: 10 years of clinical studies using an online platform for patients and physicians. *Italian Journal of Pediatrics, 46*, 105. https://doi.org/10.1186/s12913-019-4238-3

WHO. (2024). *WHO calls for safe and ethical AI for health*. https://www.who.int/news/item/16-05-2023-who-calls-for-safe-and-ethical-ai-for-health. Accessed 30 Sept 2024.

Willgerodt, M. A., Brock, D. M., & Maughan, E. D. (2018). Public school nursing practice in the United States. *The Journal of School Nursing, 34*, 232–244.

Yoon, E., Hur, S., Opsasnick, L., et al. (2024). Disparities in patient portal use among adults with chronic conditions. *JAMA Network Open, 7*, e240680.

Zhang, X., & Saltman, R. (2022). Impact of electronic health record interoperability on telehealth service outcomes. *JMIR Medical Informatics, 10*, e31837.

Zimmanck, K., Kelly, S., Kagan, D., & James, J. (2024). *FARE summit session: Taking the reigns: How and when to take control of your own medical care.*

Public Policy and Advocacy for People with Food Allergy

Kathyrn Osborne and Josie Howard-Ruben

Introduction

IgE-mediated food allergies affect every aspect of daily living, from accessing safe food, traveling, attending school and work to ensuring access to health care and emergency medications. Policies and best practices to avert allergen exposure in these settings are often the purview of government, legislative bodies, and expert advisory groups. In order to mitigate the health risks associated with food allergies, implementation of policies and regulations to minimize risk has been adopted to help people avoid allergens and to manage their environments to keep them safe. In addition to health risks, the total economic burden associated with pediatric food allergies is close to $25 billion per year, $4.3 billion of which is spent on direct medical costs (Richardson et al., 2024). Mitigating the risks associated with food allergies to keep people safe and avoid adverse outcomes and medical spending requires engagement by larger society and governing bodies. The purpose of this chapter is to describe public policies that may influence the identification and management, both acute and long term, of food allergies in children and adults diagnosed with food allergies, and to encourage nurses to advocate at the local, state, and federal level for policies that improve the lives of those with food allergy.

K. Osborne (✉)
College of Nursing, Rush University, Chicago, IL, USA
e-mail: kathryn_osborne@rush.edu

J. Howard-Ruben
Rush University College of Nursing, Chicago, IL, USA
e-mail: josie_howard-ruben@rush.edu

J. Doucette, J. Howard-Ruben (eds.), *Comprehensive Food Allergy Management for Nurses*, https://doi.org/10.1007/978-3-032-28647-5_12

Historical Background in the United States

Government regulation of the food supply and food safety in the U.S. began in 1902 with a Congressional appropriation of funds to study the safety of chemicals added to preserve the shelf life of foods (Meadows, 2006). The first Pure Food and Drugs Act was signed into law in 1906 and implemented by the Bureau of Chemistry, housed within the Agriculture Department; in 1930, the Bureau of Chemistry became what we know today as the Food and Drug Administration (Meadows, 2006). During the next 100 years a variety of public policies were enacted, most of which were aimed at regulating additives, improving food safety, setting standards for food quality and packaging, and ensuring truth in labeling. It was not until 2004 that Congress passed the Food Allergen Labeling and Consumer Protection Act (FALCPA), and in 2006 the Act was fully implemented (FDA, 2022). A list of federal public policies that followed, to improve health outcomes for people with food allergies, can be found in Table 1.

Table 1 Public policies related to food allergies

Title of the act/public law number	Signed into law	Key provisions
FDA (2022) Public Law No: 108-282, Title II 21 U.S.C. chapter "Food Allergy Management in the Hospital Setting"	8-3-2004	Amended the Federal Food, Drug, and Cosmetic Act to: Identify eight major food allergens (milk, eggs, fish, crustacean shellfish, tree nuts, wheat, peanuts, and soybeans) Describe labeling requirements for foods/food products that contain any of the eight major food allergens Require the Secretary of DHHS to submit to congress, a report on implementation of food allergen, labeling, and research Fully implemented 1-1-2006
Food Allergy and Anaphylaxis Management Act of 2011, 21 U.S.C. § 2205 and 21 U.S.C. § 321(qq), (2005) Public Law 111-353—Section 112 of the Food Safety Modernization Act 21 U.S.C. §2205	1-4-2011	Requires the Secretary of Health and Human Services to: Develop guidelines for the management of food allergy-related anaphylaxis in schools and early childhood learning programs Make these guidelines available to schools for use on a voluntary basis (Voluntary Guidelines for Managing Food Allergies in Schools and Early Care and Education Programs) https://www.cdc.gov/school-health-conditions/media/pdfs/20_316712-A_FA_guide_508tag.pdf) $30,000,000 was appropriated for fiscal years 2011–2015 to be awarded as grants to individual schools Fully implemented 1-4-2012

(continued)

Table 1 (continued)

Title of the act/public law number	Signed into law	Key provisions
School Access to Emergency Epinephrine Act 42 U.S.C. § 280g(d), (2013) Public Law No: 113-48 42 U.S.C. § 280g	11-13-2013	Amends the Public Health Services Act to give preference—for grant consideration—to states that allow self-administration of asthma and anaphylaxis medications, and provide protections for trained school employees from civil liability Requires schools in states who receive these grants to permit trained staff to maintain a supply of epinephrine, administer epinephrine to a student having a reaction, and establish a plan for properly trained staff to administer epinephrine
School-Based Allergies and Asthma Management Program Act (2021) Public Law 116-292 42 U.S.C. § 201	1-5-2021	Amends the Public Health Services Act to give preference—for grant consideration—to states that require public schools to implement allergy and asthma management programs Describes essential components of allergy and asthma management programs
The Food Allergy Safety, Treatment, Education and Research (FASTER) (2021) Act Public Law No: 117-11 21 U.S.C. § 321	4-23-2021	Identifies sesame as the ninth major food allergen with mandated labeling under the Federal Food, Drug, and Cosmetic Act Requires all packaged foods and dietary supplements that contain sesame to be labeled as such Requires DHHS to submit to congress, a report on food allergy research and data collection related to surveillance, diagnostics, prevention, treatment, and recommendations for improved outcomes Fully implemented 1-1-2023

Note. Table created by Kathryn Osborne CNM, PhD, RN from references (Food Allergen Labeling and Consumer Protection Act, 2022; Food Allergy and Anaphylaxis Management Act of 2011, 21 U.S.C. § 2205 and 21 U.S.C. § 321(qq), 2005; School Access to Emergency Epinephrine Act 42 U.S.C. § 280g(d), 2013; School-Based Allergies and Asthma Management Program Act, 2021; FASTER Act, 2021) on the table

FDA Food Code

In 1993, the U.S. Food and Drug Administration (FDA) began publishing the FDA Food Code (FDA, 2023a). The purpose of the Food Code is to provide uniform, evidence-based guidance to state, tribal, and local jurisdictions for use in the development of policies that regulate the sale of food and food products in grocery stores, restaurants, and other establishments that prepare food for direct consumption (FDA, 2024). Until 2001 the Food Code was published every 2 years; since 2005, it has been published every 4 years, with yearly supplements published as necessary (FDA, 2023a). The goal of the FDA is nationwide adoption of the Food Code to ensure the consistent use of best evidence, across states, in the mitigation of risks associated with food-related illnesses (FDA, 2024). As of the writing of this chapter,

36 states have adopted one of the versions published since 2013 (FDA, 2024), with more pending rulemaking.

The Food Code covers many topics, including food storage and preparation, handwashing and employee hygiene, safe food handling, consumer advisories, including those for food allergies, and other information essential to food safety. Although adoption of the FDA Food Code is optional, versions or parts of the Code have been adopted voluntarily by most states (FDA, 2024). It is important for policy advocates to remain aware that the document exists and that many states have statutes and regulations that reflect elements of the Code. For example, included in the Code are recommendations for employees of food service establishments. The supplement to the 2009 edition (Section 2—103.11, Annex 3) added recommendations that all employees of food service establishments receive training in food safety and instruction regarding allergy awareness (FDA, 2011). The 2022 edition added sesame as a major food allergen in the FASTER Act, which will be discussed below, effective January 1, 2023 (FDA, 2023b). Other changes in the 2022 edition are noted in C Code § 3602.12(C), which for the first time, now references that unpackaged food sold to consumers should be accompanied by written notice, with a number of disclosure options stated (e.g., card, sign, or other method). In addition, labeling for bulk foods is also recommended in 3602.11(C) (2) (FDA, 2023b).

Historically, the FDA has coordinated several initiatives to help protect consumers with food allergies, including offering guidance documents and formulating regulations, surveillance activities, and exercising regulatory powers. Recently the FDA issued a new Guidance Document (https://www.fda.gov/regulatory-information/search-fda-guidance-documents/guidance-industry-questions-and-answers-regarding-food-allergen-labeling-edition-5), (USFDA, 2025) which addresses very specific questions about food labeling in the US. It is noteworthy that guidance documents are recommendations, rather than legal requirements.

However, the Current Good Manufacturing Practice, Hazard Analysis, and Risk-Based Preventive Controls for Human Food rule (CGMP & PC rule, 21 CFR part 117) addresses the standards for preventing allergen cross-contact and undeclared allergens, among other issues, for entities that "manufacture, process, pack or hold human food" and is part of federal law. Allergen cross-contact refers to an allergen being added to a food unintentionally, which can occur during any point in the food supply and delivery process, from farm to factory and manufacturing lines to inadequate cleaning practices, and to where most recognize "cross-contact," in food preparation. In the manufacturing stage, good manufacturing practices are procedures designed to prevent cross-contact, through cleaning, production, and process controls (USFDA, 2024). As a component of its surveillance activities, the FDA operates a consumer complaint system and a food report registry, which may culminate in communications about safety concerns and recalls or other regulatory actions. Foods are also periodically evaluated to determine compliance through laboratory testing. Recalls are reported on the FDA website and are also shared by FARE and others.

Readers who are interested in implementing components of the FDA Food Code through legislation and changes in state statute can contact Food Allergy Research and Education (FARE) (https://www.foodallergy.org/our-initiatives/advocacy/know-your-rights), Food allergy & Anaphylaxis Connection Team (FAACT) (https://www.foodallergyawareness.org/living-with-food-allergies/statewide-restaurant-legislation/statewide-restaurant-legislation), or the Asthma and Allergy Foundation of America (AAFA) (https://aafa.org/advocacy/key-issues/food-allergies-advocacy/) which publishes a State Honor Roll™ (https://aafa.org/advocacy/state-honor-roll/) for policies relevant to allergic disease, including food allergy.

International Food Allergy Laws

Laws governing food allergy labeling and other allergy-related legislation vary across the globe. The University of Nebraska-Lincoln Food Allergy Research & Resource Program maintains a list of regulatory labeling (https://farrp.unl.edu/IRChart/) that reflects allergen labeling in various countries (UNL-FARRP, 2005). Overall, as many as two dozen allergens may be labeled; while nine allergens must be labeled on packaged food in the US, some locations, such as Australia, New Zealand, Canada, and the European Union, require more to be labeled, and in others, fewer are labeled. Knowing this information would be beneficial for people with food allergies traveling internationally. A sample of international advocacy efforts can be found in Table 2.

Table 2 Advocacy efforts Examples from state-specific to international

Title of the work	Focus
Resources available online	
Allergen labeling regulations by country	Provides an up-to-date, online listing of labeling regulations Web resource: https://farrp.unl.edu/IRChart/
Managing Food Allergy: GA²LEN Guidelines	Recommendations for managing food allergy provided by the Global Allergy and Asthma European Network Web resource: https://pmc.ncbi.nlm.nih.gov/articles/PMC9467869/
International Codex Alimentarius	Provides international food standards that have been adopted by the Codex Alimentarius Commission (CAC). CAC is part of the Joint Food and Agricultural Organization of the United Nations/World Health Organization. The purpose of the codex is to promote fair food trade practices and protect consumer health Web resource: https://www.fao.org/fao-who-codexalimentarius/codex-texts/list-standards/en/
Red Sneakers for Oakley	Headquartered in the United States, this 501(c)3 was established in the memory of Oakley Debbs who died following an anaphylactic allergic reaction to food allergens. The aim of the organization is to raise awareness of the dangers of food allergies, which is done through the delivery of face-to-face and online education delivered across the globe Web resource: https://www.redsneakers.org/what-we-do

(continued)

Table 2 (continued)

Title of the work	Focus
Legislation	
ADDE Act	Signed into law in California in 2025, the Allergen Disclosure for Dining Experiences (ADDE) Act requires written notification of major top 9 allergens in restaurants with 20 or more national (US) locations. While the original bill called for this notification for all restaurants, concerns about the impact on smaller restaurants led to adjustments, and passage of the current legislation. Allergen information can appear on the written menu or on digital menus (e.g., QR codes) as long as other non-digital access is available. The advocacy efforts for this bill were lead by Robyn Huey Lao and Addie Lao (the inspiration for the bill), along with the Asthma and Allergy Foundation of America Web resource: https://aafa.org/aafa-bill-to-require-allergen-labeling-in-california-restaurants-becomes-law/ Web resource: https://www.addietellsall.com
ADINA Act	There are ongoing efforts at the federal level in the US advocating for passage of the ADINA Act (the Allergen Disclosure In Non-food Articles Act). This Act would require plain-language labeling on over-the-counter and prescription medications that contain major food allergens and gluten-containing grains. The legislation was inspired by the experience of Adina, who experienced a reaction to a medication containing one of her allergens. Many medications include allergens or gluten as inactive ingredients that are not labeled; passage of this law would help mitigate risk for people with food allergies Web resource: https://www.adinaact.com
Elijah's Law Requiring Schools and Childcare Programs to Stock Epinephrine Devices Law	Elijah-Alavi Silvera experienced a fatal anaphylactic reaction after exposure to a food allergen in a daycare setting. A foundation in his name has promoted legislation to improve safety for children with food allergies in the childcare environment. Elijah's Law was first passed in New York state and has been adopted in several other states (Illinois, Virginia, Maryland, California, and Arkansas, at present) and cities with other advocacy efforts ongoing. A toolkit for implementation of the law in other states is on the website Web resource: https://www.elijahalavifoundation.org/elijah-s-law-toolkit Elijah-Alavi Foundation also contributed to the advocacy efforts for a law that requires all schools and childcare programs to stock epinephrine devices in New York City Web resource: https://www.elijahalavifoundation.org/post/protecting-kids-citywide-nyc-passes-bill-to-ensure-epinephrine-in-every-school-and-daycare
Labeling Law New York State	Packaged food requires labeling for the top nine allergens Web resource: https://www.allergicliving.com/2025/11/13/ny-law-brings-allergen-labeling-to-deli-bakery-packaged-foods/

(continued)

Table 2 (continued)

Title of the work	Focus
FAA Reauthorization Act of 2024	Signed into law in 2024, this reauthorization included a new clause that requires the Federal Aviation Association (FAA) to consider whether emergency medical kits (EMKs) include the appropriate equipment and medications used to treat anaphylaxis. In essence, this change could allow the FAA to require that EMKs carried on airplanes include epinephrine autoinjectors/devices, which it currently does not. The FAA has posted a notice of proposed rulemaking with a comment period ending in October, 2026. Web resource: https://www.allergicliving.com/2024/05/16/new-faa-act-will-make-airplane-medical-kits-anaphylaxis-ready/
Natasha's Law	UK Law enacted October 1, 2021, requires labeling of all prepackaged for direct sale foods (PPDS) to include a list of all ingredients, with the top 14 allergens clearly highlighted. This change in labeling is now required in Wales, England, and Northern Ireland. Prepackaged food for direct sale includes anything made on site and sold for consumption (sandwiches, cookies, salads, desserts, etc.) Web resource: https://www.food.gov.uk/business-guidance/introduction-to-allergen-labelling-changes-ppds#natasha-law-why-the-changes-to-allergen-information-were-introduced
Owen's Law	A grassroots organization started by a family following the death of their son, Owen, who died as a result of an anaphylactic reaction while out to eat in a restaurant. The goal of the organization is to seek legislation in the UK, that requires restaurants to provide—in writing, for patrons—any of the 14 major allergens recognized in EU law that were used in food preparation Web resource: https://owens-law.co.uk/
Protecting Children with Food Allergies Law	Augments current law requiring school food service staff working in the US National School Lunch and Breakfast programs to have yearly training in nutrition and food safety. This legislation amends the Child Nutrition Act of 1966 to also require food allergy training Web resource: https://snacksafely.com/2026/01/federal-protecting-children-with-food-allergies-bill-signed-into-law/

Note. Table developed by Kathryn Osborne from resources available online

Additional Considerations: The Politics of Advocacy Efforts and Policy Changes

Maintaining an awareness of the political environment and the "politics" of policy-making is a critical component of effective engagement in advocacy efforts. It is essential that nurses who are advocating for public policies that promote the health and wellness of the patients they serve can identify the groups and individuals with the power and influence to get a bill moving through Congress (or a state legislature or other legislative body) and signed into law. Identifying individuals and groups with the power to influence the passage of legislation, as well as the values and priorities of those in power, can help nurses plan a policy agenda and identify the key figures with whom to engage in order to improve the likelihood that the policies of interest will succeed as they move through the legislature.

One example of the way that politics influences policymaking (and the policies that nurses may be interested in) can be seen with recent changes at the Department of Education (DOE), the agency responsible for the administration and enforcement of many of the laws that provide protection for children with food allergies in public schools. Involvement of the DOE in this regulation stems from the passage of the Rehabilitation Act of 1973 (29 U.S.C. § 701 et seq.), which resulted in the enactment of the first significant disability rights law in the United States (U.S. Equal Employment Opportunity Commission, n.d.). The law, which served as a framework for the Americans with Disabilities Act (ADA) of 1990, prohibits discrimination against an individual based on disability in programs, activities, and organizations that receive federal funding. More specifically, Section 504 of the Rehabilitation Act prohibits discrimination based on disability in programs or activities that receive federal funding, including individuals with visibly apparent disabilities and those with hidden disabilities. It is this section of the United States Code (U.S.C. § 794) that provides protections for the civil rights of students with disabilities, which is enforced primarily by the Department of Education (DOE) Office of Civil Rights (U.S. Department of Education, 2025).

Policy advocates for students with severe food allergies will need to watch closely as the US administrations evolve. Any changes in the DOE or in the Office of Civil Rights may impact the civil rights of students with food allergies. Protecting the rights of children with food allergies in public schools requires that these changes should be monitored on an ongoing basis. Moreover, the individuals with the power and influence to create or amend public policies change frequently, particularly when an election results in a change in the political party that holds the majority (and therefore the political power). As a result, it is essential that those engaged in policy work remain aware of the contemporary political landscape. For now, in addition to the anticipatory advocacy efforts that must be undertaken with changes in the policy agenda of a new administration, advocacy groups working on behalf of children with food allergies continue their work to increase funding for research, improve labeling laws to ensure labeling that is accurate and truthful, and improve airline travel safety (FARE, 2025). A brief summary of these advocacy groups and the resources they provide for patients and health professionals can be found in Table 3.

Table 3 Advocacy groups for children with food allergies; resources for patients and health professionals

Organization/contact information	Key advocacy efforts of the organization
Asthma and Allergy Foundation of America (AAFA) https://aafa.org/ *Download* AAFA's Guiding Principles for Patient-Centered Public Policy	Provides public policy advocacy at the state and federal level for individuals living with allergies and asthma. Advocacy efforts are focused on improving access to high quality, evidence-based, affordable treatment and care for people with allergies and asthma, including access to medications necessary to improve food safety for school children with allergies and asthma. Additional legislative priorities include: Continued federal funding for research as well as screening and preventive services for people with allergies and asthma Promoting improved air quality (indoors and out) Securing funds for food allergy research Improved food labeling Reference: Asthma and Allergy Advocacy Action Center. https://aafa.org/advocacy/
Food Allergy Research & Education (FARE) http://www.foodallergy.org	This organization provides advocacy efforts to: Ensure access to existing treatments and improve efforts to create new ones Secure research funding Distribute allergy alerts for product recalls and label changes Respond to questions and concerns from members of the Allergy Community Encourage the airline industry to ensure epinephrine devices are carried on all commercial flights and on pharmaceutical companies to ensure that emergency medications are easily accessible and user-friendly Provide advocacy education FARE is currently working with US Airlines to ensure that they allow pre-boarding of all passengers with severe food allergies so that their seats may be adequately cleaned (as ordered by the Department of Transportation)
Food Allergy and Anaphylaxis Connection Team (FAACT) https://www.foodallergyawareness.org/	The mission of FAACT's is to "educate, advocate, and raise awareness for all individuals and families affected by food allergies and life-threatening anaphylaxis." Their efforts to accomplish this mission include advocacy and education to: Keep children safe at school Address food allergy bullying Ensure safe travel for people with food allergies Ensure a safe workplace for people with food allergies Help students with food allergies prepare for college Promote safe dining out experiences for families with food allergies FAACT provides education and support for families across the US, through face-to-face programs. Social media, and a monthly e-newsletter. Reference: FAACT https://www.foodallergyawareness.org/

(continued)

Table 3 (continued)

Organization/contact information	Key advocacy efforts of the organization
Kids with Food Allergies (KFA) https://kidswithfoodallergies.org/	KFA is the food allergy division of the Asthma and Allergy Foundation of America (AAFA). They are dedicated to improving the health status and quality of life for people with food allergies by providing support, advocacy, research, and education. Their legislative priorities are similar to the priorities of AAFA, with a focus on advocacy efforts for children with food allergies Reference: KFA https://kidswithfoodallergies.org/advocacy/
Mothers of Children Having Allergies (MOCHA)-Chicago based https://mochallergies.org/	MOCHA (Mothers of Children Having Allergies) is a parental support group whose mission is to "help parents and caregivers of children with food allergies." The organization "aims to make living with allergies just a little bit easier" and believes it is the job of parents and caregivers "to give our children the education, encouragement, experience, and enthusiasm to get out into the world and safely live their lives to the fullest." MOCHA reaches members from across the United States; they work to achieve their goals by offering: A regular newsletter that provides information, news, and policy updates A website that includes information and a variety of resources to help families live with and manage severe food allergies Educational opportunities Support and opportunities for food allergy families to connect Public policy advocacy Reference: MOCHA: About US. https://mochallergies.org/about-us/
Allergy UK https://www.allergyuk.org/about-allergy/	Provides education and support for organizations and individuals who live with severe food allergies. Their mission is that "everyone in the UK takes allergy seriously" The *Allergy UK Impact Report 2024/25* showcases the difference this organization has made for people who live with food allergies Reference: Allergy UK. https://www.allergyuk.org/
Allergy & Anaphylaxis Australia https://allergyfacts.org.au/living-with-allergies/	Provides multiple resources for living with allergies including allergen cards, posters, and webinars. Resources for daily management of allergies, different environments, as well as resources for young people
US Department of Education https://www.ed.gov/laws-and-policy/individuals-disabilities/section-504/civil-rights-of-students-hidden-disabilities-and-section-504	Protects the rights of children in public schools in the United States who are living with disabilities, including disabilities that are not visible, which includes children with severe food allergies

Implications for Nurses

Nurses are uniquely positioned to lead advocacy efforts for the patients they serve. They have extensive healthcare knowledge, they are highly trusted professionals, and as they care for patients, they see, firsthand, the effect of policies passed in Congress and in state legislatures. Moreover, nurses are keenly aware of the extent to which those policies affect the lives of their patients, which makes them well suited to speak with policymakers about legislation they are considering. Finally, nurses are skilled advocates; they advocate for their patients each time they interact with members of the healthcare team on a patient's behalf. Advocating for passage (or defeat) of health policies is much like advocating for patient care services. The audience and the message may be different, but the goals are the same: improved patient safety, improved access to care, and improved health outcomes. It is incumbent upon nurses to advocate for changes in health policy that can lead to improvements in the health status of their patients and the communities in which they live and work.

Becoming a Change Agent

An important first step in becoming a change agent is to remain informed about health policy issues that present themselves in various settings. In the public sector, health policy decisions are often made by state and local policymakers. State and national nurses' associations usually have staff in place to monitor the introduction and movement of bills and amendments through the legislature. These organizations keep their members informed about important health policy issues, provide representation of their members at policymaking tables, and offer support for members who take on the role of policy advocate.

There are several ways that individual nurses can support the efforts of local, state, and national nursing organizations. The first is to consider membership or participation in the organizations that represent nurses, and the patients and communities they serve, in the legislature. The most effective organizations are able to quickly mobilize their members to engage in advocacy efforts. One such strategy that is often used by advocacy groups is to send out an *action alert*. Action alerts are used to inform members that something is happening in the policymaking realm that requires some sort of action, usually contact with members of Congress or a state legislature. Having individual members reach out to their own elected official is an effective way for organizations to contact members of a legislative body. In fact, it is the desired approach since most lawmakers are inclined to listen more closely to the people who put them in office than those who live outside the regions they represent. When an action alert goes out, the organization often provides background information on the policy topic, a brief summary of the problem that needs to be addressed, and then a call to action, which is usually a request for contact with a policymaker. There are three ways to contact policymakers: by telephone, in writing, or in person.

Telephone contact is a quick and easy way to contact a legislator. When planning a phone contact, it is advised to prepare remarks ahead of time, and to be prepared to talk with a member of the legislator's staff. Staff members are knowledgeable about policy issues and committed to getting constituent information to their employer. Speaking with a staff member is no less valuable than speaking to the elected official. In order for the call to go smoothly there are a few points to remember. Callers should:

- Begin by introducing themselves and identifying whether they are a constituent.
- Briefly summarize the reason for the call; identify the bill number and describe the reasons they support or oppose the bill.
- Provide the elected official with a call to action, to join them in their support or opposition. If the bill needs a sponsor or bill author, this is a good time to ask for that level of support.
- Conclude by thanking the listener for their time and be sure to leave contact information so that they can reach out if they have any questions or concerns.
- Be prepared to leave a phone message. Busy legislators often use phone messages to triage and respond to constituent contacts. If asked to leave a message, the message should briefly and concisely summarize the points above.

Conveying a message through *written communication* is also acceptable. Written communication can take the form of e-mail messages or hard copy letters sent through the mail to an elected official's office.

There are also a few important points to remember regarding written communication:

- Formal letter format should be used; always use the recipient's formal title in the opening salutation (for example, Senator Smith or Representative Jones).
- The message should begin with an introduction and explanation regarding concern about the policy issue.
- The writer should summarize their position on the issue and describe why the issue matters to the policymaker's constituents.
- Keep the letter to one page in length.
- Close with a call to action—request support for the writer's position on the matter. Provide contact information, and if possible, offer to meet with the policymaker to discuss the matter further.
- As is true with telephone contact, it is important to personalize the message. Nurses can explain why this issue is important to their nursing practice, their community, and the patients they serve.

The most personal way to contact a legislator is with a *face-to-face visit*. Meeting with policymakers in this way allows elected officials and constituents to meet in real time and get to know one another. It also provides an opportunity for the open exchange of ideas. Here are some points to keep in mind when planning a visit:

- Visits of this nature should be scheduled rather than impromptu.
- Business-professional attire should be worn.
- Arrive on time and begin with a brief description of the bill and topic that will be discussed.
- The nurse should outline their position on the bill and provide evidence that supports their position.
- Offer to answer any questions the legislator might have. The nurse should only answer questions about which they are certain of the answer. When a legislator asks a question that the nurse is uncertain about, they should answer honestly and tell the legislator they will get back to them with the answer to their question as soon as possible.
- Conclude the discussion with a call to action. Nurses should ask the legislator if they can count on the legislator's support for their position. Leave a set of talking points and a business card.
- An example of talking points that can be left with a policymaker can be seen in Fig. 1.
- Thank the legislator for their time before leaving and follow up with a written note of thanks after the visit. Sending a note of thanks provides one final opportunity to remind the policymaker of the importance of this issue for their constituents and ask for their support on the matter.

Testifying at a Legislative or Congressional Committee Hearing After a piece of legislation has been introduced in one house of the legislature or Congress it is assigned to a committee. If the committee chair is compelled to bring the bill up for consideration, they will schedule the bill for a public hearing. Among those invited to speak at a public hearing are members of advocacy groups who have been asked to testify. Testimony like this can be presented in writing or orally, directly in front of a legislative or Congressional committee; the purpose of the testimony is to provide expert opinion on the substance of the bill. While this may feel like a daunting request, providing expert testimony at a public committee hearing can be one of the most exciting ways to engage in advocacy efforts. Moreover, it is an effective way for nurses to influence the development of health policy by providing a body of policymakers with evidence that supports their position on a policy matter of importance to the profession or the patients they serve. Here are some important points for nurses planning to testify at a public committee hearing to remember:

- Nurses may only speak on behalf of an organization or group if they have been asked to do so and have the endorsement of the group. Without that request and endorsement, nurses may speak only on their own behalf.
- Prepare enough printed copies of the testimony to leave a copy with each member of the committee. Deliver the copies to the committee clerk for distribution before the hearing begins.
- Dress in business-professional attire.

[Date]

The organization [name of the organization] OR individual nurse advocate [your name] is seeking support for H.R. 4019, a bill that would make grants available for law enforcement epinephrine device training and access. Gio's Law is named for a 14-year-old boy who did not receive timely epinephrine during a severe allergic reaction.

Talking Points

Why is access to epinephrine important?

- Epinephrine is the only first-line treatment for serious food allergy reactions
- "Epinephrine product" refers to epinephrine auto-injectors or any other device for epinephrine administration other than an injectable device (e.g., nasal spray or other).
- There is good evidence that delayed epinephrine is a significant predictor of poor outcomes in food allergy reactions

Under current law:

- First responders do not always have access to emergency epinephrine
- Law enforcement may not have the training to use epinephrine in emergency situations
- Delays in timely administration of epinephrine can result in poor outcomes in people with severe food allergies.

H.R. 4019 – Gio's Law

- Introduced by Rep. Lauren Gillen (D-NY4) and Rep. Andrew Garbarino (R-NY2)
- Has bipartisan support with 9 co-sponsors
- Would amend the *Omnibus Crime Control and Safe Streets Act of 1968* "to establish a grant program for provide access to, and training on the administration of, epinephrine products for law enforcement officers, and for other purposes."
  - Provide or identify training for law enforcement officers to recognize symptoms of anaphylaxis and to safely administer epinephrine devices
  - $25 million annually would be available in grants administered by the Department of Justice through 2030.

Thank you for considering this issue, which is critically important for individuals with food allergies. Please consider co-sponsoring H.R. 4019.

[In addition to the points listed here, policy advocates are encouraged to individualize their talking points with personal stories, information, and data specific to the policy-maker's district and constituents. Policy advocates are also encouraged to leave their contact information with the policy-maker.]

GovTrack.us. (2026). H.R. 4019 — 119th Congress: Gio's Law. Retrieved 6/22/2026 from https://www.govtrack.us/congress/bills/119/hr4019

Allergy & Asthma Network (2026). Support Gio's Law. Retrieved 6/22/2026 from https://advocacy.allergyasthmanetwork.org/take-action/support-gios-law/

Fig. 1 Sample talking points. (These talking points were developed by Kathryn Osborne)

- Be sure to inquire about a time limit for public comments and prepare remarks that fall within the limit. If no limit is provided, attempt to limit remarks to no longer than 3–4 min.
- Plan to arrive in the hearing room at the beginning of the day's session. Committees often hear several bills during a single session, and the order in which bills are heard is likely to differ from the agenda established by the committee chair.
- Begin the testimony by thanking the committee chair and members of the committee for allowing you an opportunity to provide comments on the bill (give the bill number and name) and briefly explain why you are qualified to provide comments.
- Explain why the key provisions of the bill are important to your organization and/or the patients you serve.
- Provide published evidence that supports your position on the bill.
- Personalize the message; without violating any individual patient's privacy, offer stories that bring a human face to the issue at hand.
- Conclude your remarks with a call to action. Favorably voting the bill out of committee and on to the full house is a reasonable request.
- Thank the committee for hearing your remarks on the bill and offer to answer any questions the members might have.
- During the Q&A period remember that you are the expert, and the members of the committee are genuinely interested in what you have to say. Remain professional and enjoy the opportunity to converse about the issue. If you aren't certain about an answer to a question, be honest and tell the committee members you'll provide the information as soon as you are able.

In addition to making direct contact with policymakers, there are a variety of ways to engage in public policy advocacy efforts. As previously mentioned, active membership in professional organizations provides nurses with an opportunity to come together and combine resources, both fiscal and human, to support the policy issues that can impact their communities and the patients they serve.

It is also important to maintain an ongoing relationship with elected officials rather than calling on them only when they are needed to carry a message to a legislative body. Use every opportunity to remind lawmakers about policy issues that are important to the profession and patients served. Offering help during a campaign is a great way to build and maintain these relationships. Consider inviting patients and the parents of children with food allergies to engage in advocacy efforts. Individuals living with food allergies can provide an impassioned point of view on these policy issues, a viewpoint that provides a face to legislation aimed at improving the lives of people with food allergies. Most importantly, remember to vote. Nurses use their voice every time they enter the voting booth. Remain aware of the issues that are important to the profession, the community, and patients served as well as the position held by every candidate on those issues. Make informed voting decisions to elect candidates who share your vision for the health of your patients and the communities in which you live and work.

Conclusion

This chapter has provided readers with information about established policies that are important to people living with food allergies, current issues under consideration, and approaches for nurses to use in advocacy efforts on behalf of children and adults living with food allergies. Existing laws address some of the problems associated with food allergies, but there is clearly more to be done to improve food safety as well as the health and well-being of those who live with serious food allergies.

There are several organizations in the US, and worldwide, that advocate for the establishment of public policies to address these concerns. These advocacy groups provide a place for individuals to come together to support changes in public policies and in private establishments to improve food safety for all. Among these advocacy groups are nursing organizations dedicated to advocacy efforts on behalf of the communities in which they live and work, as well as the patients they serve. Nurses are well situated to provide policymakers with evidence that supports passage of legislation that could improve food safety and the health status of people with food allergies, including information about the day-to-day challenges faced by this vulnerable population. As more nurses engage in advocating for public policies and gain comfort with the political process, they may consider serving on policymaking boards, working for government agencies that implement and regulate health policies, and running for office.

Nurses have a long history of engaging in patient advocacy in health systems. Advocating for public health policies aimed at improving the health of the nation is similar to advocating for safe care practices in a healthcare facility—both are actions that nurses are prepared to take as a component of high quality nursing care; both are essential to maintain healthy communities and the individuals served by nurses.

Conflict of Interest The authors declare no conflict of interest.

References

FASTER Act. (2021). https://www.congress.gov/bill/117th-congress/senate-bill/578/text

FDA. (2011). *FDA Food Code 2009*. https://www.fda.gov/food/fda-food-code/food-code-2009

FDA. (2023a). FDA Food Code. https://www.fda.gov/food/retail-food-protection/fda-food-code

FDA. (2023b). Summary of changes in the 2022 FDA Food Code. https://www.fda.gov/food/fda-food-code/summary-changes-2022-fda-food-code

FDA. (2024). *Adoption of the FDA Food Code by state and territorial agencies responsible for the oversight of restaurants and retail food store*. https://www.fda.gov/food/fda-food-code/adoption-fda-food-code-state-and-territorial-agencies-responsible-oversight-restaurants-and-retail#:~:text=In%20the%20current%20format%2C%20the,published%20in%20December%20of%202022

Food Allergy and Anaphylaxis Management Act of 2011, 21 U.S.C. § 2205 and 21 U.S.C. § 321(qq). (2005). https://uscode.house.gov/view.xhtml?req=granuleid:USC-prelim-title21-section2205&num=0&edition=prelim#:~:text=21%20USC%202205%3A%20Food%20allergy%20and%20anaphylaxis%20management

Food Allergy Research and Education (FARE). (2025). *Advocacy: Food allergy issues*. https://www.foodallergy.org/our-initiatives/advocacy/food-allergy-issues
Food and Drug Administration (FDA). (2022). *Food Allergen Labeling and Consumer Protection Act of 2004 (FALCPA)*. https://www.fda.gov/food/food-allergensgluten-free-guidance-documents-regulatory-information/food-allergen-labeling-and-consumer-protection-act-2004-falcpa
Meadows, M. (2006, Jan–Feb). A century of ensuring safe foods and cosmetics. In *FDA Consumer Magazine* (Centennial Edition). https://www.fda.gov/files/A-Century-of-Ensuring-Safe-Foods-and-Cosmetics.pdf. Accessed 6 Jan 2005.
Richardson, T., Vickery, B., Gupta, R., Goldstein, F., Kobernick, M., Chan, V., Wescott, S., Gandhi, G., & Winders, T. (2024). Navigating the landscape of food allergies: Insights and perspectives from the AMCP Market Insights Program. *Journal of Managed Care and Specialty Pharmacy, 30*(8-a), S1–S9.
School Access to Emergency Epinephrine Act 42 U.S.C. § 280g(d). (2013). https://www.congress.gov/bill/113th-congress/house-bill/2094/text
School-Based Allergies and Asthma Management Program Act. (2021). https://www.congress.gov/bill/116th-congress/house-bill/2468/text
U.S. Department of Education. (2025). *The civil rights of students with hidden disabilities and Section 504*. https://www.ed.gov/laws-and-policy/individuals-disabilities/section-504/hidden-disabilities
U.S. Equal Employment Opportunity Commission. (n.d.). *Employment protections under the Rehabilitation Act of 1973: 50 years of protecting Americans with disabilities in the workplace*. https://www.eeoc.gov/employment-protections-under-rehabilitation-act-1973-50-years-protecting-americans-disabilities
University of Nebraska-Lincoln. (2005). *Food Allergy Research and Resource Program (FARRP) food allergens—International regulatory chart*. Retrieved on August 21, 2025 at https://farrp.unl.edu
USFDA. (2024). *Current good manufacturing practices (CGMPs) for food and dietary supplements*. FDA. https://www.fda.gov/food/guidance-regulation-food-and-dietary-supplements/current-good-manufacturing-practices-cgmps-food-and-dietary-supplements. Accessed 21 Aug 2025.
USFDA. (2025). *Guidance for industry: Questions and answers regarding food allergen labeling (edition 5)*. https://www.fda.gov/regulatory-information/search-fda-guidance-documents/guidance-industry-questions-and-answers-regarding-food-allergen-labeling-edition-5. Accessed 9 Dec 2025.

Advancing Food Allergy Care: The Role of the Certified Allergy Nurse Educator

Susan Kelly, Josie Howard-Ruben, and Julianne Doucette

Introduction

With the increasing prevalence of IgE-mediated food allergies, there is an urgent need for more support for those managing life with this chronic disease. People with food allergies depend on the acquisition of new knowledge, skills, and perspectives to fully embrace life despite this potentially life-threatening diagnosis. The learning curve is steep. A food allergy diagnosis often requires the individual and their family to quickly adapt to safety measures and lifestyle changes (Warren et al., 2024). One must learn about food allergen avoidance and reading food ingredient labels, as well as practical considerations in food preparation, emergency management of allergic reactions, and food allergy treatment options.

Everyday activities require a different approach when living with a food allergy diagnosis. Warren et al. (2024) emphasizes the need for increased support to improve quality of life for individuals living with food allergies. Suddenly, everyday activities like food shopping, cooking, dining out, and traveling feel unfamiliar and overwhelming. Eating, drinking, and socializing around food requires behavior modifications that may feel uncomfortable and fastidious. Notably, this new approach to living life begins immediately upon diagnosis, when stress levels are high. According to Leung and Sampson (2021), education helps patients and

S. Kelly (✉)
Happy and Healthy Pediatrics, Mineola, NY, USA

J. Howard-Ruben
Rush University College of Nursing, Chicago, IL, USA
e-mail: josie_howard-ruben@rush.edu

J. Doucette
College of Nursing, Rush University, Chicago, IL, USA
e-mail: Julianne_Doucette@rush.edu

J. Doucette, J. Howard-Ruben (eds.), *Comprehensive Food Allergy Management for Nurses*, https://doi.org/10.1007/978-3-032-28647-5_13

families navigate food choices and social activities more confidently, reducing fear and isolation.

The American Nurses Association Code of Ethics (2025) states that "optimal nursing care enables recipients to live with as much physical, emotional, social, religious, and/or spiritual well-being as possible, aligning with their preferences, values, and determination of quality of life. Nurses lead the implementation of responsible and appropriate evidence-based interventions across the lifespan to optimize the health and well-being of those in their care." Based on the ethical underpinnings of nursing practice, the role of the allergy nurse educator is consistent with these obligations, and aims to promote the health and well-being of patients and families contending with a food allergy diagnosis.

According to the American Association of Colleges of Nursing's framework for nursing education called *The Essentials: Core Competencies for Professional Nursing Education* (AACN, 2021), nurses have a responsibility to engage in lifelong learning. Continuing to learn and master content related to food allergies through various educational strategies is necessary for the nurse working with this patient population. Although the AACN addresses these requirements for continuing education of nurses at the baccalaureate, master, and doctoral level to meet the health care needs of the public (Yoder-Wise, 2021), she states that continuous learning, self-reflection, and professional development are essential for all levels of nursing, including licensed practical nurses and associate degree nurses.

The Value of Health Care Partners

Research shows that when chronic disease management includes collaboration with health care partners, patient outcomes improve (Tandan et al., 2024). Health care partners may include not only registered nurses, but also advanced practice providers (advanced practice registered nurses [APRNs] and physician associates [PAs]), registered dietitians, licensed mental health providers, pharmacists, social workers, and physicians, as well as support groups and other resources. Registered nurses (RNs), however, play a pivotal role in the allergy care journey. RNs provide patient education, advocate for new health policies and health policy changes, and reassure and support patients and families. Because of their comprehensive training, education, and critical thinking skills, RNs help people navigate the complex health care system and coordinate individualized health care needs, and through their commitment to lifelong learning, RNs can continuously enhance their expertise in food allergy care and offer community referrals to available resources.

Allergy Care Workforce

While there is no available workforce projection in the United States for registered nurses in the specialty area of food allergy, including allergy and immunology, the number of board-certified physicians needed exceeds the number of allergists

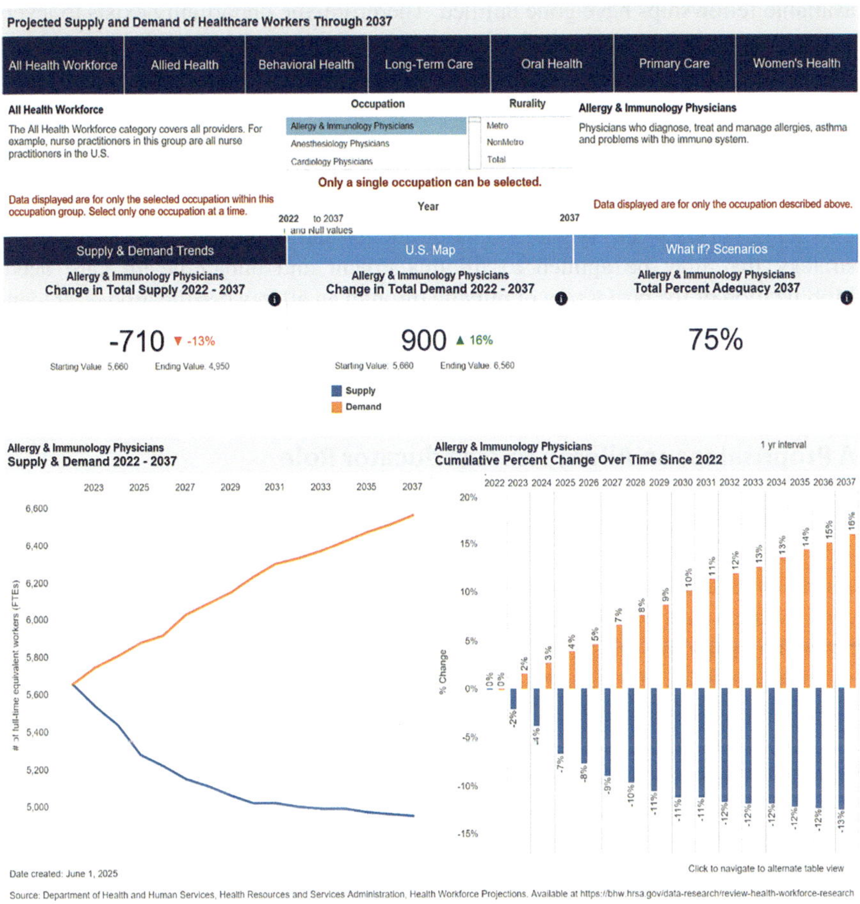

Fig. 1 Allergy and immunology physician supply and demand. (*Note.* Workforce projections. Used with permission from: Health Resources and Services Administration Data Warehouse (2025). Public Domain. https://data.hrsa.gov/topics/health-workforce/nchwa/workforce-projections)

available for this growing population, so there is a shortfall in personnel. US government projections from the National Center for Workforce Analysis (https://data.hrsa.gov/topics/health-workforce/nchwa/workforce-projections) suggest that this trend will continue (see Fig. 1) (Health Resources and Services Administration Data Warehouse, 2025). Others have cited that the number of practicing allergists available in clinical care settings is insufficient for the current needs of the allergic population (Malick & Meadows, 2021).

Further contributing to this projected shortage, Scherzer (2018) observed a decrease in the number of applicants for allergy and immunology fellowships over the previous decade. Others have also observed this (Malick & Meadows, 2021). Izadi and Saff (2022) documented no improvement in this trend, noting that some available fellowships have gone unfilled. Therefore, the opportunity exists to leverage registered nurses (RNs) and advanced practice nurses (APRNs) to better serve people and families living with food allergies and other allergic diseases.

A Role for Nursing as the Allergy Care Partner

Educating nurses in the specialty area of allergy and immunology is an untapped strategy that may be applied to fill this urgent and unmet health care need. Mobilization of the profession of nursing through an allergy certification or credentialing process may help meet the burgeoning need for comprehensive care for the food-allergic population and their caregivers.

A Proposal for an Allergy Nurse Educator Role

While allergy care teams in major research centers include expert nurses who provide excellent care and guidance, not all sites employ RNs or APRNs with allergy experience. Support and resources across care settings vary widely, as some allergy care settings may not have the funds necessary to hire additional staff to fully address patients' psychosocial, educational, and other needs. Imagine, however, if an allergy practice offered access to a certified or credentialed allergy nurse educator to help guide patients and families through the complexities of a food allergy diagnosis from the start. The allergy nurse educator, ideally, would be available on an ongoing basis to answer the myriad questions that regularly arise. The allergy nurse educator (ANE) can implement important care interventions, prioritize learning goals for patients and families, and provide guidance on activities of daily life for people with food allergies. The proposed role of the ANE would complement the services provided by other members of the allergy care team, filling the education and support gaps of this population, their caregivers, and communities (Kelly et al., 2022). The ANE role could bridge the gap in implementation of evidence-based recommendations for food allergy prevention, management options, education, and anaphylaxis preparedness and response.

In the emerging landscape of new food allergy treatment options, nurses must stay at the forefront of food allergy care to ensure patients receive up-to-date, evidence-based education and support. The ANE might also serve as a clinical support person for those undergoing food allergy treatment. As a trusted expert, the ANE could curate information tailored to the specific needs (e.g., avoidance and nuances of label reading, management of allergic symptoms, managing oral immunotherapy (OIT), treatment with omalizumab) of the patient and caregivers, be available to answer questions, and help navigate the maze of living safely with food allergies.

The ANE could also serve as a knowledgeable nursing resource not only for patients, but also for communities, such as schools, hospitals, and the workplace, as well as for other members of the health care team, including other nurses, by sharing tools, best practices, and educational strategies.

The ANE role could be deployed in a variety of healthcare settings, and virtually, via secure, HIPAA-compliant systems for those sites that would not be able to support a full-time role. Such a role could have a meaningful impact on patient outcomes, enhancing the quality of life of those living with food allergies and their caregivers. Integrating allergy nurse educators into various health care settings could enhance patient outcomes, reduce anxiety associated with food allergies, and reduce health care disparities by improving access to specialized care. Expanding the nursing role to include certification or credentialing in allergy and immunology aligns with the profession of nursing's mission to provide holistic, patient-centered care.

Maximizing the Nurse's Role in Food Allergy Management

Nurses with specialized training offer the opportunity to significantly improve patient outcomes and to help patients develop confidence in managing their food allergies. Nurses are uniquely positioned to fill this role due to their expertise in patient education, advocacy, and interdisciplinary collaboration in care management.

Currently, patients diagnosed with food allergies may wait weeks or months to see an allergist. Once diagnosed, they are given:

- allergen avoidance guidelines;
- epinephrine auto-injector/device training and a prescription;
- anaphylaxis emergency action plans;
- possible treatment options.

Many patients leave the allergist's office feeling overwhelmed and unprepared to incorporate these changes into their daily lives. Nurses can fill this gap by providing structured, evidence-based food allergy education and support.

How Can an Allergy Nurse Educator Help?

A credentialed or certified allergy nurse educator could assist patients and caregivers in several key areas:

- *Early Allergen Introduction*: The ANE can guide families on introducing allergens early to prevent food allergies. Recent studies have changed the approach to allergen introduction, and parents may require coaching and specific guidance to help manage early complementary feeding with confidence (see chapters "Early Introduction of Food Allergens" and "Food Allergy Management in Early Childhood Settings").
- *Management in Various Settings*: The ANE can assist patients in navigating food allergies in daycare, schools, workplaces, dining at restaurants, travel, and social environments. Voluntary guidelines for allergy management in school settings have been published, and the ANE could facilitate their translation to practice. As new research emerges, the ANE could critically assess new information and help patients and families to apply this knowledge when appropriate to their unique situation.

- *Label Reading*: The ANE can coach on how to read labels, including what is required labeling and what is voluntary and the significance of this information. While there is guidance for food allergen labeling, some products will also include precautionary labeling. The ANE can provide guidance on how to read specific label elements in order to avoid allergen exposure.
- *Identifying Hidden Allergens*: The ANE can educate on potential hidden allergens in products like medications, pet foods, and personal care items. People with allergies and their caregivers may not recognize all the non-food products that could contain potential allergens. Also, some patients are susceptible to exposures beyond ingestion, and the ANE can offer guidance.
- *Comprehensive Support*: The ANE can address the mental health impacts of food allergies and provide ongoing support. Mental and behavioral health resources are not always readily available, and the ANE can offer referrals and coach on self-care strategies for managing stress and anxiety.
- *Emerging Treatments*: The ANE can educate patients about new treatments such as OIT, sublingual immunotherapy (SLIT), omalizumab, and other emerging treatments while engaging in shared decision-making regarding these options that considers personal values, available options, treatment goals, risks and benefits, and available supports (Greenhawt et al., 2020).

Value of Additional Credentials or Certification in Nursing

Many specialty nursing roles either require additional credentials or a formal certification. For example, the Certified Diabetes Care and Education Specialists (CDCES) support patients with diabetes self-management (American Association of Diabetes Educators, n.d.) and the Oncology Nurse Navigator-Certified Generalist (ONN-CG), offered by the Academy of Oncology Nurse and Patient Navigator and Foundation for Learning, assists patients with navigating cancer care (AONN, 2025). Available evidence suggests that additional education and credentials, including certification, provide benefits to patients in a variety of health care settings. The literature reveals how specialty certification is associated with improved patient outcomes, increased nurse confidence, and enhanced quality of care across clinical settings (Shepherd et al., 2019; Kaplow, 2022; Fights, 2012). Despite the growing prevalence of food allergies, a formal role, certification, or structured training for nurses specializing in allergy and immunology in the United States does not currently exist. The allergy nurse educator role could bridge this gap in care.

International Allergy Nursing Roles

Internationally, several initiatives are in place to help nurses caring for patients with food allergies to develop their knowledge and skills. When comparing countries, Australia has the most comprehensive and structured program for nurses to obtain advanced training in allergy and immunology. In Australia, nurses have access to an online Professional Certificate in Allergy Nursing (https://adelaide.edu.au/study/degrees/professional-certificate-in-allergy-nursing/dom/) formerly offered by the University of South Australia in collaboration with the Australasian Society of Clinical Immunology and Allergy Incorporated (ASCIA), and now provided by Adelaide University. This program provides evidence-based education on the clinical management of allergic conditions, including food allergy, anaphylaxis, and atopic diseases. It equips nurses with the foundational knowledge to confidently support patients and families navigating the complexities of allergy care. By integrating this specialized education along with practical support, these specialized nurses take a more active role in allergy prevention, early recognition, and management, particularly in underserved or rural areas in Australia, where access to allergists may be limited. Nurses trained through this model are better equipped to conduct patient education, implement anaphylaxis management plans, and serve as key care coordinators between families, schools, and specialist services, thereby reducing the burden of allergic disease and improving quality of life for patients.

While Australia is leading the way, other countries have taken somewhat of a similar approach to develop nurses in the specialty of allergy. The United Kingdom's BSACI Allergy Nursing Mentorship Program (https://www.bsaci.org/workforce/bsaci-allergy-nursing-mentorship-program/), sponsored by the British Society for Allergy & Clinical Immunology (BSACI, 2025), is another example. This program will match mentors with mentees to help nurses with less experience in allergy care learn from mentors working in their specific area of interest.

Alternative Models for Professional Development

However, there are pathways for nurses to develop advanced knowledge in allergy care as shown in Table 1. The national non-profit patient advocacy organization, Food Allergy Research and Education (FARE, 2024), has a Food Allergy Academy (https://www.foodallergyacademy.org/) that provides a selection of courses available for the public. Also listed is a 9-month Pediatric Food Allergy Training, Pediatric Food Allergy Course, designed for "healthcare professionals working in food allergy. This may include registered dietitians, pediatricians, other physicians and researchers."

The Asthma Educator Specialist (AED-C) (https://www.nbrc.org/examinations/certified-asthma-educator-ae-c/) is one allergy-related role that is available to health care professionals, including physicians, nurses, physician associates, respiratory therapists, pulmonary function technologists, pharmacists, social workers, health educators, physical therapists, occupational therapists, emergency medical technicians, paramedics, speech-language pathologists, or others with over 1000 hours in asthma care (NBRC, 2025). As demonstrated by these expanded nursing roles in diverse clinical areas, precedents exist for leveraging nursing knowledge to assist patients manage complex and chronic health conditions.

Table 1 Organizations providing food allergy education

Organization	Description	Website
Adelaide University	Postgraduate professional certificate in allergy nursing—online course	https://adelaide.edu.au/study/degrees/professional-certificate-in-allergy-nursing/dom/ ttps://adelaide.edu.au/study/degrees/professional-certificate-in-allergy-nursing/dom/
American Academy of Allergy, Asthma, & Immunology (AAAAI)	Professional organization providing allergy education, tools, resources	www.aaaai.org
American College of Allergy, Asthma & Immunology (ACAAI)	Professional organization providing allergy education, guidelines, and advocacy	Acaai.org/allergies/allergic-conditions/food/
American Society of Allergy Nurses	Organization that provides continuing education for nurses in the area of allergy, asthma, and immunology. They host yearly conferences in the US northwest	https://www.allergynurses.org
Asthma and Allergy Foundation of America (AAFA) & Kids with Food Allergies (KFA)	Not-for-profit organization providing education, community services, and promotion of health equity among those with asthma and allergy	www.aafa.org www.kidswithfoodallergies.org
Asian Alliance for Food Allergy & Anaphylaxis (AAFAA)	Professional organization that shares food allergy issues and education on epinephrine	www.fa-asian-alliance.org
Asian Pacific Association of Allergology and Clinical Immunology (APAAACI)	Regional allergy organization of Asia which provides allergy education for health professionals	www.apaaaci.org
Australasian Society of Clinical Immunology and Allergy (ASCIA)	Non-profit professional organization providing education for health professionals, patients, and community on clinical immunology and allergy in Australia and New Zealand	www.allergy.org.au
British Society for Allergy & Clinical Immunology (BSACI)	Professional organization for health care professionals caring for patients with allergy	www.bsaci.org
European Academy of Allergy and Clinical Immunology (EAACI)	Non-profit organization of health professionals providing professional and patient education for patients—list of organizations by country	www.eaaci.org https://eaaci.org/patients/patient-organisations/
Food Allergy and Anaphylaxis Connection Team (FAACT)	Provides health care professions, education offerings, and resources on many food allergy topics	www.foodallergyawareness.org
Food Allergy Nurses Association (FANA)	International organization focused on food allergy nursing providing education and resources	www.foodallergynursing.org

(continued)

Table 1 (continued)

Organization	Description	Website
Food Allergy Research & Education (FARE)	Non-profit organization providing food allergy education research and advocacy	www.foodallergy.org
National Association of School Nurses (NASN)	Education for school nurses on many topics including an allergy and anaphylaxis toolkit and clinical practice guidelines	www.nasn.org/home
National Asthma Educator Certification Board (NAECB)	Non-profit organization that certifies health professionals in asthma care	www.nbrc.org
World Allergy Organization (WAO)	International organization that provides allergy education to many regional and national societies in various countries	www.worldallergy.org

Note. Table developed by chapter authors

Implementing the Certified Allergy Nurse Educator Role

A certified allergy nurse educator could be integrated into allergy clinics, primary care settings, hospitals, schools, and as a trusted community resource, with roles including:

- providing direct patient education in allergist offices, primary care, inpatient and outpatient care, and community health settings;
- offering virtual care and coaching appointments to address patient questions;
- training school nurses and hospital staff on food allergy management;
- advocating for food allergy policies in schools, workplaces, and public spaces;
- supporting allergists in patient education and care coordination.

Several options could be explored for implementation of this role. One option, probably more realistic in the short term, is to describe an additional educational credential earned through nursing continuing professional development in a continuing education format or in an academic setting. Credentialing suggests some qualification or assessment indicating that a person has met certain criteria (Institute for Credentialing Excellence, 2020), an outcome that could be achieved through the successful completion of an educational program and assessment of knowledge.

A longer-term option would be to formalize a certification for food allergy nursing, or perhaps more broadly in allergy and immunology. If there is an interest in this certification among allergy nurses, pursuing this option would require role delineation studies, funding, and a separate entity for certification, such as exists in the American Nurses Credentialing Center, the Oncology Nursing Certification Corporation for oncology nursing certifications, or the Foundation for Learning for nurse navigator certification, as examples. Collaboration with test development experts would also be necessary. The Institute for Credentialing Excellence provides background on this process, and the American Nurses Credentialing Center offers a process for the development of new certifications (Myers et al., 2024).

See the proposed preliminary blueprint for the food allergy component of a credential or certification for the allergy nurse educator (Fig. 2).

Preliminary Blueprint for FANE or ANE

I) Food Allergy Awareness
   a) Identify resources about food allergy—local, state and national
   b) Identify opportunities in the community to improve awareness of food allergy management
   c) Advocate for food allergy friendly policies
   d) Provide culturally aware resources for the community
   e) Educate patients, families and the community about food allergy

II) Prevention of Food Allergy
   a) Educate about early introduction of food allergens in the infant's diet to prevent food allergy
   b) Current information on infant skin care and allergies
   c) Educate about prevention of allergic reactions
   d) Dispel myths and provide evidence-based information about the evolving theories on how food allergies develop

III) Support for Diagnosis and Management
   a) Education on diagnostic testing (skin prick, serum testing, oral food challenge, component testing, etc.)
   b) Guidance on medication avoidance prior to skin prick testing
   c) Provide education on allergic response and anaphylaxis
   d) Provide education and care plans for symptom management related to allergic disease
   e) Provide education on administration of epinephrine devices
   f) Review emergency action plan
   g) Provide anticipatory guidance on other-allergic conditions (e.g., eczema, asthma, allergic rhinitis)
   h) Assist patient and family with nutrition counseling and referral to dietitian as needed
   i) Assess understanding and educate on avoidance strategies (reading labels, alternate names for allergens, cross contact, tips for dining out, etc.)
   j) Participate in shared decision making regarding available treatment options beyond avoidance
   k) Educate patient and family through treatment (e.g. avoidance, immunotherapy options, emerging therapies)

IV) Barriers to Care
   a) Social determinants of health and health care disparities such as access to healthy allergy appropriate foods, transportation needs, access to care, access to emergency medications, etc.
   b) Financial and insurance issues
   c) Cultural issues

Fig. 2 Preliminary blueprint for FANE or ANE. (*Note*. Blueprint developed by Josie Howard-Ruben RN, PhD and Julianne Doucette DNP, APRN, CPNP-PC. We acknowledge the intervention examples provided in Russell et al. (2022))

V) Psychosocial Issues Related to Food Allergy
  a) Mental health and wellness, including screening for anxiety and depression
  b) Coping strategies and self-care behaviors to alleviate anxiety
  c) Review quality of life issues associated with food allergies
  d) Family dynamics associated with food allergy (e.g., parental conflict over management)
  e) School issues and risk for bullying for children
  f) Body image issues related to food allergy
  g) Employment and workplace issues
  h) Sexuality and food allergies
  i) Resources for referral for support, medication, treatments such as cognitive behavioral therapy

VI) Food Allergy Advocacy
  a) Identify barriers to care and formulate plans to mitigate
  b) Foster problem solving skills for daily self-management of food allergy
  c) Engage in shared decision- making with patients and families for ongoing care
  d) Encourage use of evidence-based food allergy resources in all settings including daycare, schools and workplaces
  e) Provide support and resources for accommodations in school and other settings
  f) Advocate at the local, state and national level for food allergy friendly legislation

Fig. 2 (continued)

Conclusion

Patients with a diagnosis of food allergy require multidisciplinary, patient-centered care, and nurses are uniquely positioned to provide personalized education, assess readiness to learn about food allergy management, and offer resources to patients and families as they develop their self management skills. Establishing a formal credential or certification for allergy nurse educators would enhance patient education, safety, and access to care, and by participating in a multidisciplinary team, allow providers more time to focus on medical management. With a relative shortage of active allergists in clinical practice (Malick & Meadows, 2021), and with geographic distribution of allergists leaving some populations in the US without adequate allergy care, an allergy nurse educator in the clinic, or who could be seen virtually, could bridge the access gap. The next time you encounter a patient with food allergies or their caregiver, consider this question: "*How would a certified allergy nurse educator help us navigate this diagnosis?*"

The allergy nurse educator (ANE) role would provide an important addition to the allergy care team. By offering support, guidance, counseling, and education, the ANE would serve as both a coach and teacher for patients and families with food allergies and could contribute to improvement.

References

Academy of Oncology Nurse & Patient Navigators (AONN+). (2025). *Certification: Become a certified oncology navigator through AONN+ foundation for learning*. Available from: https://www.aonnffl.org

American Association of Colleges of Nursing. (2021). *The essentials: Core competencies for professional nursing education*. Available from: https://www.aacnnursing.org/Portals/0/PDFs/Publications/Essentials-2021.pdf

American Association of Diabetes Educators. (n.d.). *Diabetes care and education specialists*. Available from: https://www.diabeteseducator.org

American Nurses Association. (2025). *Code of ethics for nurses. Provision 1.3: The nature of health*. [cited 2025 Sep 25]. Available from: https://codeofethics.ana.org/provision-1-3

British Society of Allergy and Clinical Immunology. (2025). *BSACI allergy nursing mentorship program*. [cited 2025 Jun 1]. Available from: https://www.bsaci.org/workforce/bsaci-allergy-nursing-mentorship-program/

Fights, S. D. (2012). Reap the benefits of certification. *The American Journal of Nursing, 112*(1), 10–11. https://doi.org/10.1097/01.NAJ.0000410166.75658.7f

Food Allergy Research & Education (FARE). (2024). *Food allergy academy*. Available from: https://www.foodallergyacademy.org/

Greenhawt, M., Shaker, M., Winders, T., Bukstein, D. A., Davis, R. S., Oppenheimer, J., et al. (2020). Development and acceptability of a shared decision-making tool for commercial peanut allergy therapies. *Annals of Allergy, Asthma & Immunology, 125*(1), 90–96. https://doi.org/10.1016/j.anai.2020.01.030

Health Resources and Services Administration Data Warehouse. (2025). *Workforce projections*. Available from: https://data.hrsa.gov/topics/health-workforce/nchwa/workforce-projections

Institute for Credentialing Excellence. (2020). *Value of certification statement*. [cited 2025 Sep 25]. Available from: https://www.credentialingexcellence.org/Portals/0/Value%20of%20Certification%20Statement%202020%20Final.pdf

Izadi, N., & Saff, R. R. (2022). Allergy and immunology interest and exposure among US medical students. *Journal of Allergy and Clinical Immunology: Global*. https://doi.org/10.1016/j.jacig.2022.08.002

Kaplow, R. (2022, March 8). The value of certification. *AACN Blog*. Available from: https://www.aacn.org/blog/the-value-of-certification

Kelly, S., Kagan, O., Howard-Ruben, J., Doucette, J., Weiss, K., Koo, L., et al. (2022, April 4). Why we need certified allergy nurse educators. *Allergic Living*. Available from: https://www.allergicliving.com/2022/04/04/why-we-need-certified-allergy-nurse-educators/

Leung, D. Y. M., & Sampson, H. A. (2021). Food allergy: A review and update on epidemiology, pathogenesis, diagnosis, prevention, and management. *The Journal of Allergy and Clinical Immunology, 147*(4), 1101–1111. https://doi.org/10.1016/j.jaci.2020.11.009

Malick, A., & Meadows, J. A. (2021). Allergy and immunology physician workforce: Where do we stand today? *Annals of Allergy, Asthma & Immunology, 127*, 522–523.

Myers, T. L., DeGarmo, S., & Horahan, M. (2024). How certification exams reflect current practice. *Journal of Continuing Education in Nursing, 55*(11), 513–516. https://doi.org/10.3928/00220124-20241011-02

National Board for Respiratory Care (NBRC). (2025). *Certified Asthma Educator (AE-C)*. [cited 2025 Jun 1]. Available from: https://www.nbrc.org/examinations/certified-asthma-educator-ae-c/

Russell, A. F., Cooke, A. J. T., Kagan, O., & Stieb, E. S. (2022). Multifaceted role of the registered nurse on an oral immunotherapy clinical team. *Journal of Food Allergy (East Providence, R.I.: Online), 4*(2), 78–85. https://doi.org/10.2500/jfa.2022.4.220014

Scherzer, R. (2018). Increasing interest in the field of allergy and immunology in medical students and residents: A critical need. *Annals of Allergy, Asthma & Immunology, 121*(6), 657–659. https://doi.org/10.1016/j.anai.2018.09.457

Shepherd, A., Harris, C., & Morey, T. (2019). The relationship between specialty nurse certification and patient, nurse, and organizational outcomes: A systematic review. *International Journal of Nursing Studies, 94*, 50–63. https://doi.org/10.1016/j.ijnurstu.2019.02.001

Tandan, M., Dunlea, S., Cullen, W., & Bury, G. (2024). Teamwork and its impact on chronic disease clinical outcomes in primary care: a systematic review and meta-analysis. *Public Health, 229*, 88–115. https://doi.org/10.1016/j.puhe.2024.01.019

Warren, C. M., Sehgal, S., Sicherer, S. H., & Nadeau, K. C. (2024). Epidemiology and the growing epidemic of food allergy in children and adults across the globe. *Current Allergy and Asthma Reports, 24*, 95–106. https://doi.org/10.1007/s11882-023-01120-y

Yoder-Wise, P. S. (2021). Lifelong learning: Part 1. *Journal of Continuing Education in Nursing, 52*(7), 303. https://doi.org/10.3928/00220124-20210611-01

Prior Authorization Recommendations

Benjamin Nick Lagunilla, Sarah Camille Emerton,
and Tina Lin

Medication Prior Authorization

Prior authorization (PA) is a process in which a treatment or medication recommended by a healthcare provider gets approval from the patient's insurance plan before officially prescribing or ordering. Insurance companies use PA to determine if a specific medical service is necessary, cost-effective, and beneficial for the patient (Warnock, 2023).

(a) Medical Necessity: Insurers determine whether the medical necessity requirements are met (For example, a patient with a history of chronic allergic rhinitis and asthma is recommended by their allergist to try allergen immunotherapy or subcutaneous immunotherapy (SCIT) to treat their environmental allergies and asthma).
(b) Cost: Insurers determine if medication or treatment is the most financially sound option for a patient's current condition (For example, recommendation of allergen immunotherapy vs utilization of oral or nasal antihistamines).
(c) Benefit: Insurers need to make sure that on-going treatment or medication benefits the patient's condition (For example, a patient with a food allergy who has been receiving Xolair (omalizumab) injections for three months has shown a reduction in allergic reactions following accidental allergen exposure).

B. N. Lagunilla (✉)
University of California San Diego, La Jolla, CA, USA
e-mail: nlagunilla@health.ucsd.edu

S. C. Emerton
Stanford Medicine Children's Health, Palo Alto, CA, USA
e-mail: semerton@stanfordchildrens.org

T. Lin
Stanford Health Care, Palo Alto, CA, USA
e-mail: tilin@stanfordhealthcare.org

J. Doucette, J. Howard-Ruben (eds.), *Comprehensive Food Allergy Management for Nurses*, https://doi.org/10.1007/978-3-032-28647-5_14

An additional three months of injections may be pre-authorized if there is measurable improvement.

Prior Authorization Workflow (Fig. 1)

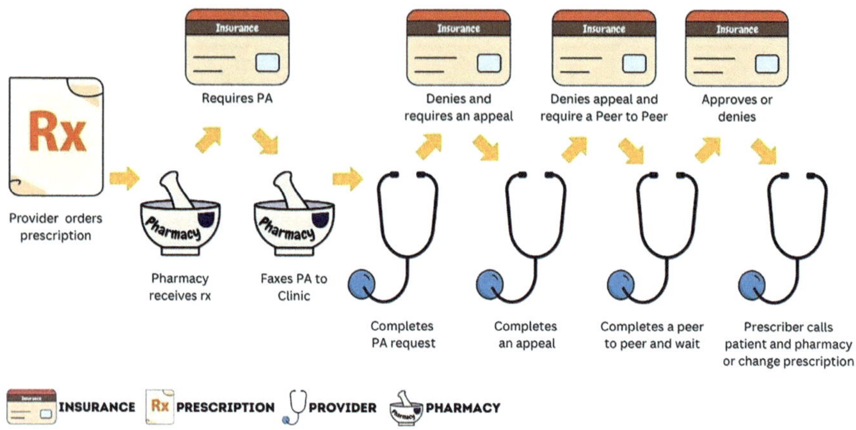

Fig. 1 Medication prior authorization: requests, appeals, and peer-to-peer review. (*Note*. Created by the authors. Adapted from Lagunilla and Morgan (2024))

Process

(a) Some procedures or medications do not require PA. To determine if a PA is required, one must check the patient's insurance website or an online PA lookup tool. An additional option is to call the insurance company and provide the member's plan information to determine necessity (American Medical Association [AMA], 2015).

(b) PA Methods

1. Fax

Manual PAs can be submitted via fax. To initiate this step, find out which required forms are needed for the specific insurance and attach necessary clinical information. The fax method may require hand-written forms to be submitted. Other insurers may require alternative authorization forms. Submission of the incorrect forms may lead to approval delays (AMA, 2015).

2. Electronic

Electronic Prior Authorization (ePA) can be done through online platforms such as CoverMyMeds or a health plan portal. An online form will require input of patient information, as well as medical conditions and needs. The advantage of ePA is quicker processing times and real-time updates.

Depending on the PA, an immediate decision may be available after submission (AMA, 2015).

3. Telephone

One can contact the insurer or pharmacy benefits plan to initiate a PA over the phone. The information required by the plan can be provided verbally. One advantage of the phone method is that you may receive an immediate decision without delay. An appeal can also be initiated immediately upon denial. However, the phone method may result in long hold times and the insurer may still require clinical documentation to be faxed before a determination is made (AMA, 2015).

(c) Check Status
1. PA turnaround can range from days to weeks. The turnaround time for the PA is dependent on whether it is routine or urgent. Routine authorization can take anywhere from 5 to 14 business days while urgent authorization will receive a decision within 72 hours. The method of PA submission can also affect average approval time (AMA, 2015).
2. Document date and method of submission to help keep track of PA status. Regular follow-up is necessary to minimize unnecessary patient care delays (AMA, 2015).
3. After the review, an approve or deny decision will be determined by the insurer. A letter will be available electronically and a printed letter will be mailed to the patient. A denial letter will specify the reason the PA is rejected.
4. Common denial reasons for procedures: not part of benefit coverage, plan exclusion, deemed not a medical necessity, service is experimental or investigational, not appropriate level of care, etc. (Patient Advocate Foundation, 2025).
5. Common denial reasons for medications: step therapy, quantity limit, non-formulary medication, generic medication coverage only, etc. (Patient Advocate Foundation, 2025).

(d) Appeals: The patient can appeal the insurer's decision through an internal or external appeal.
1. Internal Appeal—an appeal is submitted to insurers to reconsider the decision (see Fig. 2). The appeal may require additional clinic documents to be submitted or a peer-to-peer review. During the peer-to-peer, the clinician will speak with the medical director of the insurer to provide additional information and explain why the prescribed procedure and medication is the best course of treatment (Patient Advocate Foundation, 2025).
2. External Appeal—it is typically filed after an internal appeal process is completed. The average turnaround time for external appeal is about 60 days. However, it can be requested urgently due to medical necessity before an internal appeal process is completed. The turnaround time for urgent external appeal is within 72 hour. An independent third party consisting of a group of doctors will review the insurance decision and will make the final decision about coverage. The insurer must comply with the third-party decision (Patient Advocate Foundation, 2025).

IgE-Mediated Food Allergy Sample Letter of Appeal

Date

Address of Insurance Company

Topic: Letter of Appeal

Patient information and reason for requesting appeal, including name, date of birth, insurance company name, ID number, group number, date in question, specify exact medication prescribed by healthcare clinician and the fact that the medication was denied. Include the medical history of the patient and reason the medication is indicated and necessary for treatment. Include any ICD codes and diagnosis codes. Specify why the patient would benefit from the medication.

Include any documents such as physician/NP/PA notes, appeal form filled out for the specific insurance company with all patient and clinician information.

Sincerely,

Physician/NP/PA and signature

Fig. 2 IgE-Mediated Food Allergy Sample Letter of Appeal. (*Note.* Letter template developed by Julianne Doucette from *IgE-Mediated Food Allergy Sample Letter of Appeal for Xolair (omalizumab)* by Genentech USA, Inc. and Novartis Pharmaceuticals Corporation (2024). Open access)

The American Medical Association (AMA) is aiming to enhance PA by challenging insurance companies to eliminate care delays, patient harm, and reduce significant costs. An AMA survey of 1000 physicians (400 primary care and 600 specialists) conducted in 2024 found that PAs significantly increase physician burnout, cause unsafe patient care delays, lead to higher overall utilization of healthcare resources, and cause unnecessary spending (such as additional medical visits, unanticipated hospital stays, and patients regularly paying out-of-pocket for care) (AMA, 2024) (Fig. 3).

In terms of patient outcomes and safety, 28% of physicians report that PAs led to patients' hospitalization, 18% of physicians report that PAs led to patients experiencing life-threatening events that required intervention to prevent permanent damage, and 8% of physicians report that PAs inevitably led to a patient's permanent impairment, congenital anomaly/birth defects, or in some cases, death (American Medical Association Physician Survey, 2024).

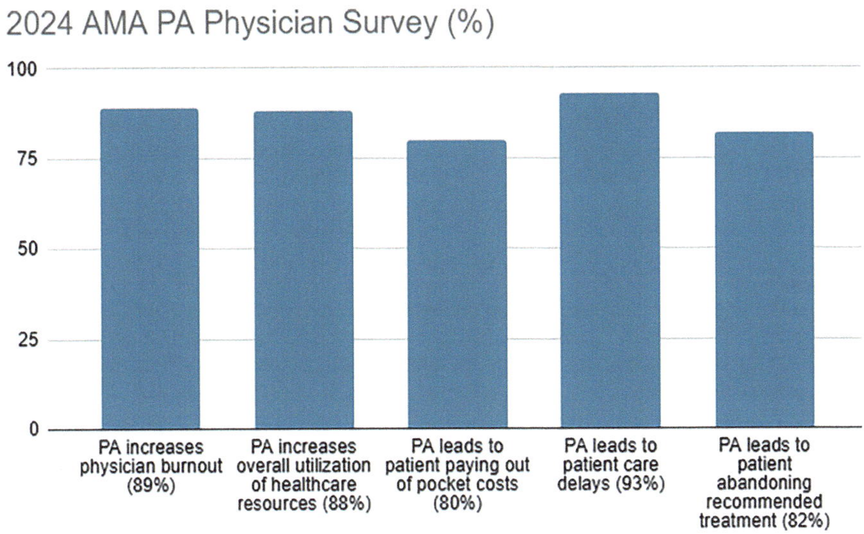

Fig. 3 2024 AMA PA Physician Survey. (*Note*. Created by the authors. Adapted from American Medical Association Physician Survey (2024))

Procedure Codes

Currently the United States uses International Classification of Diseases, Tenth Revision (ICD-10) coding while the World Health Organization (WHO) has adopted the International Classification of Diseases, Eleventh Revision (ICD-11) as of January 1, 2020 (YES HIM Consulting, n.d.). The rollout date of ICD-11 in the United States has not been set; however, some hospital systems are starting to plan for this transition (YES HIM Consulting, n.d.). The coding system is updated periodically to improve care and reporting mechanisms. The food allergy and environmental allergy codes include ICD-10 diagnosis codes used for medical billing and tracking, CPT codes for allergy testing procedures, and specific FDA code numbers for defining major food allergens requiring labeling. Nurses should understand these codes specific to food allergy and the subtle nuances between various codes such as coding for an initial encounter of anaphylaxis to an allergen, tolerance or reactivity to baked allergen, or other adverse food reaction due to a particular allergen (American College of Allergy, Asthma, & Immunology, 2025). Understanding the various codes can improve the accuracy of documentation for the PA process (Tables 1 and 2).

Table 1 Food allergy ICD-10-CM codes

Anaphylaxis/Other adverse food reaction	Allergy status
T78.00XA Anaphylactic reaction due to unspecified food, initial encounter	Z91.01 Food allergy status
T78.01XA Anaphylactic reaction due to peanuts, initial encounter	Z91.010 Allergy to peanuts
T78.02XA Anaphylactic reaction due to shellfish (crustaceans), initial encounter	Z91.011 Allergy to milk products, unspecified
T78.03XA Anaphylactic reaction due to fish, initial encounter	Z91.0112 Allergy to milk products with reactivity to baked milk
T78.04XA Anaphylactic reaction due to fruits and vegetables, initial encounter	Z91.0120 Allergy to eggs, unspecified
T78.05XA Anaphylactic reaction due to tree nuts and seeds, initial encounter	Z91.0121 Allergy to eggs with tolerance to baked egg
T78.070X Anaphylactic reaction due to milk and dairy products with tolerance to baked milk	Z91.0122 Allergy to eggs with reactivity to baked egg
T78.071X Anaphylactic reaction due to milk and dairy products with reactivity to baked milk	Z91.013 Allergy to seafood
T78.080X Anaphylactic reaction to milk and dairy products, unspecified	Z91.014 Allergy to mammalian meats
T78.08X Anaphylactic reaction due to egg with tolerance to baked egg	Z91.018 Allergy to other foods
T78.081X Anaphylactic reaction due to egg with reactivity to baked egg	
T78.089X Anaphylactic reaction due to eggs, unspecified	
T78.110X Other adverse food reactions due to milk and dairy products with tolerance to baked milk	
T78.111X Other adverse food reaction due to milk and dairy products with reactivity to baked milk	
T78.119X Other adverse food reaction due to milk and dairy products with baked tolerance/reactivity, unspecified	
T78.120X Other adverse food reaction due to egg with tolerance to baked egg	
T78.121X Other adverse food reaction due to egg with reactivity to baked egg	
T78.129X Other adverse food reaction due to egg with baked egg tolerance/reactivity, unspecified	
T78.19XX Other adverse food reactions, not elsewhere classified	

Note. Created by the authors. Adapted from American Academy of Professional Coders (2025) and American College of Allergy, Asthma, and Immunology (2025)

Table 2 CPT codes for allergy testing

Skin testing	Ingestion challenge testing
95004 Percutaneous tests	95076 Ingestion challenge test; initial 120 min of testing
95024 Intracutaneous tests	95079 …each additional 60 min of testing
95027 Patch Tests	

Note. Created by the authors. Adapted from Medi-Cal (2020)

Nursing Roles

Clinical documentation is often required by insurance companies to justify the medical necessity of the medication or procedure. Nurses can ensure all required information is complete and error free. Inaccurate or incomplete requests may result in delays or PA denial. Required clinical documents may include clinician orders, progress notes, lab results, prescribed medications, and more. If a PA is denied, then an appeal process can be initiated. The case should be discussed with the clinician to decide if an appeal process is warranted. Nurses can help facilitate the following:

(a) Assessment and Evaluation of Clinical Documents—Nurses participate in assessing patient medical records, collecting pertinent documents and reviewing recommendations by clinicians to support authorization decisions.
(b) Initiation of Documentation Needed for Step Therapy—Step therapy is a common strategy insurance companies use for cost-control.

Step therapy requires the patient to try and fail after using a lower cost alternative before coverage is approved for a more expensive medication or therapy. Evidence suggests that such protocols reduce spending for targeted therapies and promote evidence-based care by following the steps modeled on consensus treatment guidelines (Sachs & Kyle, 2022).

Food allergy brand name drugs can be affected by the "try-fail" protocol. One example includes Xolair (omalizumab) which is a biological injection that was approved by the FDA in February 2024 to reduce anaphylaxis in patients with food allergies. Insurance companies sometimes require patients to prove they failed lower cost treatments, such as oral antihistamines (e.g., cetirizine, fexofenadine) before covering this more specialized and expensive drug, although some insurance companies do recognize this medication as a first-line medication.

Allergy treatments such as allergen immunotherapy or subcutaneous immunotherapy (SCIT) are recommended by allergists to treat patients who suffer from multiple environmental triggers, such as animal dander, dust, tree, and grass pollen, or asthma. SCIT is a more costly and long-term treatment, so insurance companies require patients to prove that they have failed the standard medical pharmacotherapy first, such as use of oral antihistamines, topical nasal antihistamines, and intranasal corticosteroid sprays, before coverage approval (Durham, 2016). Overall, nurses play a role in documenting when a patient has tried a therapy and failed when requesting the step up in therapy.

Follow-Up

Nurses conduct follow-ups with pharmacies and insurance plans to support documentation and assessment for continuity of approval. Insurance authorization is typically valid for a specific time period—most commonly 6 months to 1 year. This allows the patient to trial the medication or procedure to determine its therapeutic effects. Follow-up healthcare appointments with prescribing physicians/nurse practitioners/physician associates are coordinated in a timely manner to ensure updated clinical documentation is available for PA renewal.

Conclusion

In summary, PA remains a complex yet integral component of modern healthcare, serving as both a safeguard for medical necessity and a barrier to timely treatment. While the process is designed to ensure cost-effectiveness and appropriate use of resources, its administrative burdens, frequent denials, and step therapy requirements often create frustration for patients and providers alike. Nurses and other healthcare professionals play a pivotal role in navigating this landscape by ensuring accurate documentation, advocating for patients, and streamlining workflows that support continuity of care. Ongoing reforms, technological advancements, and collaborative efforts between insurers and healthcare teams are essential to minimize delays, reduce provider burnout, and ultimately enhance patient safety and outcomes.

References

AMA. (2024). *2024 AMA prior authorization physician survey.* https://fixpriorauth.org/sites/default/files/2025-02/2024_AMA_Prior-Authorization-Physician_Survey.pdf

American Academy of Professional Coders (AAPC). (2025). *ICD-10 CM code for food allergy status Z91.01.* https://www.aapc.com/codes/icd-10-codes/Z91.01?msockid=3dc3194a981160fe33dd080c9995618d

American College of Allergy, Asthma, & Immunology. (2025). *2026 code updates.* https://college.acaai.org/2026-code-updates/

American Medical Association [AMA]. (2015). *Tips to help physicians reduce the prior authorization burden in their practice.* https://www.ama-assn.org/sites/ama-assn.org/files/corp/media-browser/premium/psa/prior-authorization-tips_0.pdf

Durham, S. R. (2016). Sublingual or subcutaneous immunotherapy for allergic rhinitis: Systematic review and meta-analysis. *Journal of Allergy and Clinical Immunology, 137*(3), 872–881. https://www.jacionline.org/article/S0091-6749(15)03112-7/fulltext

Genentech Inc., & Novartis Pharmaceutical Corporations. (2024, February). *IgE-Mediated Food Allergy Sample Letter of Appeal for XOLAIR (omalizumab) for subcutaneous use.* Retrieved from https://www.xolairhcp.com/food-allergies/resources/practice-forms-and-documents.html

Lagunilla, B., & Morgan, M. C. (2024, June). Optimizing prior authorization workflows in outpatient clinics: A comprehensive approach [Conference presentation abstract]. Sigma Region 1 International Nursing Conference 2024, Honolulu, HI, United States.

Medi-Cal. (2020, August). *Allergy testing and desensitization.* (Part 2). https://mcweb.apps.prd.cammis.medi-cal.ca.gov/assets/BB28488B-0B15-4CCA-AD91-9F9C2AC02899/allergy.pdf?access_token=6UyVkRRfByXTZEWIh8j8QaYylPyP5ULO

Patient Advocate Foundation. (2025). *Engaging with insurers: Appealing a denial.* https://education.patientadvocate.org/wp-content/uploads/2022/07/Appeals-Guide-2025.pdf

Sachs, R. E., & Kyle, M. A. (2022). Step therapy's balancing act – Protecting patients while addressing high drug prices. *The New England Journal of Medicine, 386*(10), 901–904. https://pmc.ncbi.nlm.nih.gov/articles/PMC9067323/

Warnock, N. D. (2023). Prior authorization: Process redesign with a focus on value-based care. *Population Health Management, 26*(S1), S-22. https://doi.org/10.1089/pop.2023.0146

YES HIM Consulting. (n.d.). *Preparing for ICD-11 codes: Steps for a smooth transition.* https://yes-himconsulting.com/preparing-for-icd-11-codes-steps-for-a-smooth-transition/

Resources Page

Food Allergy Resources for Nurses, Nurse Practitioners, Other Clinicians, Patients, and Caregivers

(*the following is not an exhaustive list of resources*)

General Food Allergy Resources

- *Allergy & Anaphylaxis Australia*
  Australian charity and allergy patient support organization featuring patient and health care professional educational resources
  Website: https://allergyfacts.org.au/
- *Allergy and Asthma Network (AAN)*
  Website: www.allergyasthmanetwork.org
- *Allergy Apps*
  Website: https://triggerbites.com/blog/best-food-allergy-apps
- *Allergy Life Australia*
  Website: https://allergylife.com.au/pages/allergy-support-group
  Email: contact@allergylife.com.au
  National non-profit with the aim of supporting those with food allergy in Australia. They provide online support groups with monthly meetings
- *Allergic Living*
  Website: https://www.allergicliving.com/
  Provides food allergy articles and recipes
- *American Academy of Allergy Asthma & Immunology (AAAAI)*
  Website: www.aaaai.org and www.aaaai.org/conditions-treatments/allergies/food-allergy
- *American College of Allergy, Asthma & Immunology*
  Website: https://acaai.org/
- *Anaphylaxis UK*
  Website: https://www.anaphylaxis.org.uk/

J. Doucette, J. Howard-Ruben (eds.), *Comprehensive Food Allergy Management for Nurses*, https://doi.org/10.1007/978-3-032-28647-5

- *Asthma and Allergy Foundation of America (AAFA)/Kids with Food Allergies (KFA)*
  Website: http://www.kidswithfoodallergies.org/
- *Australasian Society of Clinical Immunology and Allergy (ASCIA)*
  Website: www.allergy.org.au
  Website for ASCIA members, health professionals and the public for education and informational purposes on allergy and anaphylaxis
- *British Society for Allergy & Clinical Immunology (BSACI)*
  Website: https://www.bsaci.org
  Website for BSACI members and the professional society for the allergy specialty
- *Center for Food Allergy Asthma Research (CFAAR)*
  Website: https://www.feinberg.northwestern.edu/sites/cfaar/index.html
  Center at Northwestern University addressing epidemiology, advocacy, and health services research on allergic disease. Provides educational resources on food allergy.
- *European Academy of Allergy and Clinical Immunology (EAACI)*
  Website: https://eaaci.org
  Non-profit organization of clinicians, researchers, and allied health professionals for people affected by allergic diseases
- *FDA Food Allergy Page*
  Website: https://www.fda.gov/food/nutrition-food-labeling-and-critical-foods/food-allergies
- *Food Allergy and Anaphylaxis Connection Team (FAACT)*
  Website: www.foodallergyawareness.org
  Public education, advocacy and awareness of food allergy.
- *Food Allergy Management and Prevention Support Tool for Infants and Toddlers (FAMP-IT)*
  Website: https://www.famp-it.org
- *Food Allergy Research & Resource Program (FAARP)*
  Industry-funded organization that collaborates with a diverse set of interest holders in food allergy, focused on improving safety of food products for people with food allergies. Offers confidential analysis of food samples.
  Website: https://farrp.unl.edu/confidential-analysis/
- *Food Allergy Research and Education (FARE)*
  Website: www.foodallergy.org and www.foodallergyprevention.org
  Website for clinician resources: https://www.foodallergy.org/resources/clinician-resources
  Charitable organization with the mission to improve the quality of life of those with food allergy through research, education and advocacy
- *Hoyt Institute of Food Allergy*
  Website: https://www.hoytallergy.com/
  Evidence-based institute lead by allergist Dr. Hoyt who developed Code Ana. She provides clinical care for patients and families and food allergy management education for physicians, nurses practitioners, and physician associates through podcasts and CME courses.

- *MedicAlert Foundation*
  Website: www.medicalert.org
  Company that keeps medical information about members and is available 24/7 for access during an emergency. They offer medical IDs, bracelets, necklaces etc.
- *National Allergy Council Australia*
  Website: www.preventallergies.org.au
  Health Direct through the Australian government providing education and information to prevent food allergies.
- *National Institute of Allergy and Infectious Disease (NIAID)*
  US government organization that supports research to prevent and manage infectious, immunologic, and allergic diseases.
  Website: https://www.niaid.nih.gov
- *World Allergy Organization (WAO)*
  Umbrella allergy specialty organization for over 115 countries
  Website: https://worldallergy.org

Diagnosis and Management

General

- *NIAID Original and Addendum Guidelines*
  Website: https://www.niaid.nih.gov/diseases-conditions/guidelines-clinicians-and-patients-food-allergy
- *EAACI Guidelines: Management of IgE-mediated Food Allergy*
  Website: https://onlinelibrary.wiley.com/doi/10.1111/all.16345
- *World Allergy Organization 2022 Guidelines*
  Website: https://www.worldallergyorganizationjournal.org/article/S1939-4551(22)00063-1/fulltext
- *Anaphylaxis: 2023 Practice Parameter Update*
  Link-https://www.annallergy.org/article/S1081-1206(23)01304-2/fulltext
- *GA²LEN Global Allergy and Asthma European Guidelines*
  Website: https://pmc.ncbi.nlm.nih.gov/articles/PMC9467869/

Diagnosis

- *Australasian Society of Clinical Immunology and Allergy (ASCIA)*
  Skin Prick Testing Guide for Diagnosis of Allergic Disease
  Website: https://www.allergy.org.au/images/hp/ASCIA_HP_Skin_Prick_Testing_Guide_2025.pdf
- *BSACI Paediatric Allergy Skin Prick Testing (Standard Operating Procedure)*
  Link: https://www.bsaci.org/wp-content/uploads/2024/10/paedSPTnew_V2.pdf
- *EAACI Guidelines: Diagnosis of IgE-mediated FA*
  Website: https://onlinelibrary.wiley.com/doi/10.1111/all.15902
- *European Academy of Allergy and Clinical Immunology (EAACI)*
  Allergy-Focused Diet History Adult Version
  Link: https://static-content.springer.com/esm/art%3A10.1186%2Fs13601-015-0050-2/MediaObjects/13601_2015_50_MOESM2_ESM.pdf

Cross-Contact & Exposure Prevention Resources

- *FAACT-How to prevent cross-contact and accidental environmental exposure*
  Website: https://www.foodallergyawareness.org/food-allergy-and-anaphylaxis/cross-contact/

Travel Resources

- *FARE Chef Cards*
  Website: https://www.foodallergy.org/resources/food-allergy-chef-cards
- *Equal Eats Cards and Equal Eats App for iOS and Android*
  Website: https://equaleats.com/?gad_source=1&gad_campaignid=15061416614&gbraid=0AAAAACUgfXktndfuwxUxXzztXcLHnLsIt&gclid=Cj0KCQjwn8XFBhCxARIsAMyH8BvXKXxEz79yaN9TL9Av12Tpw5d1nx5G3ifFR9LTuBKvxzhhuaqMxEsaAnsFEALw_wcB
- *Australian Allergy Life-My Allergy Card*
  Website: https://allergylife.com.au/pages/my-allergy-card?gad_campaignid=17429429501&gad_source=1&gbraid=0AAAAABIpBeqpaWC-VjJgowobUJVFYztwJU&gclid=Cj0KCQjwn8XFBhCxARIsAMyH8BsnIc7CczlW7tdTz1bLwNIiyU2EigPOS9GybISjJVksYJgJDyzV89oaAkS8EALw_wcB
- *Allergic Living-Airline Resources*
  Airlines & Allergies Guide Domestic (2025)
  Website: https://www.allergicliving.com/2025/07/11/allergic-livings-airlines-allergies-guide-domestic/
  Airlines & Allergies Guide International (2025)
  Website: https://www.allergicliving.com/2025/07/11/allergic-livings-airlines-allergies-guide-international/
- *Australasian Society of Clinical Immunology and Allergy (ASCIA) Action Plan for Anaphylaxis*
  Website: www.allergy.org.au/images/stories/anaphylaxis/2025/ASCIA_Action_Plan_Anaphylaxis_General_2025.pdf
- *Food Allergy & Anaphylaxis Emergency Care Plan*
  Website: https://www.foodallergy.org/living-food-allergy/food-allergy-essentials/food-allergy-anaphylaxis-emergency-care-plan
- *Food Allergy Canada Anaphylaxis Emergency Plan*
  Website: https://foodallergycanada.ca/tools-and-downloads/downloads/emergency-plan-forms/
- *Canadian Anaphylaxis Action Plan for Kids*
  Website: https://cms.trekk.ca/wp-content/uploads/2023/11/Anaphylaxis_Action_Plan_Redesign7_-_school_daycare_002_2.0.pdf
- *Immune Tolerance Network*
  Website: https://www.leapstudy.co.uk/about-peanut-allergy.html

Reading Labels Resources

- *USFDA food label examples and video*
  Website: https://www.fda.gov/food/food-allergies/faster-act-sesame-ninth-major-food-allergen
- *US FDA Guidance Questions and Answers Regarding Food Allergen Labeling*
  Website: https://www.fda.gov/regulatory-information/search-fda-guidance-documents/guidance-industry-questions-and-answers-regarding-food-allergen-labeling-edition-5
- *Food Allergy Videos*
  Website: https://www.aaaai.org/tools-for-the-public/video-library/food-allergy-videos
- *How to Read a Food Label*
  Website: https://www.stlouischildrens.org/fame/how-read-food-label

Training

- *MenuTrinfo AllerTrain & AllerTrain U*
  Website: https://menutrinfo.com/training/allertrain-allertrain-u/

Medication and Treatment Resources

- *FAACT Epinephrine Options Poster*
  Website: https://www.foodallergyawareness.org/food-allergy-and-anaphylaxis/treatment-and-management/epinephrine/
- *Nasal epinephrine device (Neffy) Healthcare Professionals Website*
  Website: https://neffypro.com/resources/#resource-library
- *Palforzia (Archis Hypogaea) package insert*
  Website: https://www.fda.gov/media/134838/download?attachment
- *Xolair (Omalizumab) package insert*
  Website: https://www.accessdata.fda.gov/drugsatfda_docs/label/2024/103976s5245lbl.pdf
- *Practice Devices*
  - Generic EAI: https://www.epinephrineautoinject.com/order-product-trainers/
  - AUVI-Q: https://www.auvi-q.com/hcp/trainer
  - Neffy IN Epinephrine: https://neffypro.com/sign-up/?demoDevices=true
  - Many options for carrying your/your child's epinephrine devices: https://www.allergylifestyle.com/product-category/allergy-shop/epipen-cases/

Disparities in Food Allergy

- *American Academy of Pediatrics Promoting Food Security for All Children*
  Link: https://publications.aap.org/pediatrics/article/136/5/e1431/33896/Promoting-Food-Security-for-All-Children?autologincheck=redirected
- *American Academy of Family Physicians*
  Link: https://www.aafp.org/fpm/blogs/quick-tips/social_determinants
- *American Academy of Pediatrics Food Research & Action Center Screen and Intervene: A Toolkit for Pediatricians for to Address Food Insecurity*
  Link: https://frac.org/aaptoolkit
- *USDA Food and Nutrition Administration WIC Benefits*
  Link: https://www.fna.usda.gov/wic/benefits

Early Introduction of Allergens & Food Allergy Prevention

- *Consensus Approach to the Primary Prevention of Food Allergy Through Nutrition: Guidance from AAAAI, ACAAI, and CSACI*
  Link: https://www.aaaai.org/Aaaai/media/Media-Library-PDFs/Allergist%20Resources/Statements%20and%20Practice%20Parameters/A-Consensus-Approach-to-the-Primary-Prevention-of-Food-Allergy-Through-Nutrition-Jan-21-(1).pdf
- *FAMP-IT (Food Allergy Management and Prevention in Infants and Toddlers)*
  Website: https://www.famp-it.org
  Offers clinician-focused guidance, handouts, and an algorithm for early allergen introduction. Includes information on skincare and eczema, IgE-mediated food allergy and non-IgE-mediated food allergy.
- *Prevent Allergies (EAACI-affiliated Public Campaign)*
  Website: https://www.preventallergies.org
  An international public health initiative promoting the early introduction of allergenic foods for allergy prevention. Professionals can order "Food Allergy Prevention Kits" and a good resource for families.
- *FARE Food Allergy Prevention Website*
  Website: https://www.foodallergy.org/research-innovation/accelerating-innovation/early-introduction-and-food-allergy-prevention
  Explains major clinical trials and offers tools like handouts for introducing peanut and egg in infancy.
- *FAACT Website*
  Website: https://www.foodallergyawareness.org/food-allergy-and-anaphylaxis/prevention/
  Public education, advocacy and awareness of food allergy.
- *National Peanut Board—Early Introduction Resources*
  Website: https://www.nationalpeanutboard.org
  Public awareness resources on peanut allergy prevention and education offering straightforward, visual guides for families, safety and dosage tips…
  Early introduction video: https://nationalpeanutboard.org/resources/videos/how-to-introduce-peanut-to-babies-early/

- *Solid Starts App & Website*
  Website: https://www.solidstarts.com
  Parent app to support Baby-led weaning and safe introduction of top 9 allergens with how to prepare each allergen at different developmental stages. Well done with lots of pictures. Includes tracker of allergens. Free version is available.
- *Food Allergy Research and Education*
  Website: www.foodallergyprevention.org
  Charitable organization with the mission to improve the quality of life of those with food allergy through research, education and advocacy
- *Australasian Society of Clinical Immunology and Allergy (ASCIA)-Prevention*
  Website: www.allergy.org.au
  ASCIA_PC_FAST_FACTS_Infant_feeding_and allergy_prevention_2026.pdf
  Allergy prevention—Australasian Society of Clinical Immunology and Allergy (ASCIA)
  Website for ASCIA members, health professionals and the public for education and informational purposes on allergy and anaphylaxis.
- *National Allergy Council Australia-Prevention*
  Website: www.preventallergies.org.au
  Health Direct through the Australian government providing education and information to prevent food allergies.

Food Allergy Management in Early Childhood Settings

- *How a Child Might Describe an Allergic Reaction*
  https://www.foodallergy.org/sites/default/files/2025-07/FPP%20Child%20Reaction%208.5%20x%2014.pdf
- *National Association of School Nurses*
  Allergy and Anaphylaxis Toolkit
  Website: https://learn.nasn.org/courses/58035
- *Centers for Disease Control and Prevention Voluntary Guidelines for Managing Food Allergies in Schools and Early Care and Education Programs*
  Website: https://www.cdc.gov/school-health-conditions/media/pdfs/20_316712-a_fa_guide_508tag.pdf
- *Food Allergy Management in Schools (FAMS): Expert Recommendations K-12*
  Website: https://www.foodallergy.org/resources/food-allergy-management-schools-fams-expert-recommendations-k-12
- *American Academy of Pediatrics Allergy and Anaphylaxis Management in Schools*
  Website: https://www.aap.org/en/patient-care/school-health/management-of-chronic-conditions-in-schools/allergy-and-anaphylaxis-management-in-schools/?srsltid=AfmBOor95jUa8Wp8rMQiwF4FR-gs43CAqDbSXLuXg6smAbz-Rocq1SE7T
- *AAFA's Recommended Language for Signs and Symptoms of Food Allergy Reactions in Infants and Toddlers*
  Website: https://aafa.org/asthma-allergy-research/our-research/food-allergy-anaphylaxis-in-infants/

- *Asthma and Allergy Foundation of America-Kids with Food Allergies Food Allergy Action Plan for the Treatment of Anaphylaxis*
  Website: https://kidswithfoodallergies.org/living-with-food-allergies/food-allergy-treatment/allergy-anaphylaxis-action-plan/
- *Code Ana*
  Website: Code Ana (2024) Code Ana | Medical Emergency Response & Epinephrine Training. https://codeana.org/
- *ASCIA Action, First Aid, Management, Transfer, Travel and Treatment Plans*
  Website: https://www.allergy.org.au/hp/ascia-plans-action-and-treatment?highlight=WyJwbGFuIl0=
- *FARE Food Allergy & Anaphylaxis Emergency Care Plan (English and Spanish)*
  Website: https://www.foodallergy.org/living-food-allergy/food-allergy-essentials/food-allergy-anaphylaxis-emergency-care-plan
- *National Allergy Council Allergy Aware*
  Website: https://allergyaware.org.au/childrens-education-and-care
- *Food Allergy and Your Kiddo*
  Website: https://foodallergyandyourkiddo.com/
- *Kids with Food Allergies*
  Website: https://www.kidswithfoodallergies.org/wp-content/uploads/2022/12/potential-food-allergens-in-preschool-daycare-activities-crafts.pdf
- *FAACT Bullying*
  Website: https://www.foodallergyawareness.org/bullying/bullying-facts-stats-and-resources/
- *Food Allergy Academy*
  Website: https://www.foodallergy.org/our-initiatives/education-programs-training/fare-training
- *FARE Free Food Allergy Downloadable Posters and Resources*
  Website: https://www.foodallergy.org/living-food-allergies/food-allergy-essentials/free-downloadable-resources
- *National Allergy Council Australia Allergy Aware*
  Website: https://allergyaware.org.au/childrens-education-and-care/best-practice-guidelines-cec.
- *School Nursing Evidence-Based Clinical Practice Guideline: Students with Allergies and Risk for Anaphylaxis*
  Website: https://learn.nasn.org/courses/58496

Food Allergy Management in Adolescents and Young Adults

Food Allergy and Anaphylaxis Connection Team (FAACT)-College Resource Center and College Toolkit

- *College Resource Center*
  https://www.foodallergyawareness.org/college-resource-center/
- *Move-In Ready*
  https://www.foodallergyawareness.org/college-resource-center/for-students/move-in-ready/

- *Move-In Ready: Student Checklist*
  https://www.foodallergyawareness.org/college-resource-center/for-students/move-in-ready/
- *Legal Considerations*
  https://www.foodallergyawareness.org/college-resource-center/legal-considerations/
- *Dining & Food Service*
  https://www.foodallergyawareness.org/college-resource-center/dining-and-food-service/
- *Signs and Symptoms of Anaphylaxis*
  https://www.foodallergyawareness.org/food-allergy-and-anaphylaxis/signs-and-symptoms/

American Academy of Allergy Asthma and Immunology Food Allergy Stages

- *Food Allergy Stages: Young Adult (18–21 years)*
  https://www.aaaai.org/Aaaai/media/Media-Library-PDFs/Tools%20for%20the%20Public/Conditions%20Library/AAAAI-0622-205-FA-09.pdf
- *Food Allergy Stages: Early Teen (11–14 years)*
  https://www.aaaai.org/Aaaai/media/Media-Library-PDFs/Tools%20for%20the%20Public/Conditions%20Library/AAAAI-0622-205-FA-07.pdf
- *Food Labels: Read It Before You Eat It!*
  https://www.aaaai.org/tools-for-the-public/conditions-library/allergies/food-labels

Food Allergy Research & Education-(FARE) Resources

- *How to Read a Food Label*
  https://www.foodallergy.org/resources/how-read-food-label
- *Preparing for College*
  https://www.foodallergy.org/resources/preparing-college
- *FARE Food Allergy College Program*
  https://www.foodallergy.org/our-initiatives/education-programs-training/fare-food-allergy college-program
- *Free Downloadable Resources*
  https://www.foodallergy.org/living-food-allergy/food-allergy-essentials/free-downloadable-resources

Social Emotional Impact of Food Allergy

- *The Food Allergy Counselor*
  Website: https://www.foodallergycounselor.com/
  Licensed Therapist providing a resource for patients and families navigating the anxiety of food allergy. Book-May Contain Anxiety: Managing the Overwhelm of Parenting Children with Food Allergies. Multiple food allergy worksheets for personal use on the website.

- *Academy of Food Allergy Counseling*
  Website: https://www.foodallergycounseling.org/directory
  Allergy informed counselors located across the US and a few internationally
- *FARE Find a Support Group*
  Website: https://www.foodallergy.org/living-food-allergies/join-community/find-support-group
  Support Group Planning Manuel: https://www.foodallergy.org/media/1185/download

Meditation Apps

- *Calm*
  Website: https://www.calm.com/
- *Headspace*
  Website: https://www.headspace.com
- *Insight Timer*
  Website: https://www.insighttimer.com

Role of Technology in the Diagnosis and Management of FA

- *AsthmaXcel*
  Website: https://www.asthmaxcel.net/
- *Professional Networking in Nursing*
  Website: https://nursejournal.org/resources/networking-in-nursing/

Public Policy and Advocacy for People with Food Allergy

- *FDA Food Code*
  Website: https://www.fda.gov/food/fda-food-code/food-code-2022
- *FDA Food Guidance*
  Website: https://www.fda.gov/regulatory-information/search-fda-guidance-documents/guidance-industry-questions-and-answers-regarding-food-allergen-labeling-edition-5
- *Food Allergy Research and Education-Know Your Rights*
  Website: https://www.foodallergy.org/our-initiatives/advocacy/know-your-rights
- *FAACT*-Statewide Restaurant Legislation
  Website: https://www.foodallergyawareness.org/living-with-food-allergies/statewide-restaurant-legislation/statewide-restaurant-legislation
- *Asthma and Allergy Foundation*
  Website: https://aafa.org/advocacy/key-issues/food-allergies-advocacy/
- *Allergen Labeling Regulations by Country*
  Website: https://farrp.unl.edu/IRChart/

Nursing Organizations

- *American Society of Allergy Nurses (ASAN)*
  Based in the northwest US, the first organization supporting nurses in allergy care that provides continuing education for nurses
  Website: https://www.allergynurses.org
- *ASCIA Nurses Page*
  Website: https://www.allergy.org.au/members/nurses
  Resources about interest groups, membership, training and conferences for nurses collated by ASCIA.
- *Food Allergy Nursing Association (FANA)*
  Website: https://www.foodallergynursing.org
  Organization with a mission to advance nursing education, research, leadership, innovation, and collaboration in the food allergy subspecialty area

Nursing Education Resources

- *ASCIA e-Training for Health Professionals*
  Allergy education training site for health care professionals in New Zealand and Australia
  Website: https://traininghp.ascia.org.au
- *Professional Certificate in Allergy Nursing*
  Course offered for allergy nurses in collaboration with the Australian Society of Clinical Immunology and Allergy Incorporated (ASCIA).
  Website: https://adelaide.edu.au/study/degrees/professional-certificate-in-allergy-nursing/dom/

Other Videos

- *The Last Bite Full Documentary Film 2025*
  https://www.youtube.com/watch?v=7vFliKqwvzk
- *Anaphylaxis Interactive Learning Guide AAAAI*
  https://www.aaaai.org/tools-for-the-public/anaphylaxis